The Praeger Handbook on Women's Cancers

Personal and Psychosocial Insights

Michele A. Paludi, Editor

Women's Psychology
Michele A. Paludi, Series Editor

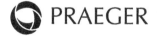 PRAEGER

AN IMPRINT OF ABC-CLIO, LLC
Santa Barbara, California • Denver, Colorado • Oxford, England

Library of Congress Cataloging-in-Publication Data

The Praeger handbook on women's cancers : personal and psychosocial insights / Michele A. Paludi, editor.

     pages cm.—(Women's psychology)

   ISBN 978-1-4408-2813-3 (hardback)—ISBN 978-1-4408-2814-0 (ebook)

1. Cancer in women—Handbooks, manuals, etc. I. Paludi, Michele Antoinette, editor of compilation.

  RC281.W65P73   2014

  616.99′40082—dc23   2013047550

ISBN: 978-1-4408-2813-3
EISBN: 978-1-4408-2814-0

18 17 16 15 14 1 2 3 4 5

This book is also available on the World Wide Web as an eBook.
Visit www.abc-clio.com for details.

Praeger
An Imprint of ABC-CLIO, LLC

ABC-CLIO, LLC
130 Cremona Drive, P.O. Box 1911
Santa Barbara, California 93116–1911 .

This book is printed on acid-free paper ∞
Manufactured in the United States of America

There Is Always Hope
–Lorene Paludi Richardson

Cancer seems such an evil word in which we all find fear;
Parent, child, husband, or wife, anyone that we hold dear.
To know a loved one suffers, breaks every human heart;
Mere mention of the word, and you don't know where to start.
More often than not a prayer begins, then longing for relief;
You pray and pray and hope for the best, clinging to your belief.
Faith in God and doctors, too; believing there's always hope;
Yet frightened that all your dreams may soon go up in smoke.
It hits everyone the same, but I feel for women it's worse,
Thinking not only of themselves, but those they may leave on Earth.
They worry about their children, or their baby's every need,
Who will comfort or correct them, when they fall or start to read.
Can she watch them leave for school, or help them with their math?
Will she see them off on their first date, or walk their wedding path?
She'll worry about her spouse, perhaps an aging mom and dad,
Anyone she's close to, and it will make her sad.
Then suddenly she'll realize that she's *NOT* giving up,
Her cup ain't runnin' over yet . . . there's still room to fill it up.
You see, a mother, any woman, has this inner strength inside;
You don't know where it comes from, but she handles it in stride.
When she's so exhausted, and feels she just can't think,
She manages to raise it up and steps back from the brink.
Whatever it takes to get it done, she finds the strength to fight;
Oh, she struggles every day . . . yet pushes with all her might.
When cancer becomes the demon, she fights with renewed grace;
She believes deep down inside that she must win this race.
Chemo, radiation, all the medicine and prayer,
It all helps just knowing . . . that she is in God's care.
Some of us are lucky, when it's not so advanced;
We may very possibly, just get another chance.
Then all those tears and worry that managed to amass
Become a well-worn part of our once saddened past.

We must go along believing that there is *always* hope;
And our family, friends, and loving God give us the strength to cope.
Medicine and prayer go often hand in hand;
But for some it may forever be so hard to understand.
I lost my mom to this disease; leukemia was its name;
I still remember where I was and the day when that call came.
Our world had just been shattered, thinking of what was to come;
But my mom lived, 15 more years, still believing she had won.
She was luckier than many, and I'm grateful as can be;
The Good Lord knew we weren't ready, especially . . . well, "me."
So hope *cannot* be abandoned . . . it just isn't right;
It's what gives that inner strength that's hidden from our sight.
A cure *WILL BE* forthcoming, somewhere out of the blue,
From some tiny little cell or gene . . . or a plant that no one knew.
So love your loved ones dearly; hug them with all your might;
And live a life worth living, not cowering from fright.
One thing is for sure . . . live it without regret;
Know that just one shred of hope, *isn't* all we get.
Hope does spring eternal; that's what the poet said;
It is hope that keeps us going . . . no matter what's ahead.
The beauty of God's world is here and in eternity,
Where He makes each decision, of just what is to be.

Lovingly dedicated to members of the Richardson/Paludi family, whose love continues from their heavenly home.

Contents

PART IV: WOMEN AND CANCER: RELATIONSHIPS AND SEXUALITY ISSUES

Series Foreword

Michele A. Paludi

Because women's work is never done and is underpaid or unpaid or boring or repetitious and we're the first to get fired and
what we look like is more important than what we do and if we
get raped it's our fault and if we get beaten we must have pro-
voked it and if we raise our voices we're nagging bitches and if
we enjoy sex we're nymphos and if we don't we're frigid and if
we love women it's because we can't get a "real" man and if we
ask our doctor too many questions we're neurotic and/or pushy
and if we expect childcare we're selfish and if we stand up for
our rights we're aggressive and "unfeminine" and if we don't
we're typical weak females and if we want to get married we're
out to trap a man and if we don't we're unnatural and because
we still can't get an adequate safe contraceptive but men can
walk on the moon and if we can't cope or don't want a pregnancy we're made to feel guilty about abortion and . . . for lots of
other reasons we are part of the women's liberation movement.

Author unknown, quoted in *The Torch*, September 14, 1987

This sentiment underlies the major goals of Praeger's book series Wom-
en's Psychology:

1. Valuing women. The books in this series value women by valuing
   children and working for affordable child care; valuing women by

respecting all physiques, not just placing value on slender women; valuing women by acknowledging older women's wisdom, beauty, aging; valuing women who have been sexually victimized and viewing them as survivors; valuing women who work inside and outside of the home; and valuing women by respecting their choices of careers, of whom they mentor, of their reproductive rights, their spirituality, and their sexuality.

2. Treating women as the norm. Thus the books in this series make up for women's issues typically being omitted, trivialized, or dismissed from other books on psychology.

3. Taking a non-Eurocentric view of women's experiences. The books in this series integrate the scholarship on race and ethnicity into women's psychology, thus providing a psychology of *all* women. Women typically have been described collectively, but we are diverse.

4. Facilitating connections between readers' experiences and psychological theories and empirical research. The books in this series offer readers opportunities to challenge their views about women, feminism, sexual victimization, gender role socialization, education, and equal rights. These texts thus encourage women readers to value themselves and others. The accounts of women's experiences as reflected through research and personal stories in the texts in this series have been included for readers to derive strength from the efforts of others who have worked for social change on the interpersonal, organizational, and societal levels.

A student in one of my courses on the psychology of women once stated:

> I learned so much about women. Women face many issues: discrimination, sexism, prejudices . . . by society. Women need to work together to change how society views us. I learned so much and talked about much of the issues brought up in class to my friends and family. My attitudes have changed toward a lot of things. I got to look at myself, my life, and what I see for the future. (Paludi, 2002)

It is my hope that readers of the books in this series also reflect on the topics and look at themselves, their own lives, and what they see for the future.

This *Handbook on Women's Cancers* provides readers with the opportunity to accomplish this goal and offers suggestions for all of us working with women cancer patients and survivors as psychotherapists, attorneys, health professionals, families, and friends. This text also assists us as advocates in guiding institutional and social policy change in medical research and in lobbying state and federal legislators on issues related to women's cancers. This text brings together scholarship, poetry, personal accounts, and biographies of women cancer survivors and victims. Gerlach, Marino, and Hoffman-Goetz (1997) noted that many gynecological cancers are not addressed in popular magazines. They note that most women obtain their education about cancer from this type of popular media. I edited this handbook to offer women and their family and friends up-to-date information on breast and gynecological cancers, including cancer treatment centers, popular books for young children as well as adults, and the American Cancer Society's guidelines for early detection of cancers in women. It is my hope that this book will bring education, healing, hope, empowerment, and sustenance for all who read it.

REFERENCES

Gerlach, K., Marino, C., & Hoffman-Goetz, L. (1997). Cancer coverage in women's magazines: What information are women receiving? *Journal of Cancer Education, 12,* 240–244.

Paludi, M. (2002). *The psychology of women* (2nd ed.). Upper Saddle River, NJ: Prentice Hall.

Foreword

Susan Strauss

> The goal is to live a full, productive life even with all that ambiguity. No matter what happens, whether the cancer never flares up again or whether you die, the important thing is that the days that you have had you will have lived.
>
> –Gilda Radner

A woman's body is a complex, intricate, and beautiful architectural feat of anatomy and physiology found within cells, tissues, organs, and systems. A woman's synchronization of hormones, with responding physiological changes of menstruation, reproduction, and menopause, is a daily miracle for women around the globe. Most women live their lives and experience the joys of womanhood without the storm that arises when she hears that dreaded word—cancer.

It is sometimes these very wondrous hormones, which have shaped her body, provided the ability to reproduce, to feed her baby, and bring her into her later life absent menstruation, that may cause the havoc of cancer. Perhaps her cancer diagnosis is due to her luck of the draw in having a genetic mutation that predisposes her to a specific cancer, or she has been exposed to environmental carcinogens, or a virus could be the culprit. Whatever the cause, the word—*cancer*—has become synonymous with the word *death*, which it need not be.

Dr. Paludi's book is a compilation of chapters examining women's cancer from a variety of perspectives and highlighting the myriad aspects of cancer. We now know that all cancer is genetic, and that cancer is not just one disease but many. Managing women's cancer from diagnosis through treatment and survivorship is an ever-evolving task. Whether the cancer is in its early or advanced stages, clinical trials are leading the way for new therapies to achieve successful outcomes. New treatments are being studied that are patient specific based on her unique tumor biology, resulting in improved quality of life.

Dr. Paludi's book examines cancer both from the perspective of the woman stricken with the disease as well as from the experience of her family. The chapters delve into the psychological impact on family members—the recognition, for example, that breast cancer in one sister may mean an increased risk in another sister—and highlights genetic counseling and genetic testing. The book deals with the difficult discussion of how cancer and its treatment impact a woman's sexuality, libido, and sexual self-esteem as well as the sexual relationship with her partner.

Discussions about treatment options, the elements to consider when determining which treatments to undergo, and the emotions that contribute to that decision-making process are examined. Included in her decision-making process is the fear of the numerous complications, some long lasting, from chemotherapy, radiation, and surgery. How do cancer survivors cope with the long-term effects of their treatment? This question is compounded if a female is diagnosed with cancer as a child, an adolescent, or a young adult; she has a longer life in which to deal with the potential untoward effects from her treatment.

A book on cancer would not be complete if it did not address the critical role that family caregivers, often the woman's children, play in supporting their family member during her cancer treatment and her healing. And, of course, not all treatment leads to healing; some treatment is not effective, and the woman dies of this devastating disease. Dr. Paludi's book does an excellent job of exploring the very difficult topic of suffering at the end of life. Death and dying do not necessarily follow linear steps, and for some of us our grief can become all-encompassing, interfering with our own life when a loved one has died. A moving chapter addresses the role of the survivor's faith and love within the web of the survivor's loss.

The topics of cancer, psychological pain, and death and dying are not pleasant to consider. The positive aspect of Dr. Paludi's book, however, is that the chapters discuss the positive changes that have occurred in cancer treatment resulting in improved health outcomes, longer life spans, and quality lives. The future of cancer treatment is exciting and hopeful. Cancer research, particularly of the genome, is suggesting a future where cancer may not be anything more than a chronic disease to be managed. Let's hope the future arrives quickly.

Foreword

Jennifer L. Martin and G. Michelle Collins-Sibley

As women approaching middle age, we look back and wish we could share the sage wisdom we have gathered over the years with our younger selves. We now have family and friends living with, surviving, and lost to cancer. Often we do not like to think about a tragedy such as cancer affecting us, or those we love, until we have no choice but to confront it directly, through the eyes of our loved ones or through our own eyes in the mirror. Because of this, it is important for us to share information that we believe would help girls and young women.

In this era of abstinence-only education, many school-aged girls are not taught to know their bodies, or to value their bodies and their sexuality. Abstinence-only programs teach girls to "wait until marriage" to explore their sexuality. Sexually transmitted infection (STI) and pregnancy rates reveal not only that young people are not "waiting," but also that they are ill equipped to protect themselves from harm that may have life-threatening consequences for them later. A recent study by the Guttmacher Institute (2013) revealed that 71 percent of U.S. teens have had sex by age 19. However, the sexual double standard is unfortunately still the standard. The label of promiscuity is pinned prominently to the chests of girls only.

Illinois may be a forerunner in sexuality education if Governor Pat Quinn signs into law House Bill 2675, which requires schools to provide sex education programs that include age-appropriate and medically accurate lessons on birth control and STIs. However, this law is not a panacea. It still allows schools to "op-out" of sexuality education altogether.

Because the question of sexuality education is so highly politicized, advocates for women and girls, such as ourselves, need to be vocal whenever we can and to encourage others to do the same. Those who promote abstinence-only sex education often do so in the name of cherishing our children and teaching them self-respect; however, this promotion of abstinence until marriage contributes to the long history of cultural objectification of and desire to control women's bodies and fertility.

Images of black women and their bodies have been understood "to represent that which could be dominated and that which could be possessed, especially sexually" (Willis & Williams, 2002, p. 3). Black bodies, women's bodies are at once invisible and hypervisible. Remember Sojourner Truth, female because she bore children yet male because of her work as a field hand? Or the tragic mulatto whose black blood is concealed by an apparently white body—a body whose beauty is linked to its whiteness?

Against the weight of that history, reinforced by centuries of New World enslavement with its mammies, Aunt Jemimas, tragic mulattos, Sapphires, or Jezebels—not to mention the double whammy of a Cartesian dualism exalting the mind and denigrating the body and contemporary objectifications of women in popular culture—what does it mean to teach young 21st-century women, whatever their heritage, to respect their bodies and learn about cancer? Cancer represents a new manifestation of the cultural double bind, so often striking women at the heart of culturally inscribed definitions of the feminine—literally the internal and external signs of womanhood: womb and breasts. Too often, for too many women, treating their disease comes at too high a price: the perceived loss of their essential womanliness. So rather than confront that fear, they may retreat into ignorance, into silence.

So where do we begin? In "Poetry Is Not a Luxury," Audre Lorde recalls for us that "[t]he white fathers told us: I think therefore I am," but "[t]he Black Mother within each of us—the poet—whispers in our dreams: I feel, therefore I can be free" (p. 38). Lorde reminds us that our strengths reside not just in our minds but also in our bodies, in our feelings—our visions. While we may mourn the loss of corporeal elements of the body, we are not merely our bodies. Rather than "decorporealizing" ourselves, to borrow Carla J. Peterson's word, as did 19th-century abolitionists with their focus on mind, soul, or rhetorical skill, we might begin by reminding ourselves of the teachings of our African ancestors that the body is never simply flesh but always flesh *and* spirit, that the boundary between the material and spiritual worlds is fluid and permeable, for "the material is just the spiritual taking on form" (Somé, qtd. in Peterson, 1998, p. ix). While we may mourn the loss of corporeal elements of the body, we are not merely our bodies.

NOTE

This foreword is dedicated to Barrie Herbold, Flo Bush, and Alice Kondraciuk.

REFERENCES

Guttmacher Institute. (2013, June). Facts on American teens' sexual and reproductive health. Retrieved from http://www.guttmacher.org/pubs/FB-ATSRH .html

Lorde, A. Poetry is not a luxury. *Chrysalis: A Magazine of Female Culture, 3.*

Lorde, A. (1978). *A litany for survival: The black unicorn poems* (pp. 31–32). New York: Norton.

Lorde, A. (1984). *Poetry is not a luxury: Sister, outsider.* Freedom, CA: The Crossing Press.

Lorde, A. (1995). *The cancer journals* (2nd ed.). San Francisco, CA: Aunt Lute Books.

Peterson, C. (1998). *Doers of the world: African American women speakers and writers in the North, 1830–1880.* New Brunswick, NJ: Rutgers University Press.

Peterson, C. J. (2001). Foreword: Eccentric bodies. In M. Bennett & V. D. Dickerson (Eds.), *Recovering the black female body: Self-representation in African American women* (pp. ix-xiii). New Brunswick, NJ: Rutgers University Press.

Willis, D., & Williams, C. (2002). *The black female body: A photographic history.* Philadelphia, PA: Temple University Press.

Acknowledgments

I thank Hamilton College, especially graduate Sarah Perdomo, for inviting me to present my work on women's cancers in 2011. It was this opportunity that led me to meet geneticist Dr. Jinnie Garrett and students committed to talking about and participating in advocacy programs on women's cancers. I had always discussed women's cancers in my courses on the psychology of women, but my work at Hamilton College during the 2011–2012 academic year led me to become more educated about women's cancers, especially about feminist revisions to the books available to women and their families.

I am especially grateful to Hamilton College for selecting Rebecca Skloot's text, *The Immortal Life of Henrietta Lacks* (2010), as the book to discuss for the 2011–2012 academic year. Learning about Ms. Lacks and the intersection of sexism and racism in medical care has made me more sensitive to these issues and fueled my passion to lobby on behalf of women's cancers and other health issues.

Henrietta Lacks, an African American woman, was the unwitting source of cells from a cancerous tumor in her cervix to create the first known human immortal cell line used in medical research. This cell line is referred to as the HeLa (He from Henrietta, and La from Lacks) cell line. As Skloot noted with respect to Ms. Lacks:

> Her cells were part of research into the genes that cause cancer and those that suppress it; they helped develop drugs for treating herpes, leukemia, influenza, hemophilia, and Parkinson's disease, and they've been used to study lactose digestion, sexually transmitted

diseases, appendicitis, human longevity, mosquito mating, and the negative cellular effects of working in sewers. (p. 4)

Neither Ms. Lacks nor any family member gave their consent for this removal of cells. Shortly before I completed writing this handbook, the U.S. National Institutes of Health and the family of Ms. Lacks agreed to the following:

The distribution and access of Ms. Lacks' cells will be restricted to scientific researchers who are funded by United States government grants. Furthermore, requests will be reviewed by a six-person panel that includes members of Ms. Lacks' family. Publications resulting from this research will reference that Henrietta Lacks was the source of the cells. (Kroll, 2013)

The topic of women's cancers is a difficult one to write about and discuss. I thank the contributors to this handbook for being willing to participate in this project. I met most of you for the first time through this handbook. I look forward to more collaborations. Thank you for the work you do on behalf of women patients and survivors.

I also thank Debbie Carvalko at Praeger for her understanding of my wanting to pursue and deal with topics that aren't the easiest but that are the most important. And finally, I thank my sisters Rosalie Paludi and Lucille Paludi.

REFERENCES

Kroll, D. (2013, August 8). Ethical justice, but no financial rewards, for the Henrietta Lacks family. *Forbes*. Retrieved from http://www.forbes.com/sites/davidkr oll/2013/08/08/ethical-justice-but-no-financial-rewards-for-the-henrietta -lacks-family/.

Skloot, R. (2010). *The immortal life of Henrietta Lacks*. New York: Crown.

Introduction

Michele A. Paludi

During the completion of writing this handbook, national news brought the issue of women's cancers to the forefront once again. In May 2013, actress Angelina Jolie announced that she had undergone a preventive double mastectomy. Jolie wrote an op-ed essay for the *New York Times* in which she discussed this surgery as "proactive" and a choice that she was "very happy I made."

Jolie had tested positive for the BRCA 1 gene (Breast Cancer Susceptibility Gene 1), which increases the risk of breast and ovarian cancer. This gene belongs to a class of genes referred to as tumor suppressors (National Cancer Institute, 2013). Women's risk of developing breast or ovarian cancer is increased if they inherit a BRCA 1 (or BRCA 2) mutation. The National Cancer Institute (2013) has noted that approximately 12 percent of women in the general population will develop breast cancer during their lifetime as compared to 60 percent of women who inherited the BRCA 1 gene. Breast or ovarian cancer is associated with a BRCA 1 or 2 mutation in families with a history of multiple cases of breast cancer or breast and ovarian cancer. Hatfield (2012) offered the following additional statistics about breast cancer:

- Estimated number of new cases of breast cancer in the United States in 2012: 226,870

- The average age a woman is diagnosed with breast cancer: 61

- Overall five-year relative survival rate for a woman diagnosed with breast cancer that has spread to other organs: 23.8%

- Overall five-year relative survival rate for women currently diagnosed with breast cancer: 89%
- Overall five-year relative survival rate for a woman diagnosed with breast cancer that has not spread but is localized: 98.4%
- The number of deaths from breast cancer in 2012: 39,510

Also important to note is the incidence of breast cancer for women of color. People of color comprise 26 percent of the total population in the United States. By 2050 it is projected that people of color will represent approximately 50 percent of the population. Approximately 6 percent of practicing physicians are Latino, Native American, and African American (Paludi, 2013b). People who share cultural norms, experiences, and values are more comfortable with one another and communicate better. Good communication leads to good care. If the medical workforce does not reflect the demographics, then the health care delivery is compromised (Paludi, 2013b).

Breast cancer is the most common cancer for Latinas (Pabst, 2012). Rivera (cited in Pabst, 2012) explained the finding that women of color in the age group of 40 and older are less likely to utilize cancer preventive services because their primary responsibility and concern is to their families.

African American women are more likely to die from breast cancer than any other racial group (Baksh, 2011). They are less likely than white women to be diagnosed with breast cancer because of unequal access to improved treatments and lack of medical coverage. African American women younger than 45 have a five-year survival rate of 76 percent as compared to white women, who have an 89 percent survival rate.

Pabst (2012) also noted that Asian immigrant women living in the United States for as few as 10 years had an 80 percent higher risk of breast cancer than new immigrants.

Breast cancer is the leading common cancer in women in the United Kingdom. The highest incidence of breast cancer is in older women, explained by the impact of screening for breast cancer. In Scotland, lung cancer has surpassed breast cancer as the most common cancer (Cancer Research UK, 2013a). Throughout the rest of the world, breast cancer is the most diagnosed form of cancer (Cancer Research UK, 2013a). Incidence rates are highest in Western Europe and lowest in Eastern and Middle Africa. Within the European Union, the highest incidence rates of breast cancer are in Belgium, with 145 cases per 100,000), and the lowest rates are in Greece (57 cases per 100,000).

With respect to ovarian cancer, lifetime risk estimates in the general population are 1.4 percent as compared to 15–40 percent of women who have inherited the BRCA 1 or 2 gene (National Cancer Institute, 2013).

Sowter and Ashworth (2005) reported that the risk of developing BRCA 1– or 2–associated ovarian cancer is related to several factors, including reproductive history, more menstrual cycles, and hormonal exposure. Additional statistics concerning ovarian cancer offered by the Ovarian Cancer National Alliance (2013) include:

- Estimated new cases of ovarian cancer diagnosed in 2013: 22,240
- Estimated number of women who will die of ovarian cancer in 2013: 14,030
- A woman's lifetime risk of developing ovarian cancer is 1 in 72
- A woman's lifetime risk of dying from ovarian cancer is 1 in 95
- Median age of diagnosis: 63
- Median age of death: 71
- Relative five-year survival rate: 44%

The incidence and mortality rates of ovarian cancer are lower for African American women than for white women. Ovarian cancer for African American women is 74 percent of white women's rates. In addition, deaths from ovarian cancer are 80 percent of the rate for white women (Ovarian Cancer National Alliance, 2013).

Latinas have the second highest rate of ovarian cancer in the United States (Gillette, 2013). One explanation of this statistic concerns the following, according to Nucatola (cited in Gillette, 2013): "a greater percentage of Latinas (37 percent) are uninsured than the women of any other racial or ethnic group, and more than a quarter of Latinas live in poverty. Latinas are also more likely to live in areas with poor access to family planning services" (p. 1).

Within the member states of the European Union, ovarian cancer rates vary, with 12 cases per 100,000 women in Southern Europe to 17 cases per 100,000 women in Northern Europe. The highest incidence rates are in Latvia and Lithuania, and the lowest in Cyprus and Portugal (Cancer Research UK, 2013b).

Angelina Jolie indicated that her physicians informed her that she had an 87 percent risk of breast cancer and a 50 percent risk of ovarian cancer. She further indicated that the surgery reduced her chances of developing breast cancer from 87 percent to less than 5 percent. As she stated:

I am writing about it now because I hope that other women can benefit from my experience. Cancer is still a word that strikes fear into people's hearts, producing a deep sense of powerlessness. But today it is possible to find out through a blood test whether you are highly susceptible to breast and ovarian cancer, and then take action. (p. 1)

Reactions to Jolie's preventive surgery were for the most part positive, citing her courage and strength. For example:

> Angelina Jolie's essay about her choice to undergo a double mastectomy . . . was brave and generous. What rings through loudest is her commitment to her children, to be alive for them many years into the future. (*New York Times,* May 14, 2013, p. 1)
>
> I admire Angelina Jolie, and think it's great that she's encouraging other women to get the test. (*New York Times,* May 14, 2013, p. 1)
>
> Kudos to Angelina Jolie for speaking openly about her risk of developing breast and ovarian cancer. Despite decades of advocacy, many women are reluctant to speak about cancer, especially below-the-belt diseases like ovarian cancer. (*New York Times,* May 14, 2013, p. 1)

Jolie joined other women in the public spotlight who made the choice to have prophylactic mastectomies, for example, Christina Applegate, Debbie Wasserman Schultz, Giuliana Rancic, Sharon Osbourne, and Wanda Sykes. These women have been advocates for early screening for breast cancer. According to Osbourne (cited in Byrne, 2013, p. 1):

> As soon as I found out I had the breast cancer gene, I thought, the odds are not in my favor. I've had cancer before and I didn't want to live under that cloud. I decided to just take everything off.

Jolie, Osbourne, and others identified the benefits of BRCA testing, including:

> Identifying high-risk women;
> Identifying noncarriers in families with a known mutation;
> Allowing early detection and prevention strategies;
> Assisting in relieving anxiety regarding having cancer.

There are noted risks and limitations to this testing as well (Garrett, 2011), including:

> Not all mutations are detected;
> There is a continued risk of sporadic cancer;
> The efficacy of the interventions have yet to be proven;
> The test may result in economic harm and psychosocial harm.

With respect to the latter, there is an enormous disparity in access to quality health care for women with breast and gynecological cancers. Many women do not have health insurance. This lack of health insurance is a severe health threat for women seeking an exam and/or diagnosed with cancer. The BRCA test costs about $3,000. Uninsured women are more likely to die of breast and gynecological cancers. Furthermore, women are less likely to obtain appropriate medical care. Ayanian, Kohler, Abe, and Epstein (1993) reported that women with Medicaid were more than twice as likely to be diagnosed with late-stage cancer than were women who were privately insured.

In addition, women may not have access to prevention. For example, women who were adopted cannot obtain approval for the BRCA test as a consequence of not knowing their family's health risk of cancer. Thus, is there really a choice that *all* women have with respect to prophylactic surgery? No.

Habermann et al. (2010) evaluated national trends in prophylactic mastectomies from 2000 through 2006. They reported that approximately 15 percent of women aged 18 to 39 chose to have this surgery. This statistic is triple the percentage in 2000. CNN reported that the percentage of prophylactic mastectomies in 2013 was 20 percent. In addition, women with unilateral breast cancer commonly elect a contralateral prophylactic mastectomy in order to prevent cancer in their opposite breast (Tuttle, Habermann, Grund, Morris, & Virnig, 2007).

Recently, Saslow (2012) addressed prophylactic bilateral salpingectomy, the removal of the fallopian tubes to prevent ovarian cancer. Fallopian tubes are small ducts that link ovaries to the uterus. They are also referred to as oviducts, salpinges, or uterine tubes. These tubes extend out from the sides of the upper end of the uterus. They are narrow and lined with hair-like projections called *cilia*. The fallopian tubes each have three layers: internal mucosa, intermediate muscular layer, and outer serosa peritoneum of the uterus. The main purpose of the fallopian tubes is to carry a fertilized egg into the uterus for implantation. They are approximately four inches long. The ends of fallopian tubes are referred to as "fimbria."

In September 2013, lyricist Kara Dioguardi reported in *People* magazine (Born to Rock, 2013, p. 82) that she tested positive for BRCA 2 and opted to have her ovaries, uterus, and fallopian tubes removed. According to Dioguardi: "Grey [her son] may not know my grandmother or mother, but I can sing the songs they sang to me and know that he'll feel connected to them through me" (p. 82). Dioguardi's mother died of ovarian cancer when she was 50 years old.

Saslow (2012) noted that to date there is insufficient prospective research that this surgery will prevent or even decrease women's risk of ovarian cancer. She also identified some potential risk factors, including earlier menopause and increased risk of stroke, heart disease, and osteoporosis as a consequence of the lack of blood supply to the ovaries. However, FORCE (2011) noted that one-third of the 333 women in her study indicated that they would be willing to undergo this surgery. Women's responses included the following:

> I made the choice to have my tubes and one ovary removed last year. For me, it felt like the right decision. It was done almost a year ago and I have zero regrets about the surgery. (p. 4)
>
> I also want to keep my ovaries for as long as possible and have been asking my gynecologist to take out my tubes as a better-than-nothing prophylactic measure for now. (p. 4)
>
> It's tempting to keep the ovaries, because undergoing surgical menopause during my sexual peak feels like another cruel, cruel hand dealt to the BRCA patient. (p. 3)
>
> Ovarian cancer is terrifying, but so is early menopause. I would love another option. (p. 3)

Parker (2010) noted that bilateral oophorectomy (surgical removal of women's ovaries) during a hysterectomy is common to prevent ovarian cancer. It is performed in 55 percent of women having a hysterectomy. Parker's research suggests that this prophylactic surgery has great risk. The procedure causes a decline in circulating ovarian estrogens and androgens. Estrogen deficiency is a contributing factor to coronary artery disease, hip fracture, and neurological conditions. Parker concluded that more women are undergoing this procedure than they should. Brawley (cited in Webber, 2013) described this increase in prophylactic surgeries as a "nightmare. . . . A lot of women are going to go to their doctor and demand this test and not really need this test" (p. 1). Brawley believes that women's decisions to be tested are in direct response to Jolie's decision to have a mastectomy, what *Time* magazine in 2013 termed "The Angelina Effect."

It is also noted that prophylactic surgery does not prevent cancer totally. For example, the American Cancer Society indicates that approximately 10 percent of the breast tissue is still present following a double mastectomy and may become cancerous. Ehrenreich (2009) also noted that mammographic screenings of women less than 50 years old fail to reduce breast cancer mortality. A breast cancer survivor herself, Ehrenreich (2009) summarized:

> I do know that biopsy was followed by the worst six months of my life, spent bald and barfing my way through chemotherapy. This is what's at stake here: Not only the possibility that some women may die because their cancers go undetected, but that many others will lose months or years of their lives to debilitating and possibly un-necessary treatments. (p. 2)

In addition, common physical changes accompanying cancer and cancer treatment include: scars from surgery, fatigue, lymphedema, loss of sensation, less endurance, changes in sexual functioning, weight fluctua-tions, and changes in body functions (Paludi, 2011). All of these physical changes impact women's body image, including feelings of insecurity, deficiency, and embarrassment (Paludi, 2011). Signs of negative body image include feelings of shame, difficulty with intimacy, overpreoccupa-tion with appearance or body changes, camouflaging or hiding aspects of their appearance, and emotional problems that interfere with women's daily living.

Psychological responses to cancer diagnoses and treatments include: severe emotional distress, major depression, suicidal ideations, general-ized anxiety disorder, and post-traumatic stress disorder (Paludi, 2011).

WOMEN'S CANCERS: FEMINIST ISSUES

An issue raised by the responses to Jolie's surgery concerns whether breasts and reproductive organs define femininity and beauty (Datan, 1989; Wilkinson & Kitzinger, 1994). Certainly racism in American culture's standard of physical attractiveness is evident (Poran, 2002). Furthermore, women with disabilities are not typically considered attractive (Paludi, 2013a). They are also less likely to undergo screening for cancer (Smith & Hutchinson, 2004; Turnbull, 2013) as a consequence of lack of access to health care prevention, inaccessible environments, and stereotypes about disabilities. Rajan (cited in Turnbull, 2013) noted: "It's really hard for healthcare professionals to think of a patient with a disability as a woman first, due to stereotypes and unknowns" (p. 1).

Other issues include emotional and cultural meanings associated with breasts and mastectomies and sexuality. As one woman noted (cited in DeLucrezia, 2013, p. 9):

In the U.S., one need look no further than a magazine rack to know that we seem to prize women's parts over the person. Sadly, no matter how much progress we've made in this area, it is still an issue. And more importantly it is an issue that is killing women, who are terrified of breast cancer diagnosis.

Women's experience of cancer is influenced by a cultural emphasis on "attractive" bodies, especially on breasts as objects of men's sexual interest (Spence, 1995). Many women diagnosed with breast cancer are concerned with being "less feminine," "damaged," and "deficient" (Paludi, 2011). Szumacher (2006) reported that even the terms used to discuss surgeries for women's cancers are negative, such as "disfigurement" or "mutilation." In addition, surgeons often describe how they can "restore" the feminine figure (Szumacher, 2006).

Such terms reinforce women's sense of bodily imperfection and reinforce their feelings of being worthless to society. Women who fear the loss of their breasts often have this fear trivialized through such comments as "Who will know?" or "You can have new ones made." Women often feel a sense of diminished femininity when diagnosed with gynecological cancers as well as when having mastectomies.

O'Connor (2013) noted that Americans are breast obsessed and that the United States is among the countries with the most cases of diagnosed breast cancer. She stated:

> Not every woman keeps her breasts. . . . But some women don't miss their breasts, and there is a power in hearing from them. . . . Jolie expresses no sorrow whatsoever. Her only nod to missing one's natural breasts comes in a brief, optimistic note about reconstruction: "There have been many advances in this procedure in the last few years, and the results can be beautiful." (p. 4)

Latteier (1998) and Wiederman and Hurst (2006) also discussed breast obsession as culturally constructed and interwoven with attractiveness, beauty standards, breast-feeding practices, and sexuality. In patriarchal cultures, breasts are a "daily visible and tangible signifier" of femininity (Young, 1992). Consequently, women with breast cancer are positioned away from femininity (Paludi, 2011; Spence, 1995). Furthermore, women with breast cancer are perceived as asexual.

Recently, Puvia and Vaes (2013) reported that sexually objectified women were significantly dehumanized, while nonobjectified women were not. There has been an overemphasis by medical personnel on "looks" and a cultural definition of "beauty" (Paludi, 2011; Szumacher, 2006). Terms include "ingenious new techniques" to enable "the exhibition of a modest degree of cleavage" and procedures to "improve" women's bodies. Women may view their breasts as belonging to their lovers and children. Thomas-MacLean's (2005) interviews with women who have had mastectomies revealed women identifying themselves as having a loss of bodily symmetry, which led to their concealing the "deformity." Manderson and Stirling (2007) reported women who have had mastectomies wearing prosthesis to appear "normal" and "whole."

Szumacher (2006) offered the following woman's account as supportive of a cultural definition of beauty:

> My . . . second mastectomy, performed at the time of breast reconstruction, was prophylactic. My surgeon said he could not offer a good match after reconstruction unless both breasts were reconstructed and

I allowed myself to be swayed to his belief. Now, I regret sacrificing my healthy left breast. . . . If I had to do it again, I would not trade a healthy, functioning breast just to try to achieve what a surgeon calls "A better match." It is a lasting regret. I could have breast-fed our son if I had resisted that surgeon's coercion.

Jolie's op-ed piece included the following comments:

I had the major surgery, where the breast tissue is removed and temporary fillers are put in place. The operation can take eight hours. You wake up with drain tubes and expanders in your breasts. It does feel like a scene out of a science-fiction film. But days after surgery you can be back to a normal life. (p. 1)

O'Connor (2013) interpreted Jolie's statement to mean "You can be a woman without natural breasts. You can be a normal woman with no breasts at all" (p. 3).

Additional forms of women's cancers elicit similar cultural concerns related to femininity when they should elicit discussion/concern about morbidity, survival rate, impact on psychological health, and so on. Findings from research by Sacerdoti, Lagana, and Koopman (2010) identified changes in sexual functioning and self-concept issues in women with fallopian tube cancers, especially those who had surgical removal of the tubes. Women reported a decrease in positive body image, distancing in intimate relationships, and decrease in self-concept. I note that few prospective studies have been conducted on prophylactic surgery for fallopian tube cancer.

REDEFINING WOMEN'S HEALTH

Paludi (2011) called for reframing women's responses to cancer diagnoses and treatment in terms of "resilience." Ehrenreich (2009) called for a new women's health movement:

one that is sharp and skeptical enough to ask all the hard questions: What are the environmental (or possibly life-style) causes of the breast cancer epidemic? Why are existing treatments like chemotherapy so toxic and heavy-handed? And, if the old narrative of cancer's progression from "early" to "late" stages no longer holds, what is the course of this disease (or diseases)? What we don't need, no matter how pretty and pink, is a ladies' auxiliary to the cancer-industrial complex. (p. 2)

A new women's health movement includes a feminist approach to deciding on treatment for cancer (Paludi, 2011; Szumacher, 2006), a movement that encourages women to:

- Make their own choices;
- Not rely on masculine-based definitions of beauty;
- Not rely on masculine-based definitions of sexuality;
- Not accept victim blaming;
- Be critical of medical advice;
- Facilitate support groups;
- Assist women with transportation to health care and treatment;
- Lobby for better health care;
- Lobby for better preventive care.

Furthermore, the literature on breast and gynecological cancers is typically not written at the appropriate reading level and is not culturally sensitive (Guidry, Fagan, & Walker, 1998). These facts play an important part in why women are not as knowledgeable as they must be about cancer (Paludi, 2002). Breast self-examination for breast cancer is used by only a fraction of the women who might benefit from it. Research has also indicated that older women, who are at a greater risk for breast cancer, are least likely to examine their breasts (Grady, 1988). The failure of women to use breast self-examination may result from being discouraged from touching their bodies (Fulmore, 1999; Helgeson, Cohen, Schultz, & Yasko, 2000).

In addition, women who ask questions of their physicians and surgeons are commonly referred to as "problem patients." Albino, Tedesco, and Schenkle (1990) concluded:

> Efforts of female patients to gain information and to take responsibility for their health are reconstructed by physicians to reflect women as emotionally dependent and hypochondriacal. . . . The maintenance of a male power advantage through withholding and reconstructing information . . . reflects . . . the white male middle class monopoly on medical knowledge and practice. The problem for women is twofold: first, it involves gaining access to health care and then, gaining full benefit from health care. (pp. 232–233)

Albino, Tedesco, and Schenkle (1990) also noted that physicians "talked down" to women patients, and they did not use technical language because they believed that women could not understand the scientific and medical terminology. In addition, Verbrugge (1984) found that when women complained of physical symptoms, they were often diagnosed as mentally disturbed.

These views are reflected in self-help books for women cancer patients (Paludi, 2011; Szumacher, 2006). Szumacher (2006) offered the following examples:

> Cancer can be broadly viewed as the result of decreasing cooperation with the natural flow of life. (Clyne, 1989)
>
> Cancer or similar diseases are illnesses of the weakened spirit which is off balance and has lost the rhythm of life, of love. (Richardson, 1988, p. 105)

These self-help books contribute to victim blaming; they imply that women are responsible for getting cancer and can cure themselves. These books will not be helpful to women in their search for meaning about their cancer and their identities, once they are survivors.

Bury (1982) noted that chronic illness is a "biographical disruption"; it undermines how we view ourselves and rethink our biography and self-concept from victim to survivor. For example, "Now that I have endometrial cancer, who am I? How have I changed? What has been the meaning of my life?" This "biographical disruption" is exemplified in the television program *The Big C*, which aired on Showtime beginning in 2010. *The Big C* chronicles the character Cathy Jamison, who is diagnosed with cancer. Her realization of this disease forces her to live differently as an adult. She initially conceals her cancer diagnosis from her family, which confuses them. She is depicted as finding freedom in new ways to express herself to her family and friends. *The Big C* has been viewed as a type of "self-help" book for cancer victims and their families. For example:

> This show was catharsis for my family and me. We've been through so many lives and deaths with cancer, and this show helped us talk about the likelihood of our own inevitable deaths. For me, especially, this show allowed me to grieve for my father, who passed away in 2010. The writers had quite the challenge to make the story relatable, and the entire cast was incredible in their portrayals of the struggles that family, friends, and the ill experience. (Hollywood Reporter, 2013, p. 1)
>
> I struggled to let go after my mother died of cancer in 2010—it was as if I wasn't allowed to cry because I knew she was dying. Thanks to Laura and the cast I have cried so much and feel as if I understood what my mom went through—from her perspective. Thank you for the healing. (Hollywood Reporter, 2013, p. 1)

The Big C is a representation of the feminist health care movement, which has provided many women with affordable, safe, and affirming medical services. The work on feminist health care for women contributes to an enlightened health care system, one that values *all* women and *all* women's bodies and minds. It is well noted that when women are provided with a choice of treatment for their cancers, their long-term adjustment to the illness is improved (Leinster, Slade, Dewey, & Ashcroft, 1989). Szumacher (2006) aptly summarizes the feminist perspectives on health care:

> Feminism involves the elimination of factors that contribute to continued systematic subordination of women . . . existing sexist oppression is wrong and must be abolished. The supremacy of medical hegemony over women patients with breast cancer is but one example of such oppression. (p. 656)

Angelina Jolie's decision was her preference, her choice. She was part of the decision-making process and offers one statement in fighting oppression. In response to Jolie's decision, Norsigian (2013) concluded:

> [I]t is now up to women's health advocates to ensure that the media coverage and public debate that follows does not offer false information or false hope . . . if women are not fully informed about all the issues involved before imagining that Jolie's decisions would be the right ones for them. (p. 1)

Zuckerman (cited in Norsigian, 2013) noted:

> As an actress whose appeal has focused on her beauty, surgically removing both her breasts when she didn't have cancer was a very gutsy thing to do. But if we care about women's health, we need to stop thinking of mastectomy as the "brave" choice and understand that the risks and benefits of mastectomy are different for every woman with cancer or the risk of cancer. In breast cancer, any reasonable treatment choice is the brave choice. (p. 2)

The contributions to this edited volume represent additional statements in fighting women's oppression with respect to breast and gynecological cancers. This handbook offers women and their friends and family up-to-date educational information for assisting them in making their brave choices.

CANCER AND THE WORKPLACE

As an organizational and forensic psychologist, my work in career psychology and discrimination also contributed to my decision to edit this handbook on women's cancers. Women have experienced discriminatory treatment by their employers because of cancer diagnosis and treatment.

In fact, I invited some women to share their stories in this handbook who refused for fear of retaliation by their employers, who did not know about the women's cancer and treatment. I respected their wishes. I break the general silence about this issue in the next section of this introduction. It is my hope that employers reading this handbook will also respect women employees who are battling cancer and not put them in the situation of also battling to keep their jobs, especially at the time when they need health insurance the most.

Consider the following:

In 2013 the Equal Employment Opportunity Commission (EEOC) sued Kyklos Bearing International for disability discrimination. Kyklos, an Ohio bearings manufacturer, fired one of their employees, Donique Price, because she had cancer. Kyklos claimed it fired Ms. Price because of her medical restrictions: she was required to lift as a condition of her employment, and no light duty work was available for her. However, the EEOC stated that Ms. Price had provided Kyklos with documentation from her physician that established she had been cleared to work without any restriction due to her being a cancer survivor. The EEOC Regional Attorney for this case, Debra Lawrence, stated: "Ms. Price bravely fought and won her battle against cancer, and now she is fighting for her employment rights.... Businesses need to view employees such as Ms. Price as the strong, resilient workers they are, not as potential weak links or future financial risks." (EEOC, 2013a, p. 1)

Also in 2013, the EEOC sued the Midwest Regional Medical Center in Oklahoma City for firing an employee as a result of her cancer and cancer treatment. The employee, Janice Withers, informed her supervisor that she had been diagnosed with cancer and would be undergoing radiation treatment. She was offered a leave of absence by her supervisor; however, Withers indicated that she wanted to work during the treatment for her cancer.

During her radiation treatment, Withers called into work ill because of nausea and fatigue. Her supervisor, Susan Milan, advised her that she was being placed on a leave of absence and told her to "get rested up from the radiation." Prior to her return to work at the mutually agreeable date, Milan fired Withers for "no call/no show." Withers was denied the opportunity to return to her job and perform her duties with or without a reasonable accommodation (EEOC, 2013b, p. 1).

In 2012 the EEOC sued The Home Depot in Towson, Maryland, on behalf of Judy Henderson, a cashier with the organization for 13 years. The Home Depot originally accommodated Henderson by granting her unpaid leave in order for her to undergo surgery to remove a tumor.

However, the company then informed Henderson that she would be terminated from her employment unless she advised the company of her health status. Henderson promptly provided The Home Depot with medical documentation confirming her medical release to return to her job. The Home Depot failed to respond to her medical documentation and fired her, presumably because the company lacked work for her. The EEOC charged, however, that the real reason was disability discrimination because of her cancer. In the past Henderson had been laid off temporarily, not terminated, when there was a seasonal lack of work. In addition, The Home Depot hired two cashiers at the same store after Henderson provided the company with her medical documentation. According to EEOC district director Spencer Lewis Jr., "It can be difficult for a major nationwide retailer the size of Home Depot to show how a few extra weeks of unpaid leave would be an undue hardship" (ADA in the Workplace, 2013).

These are but a few examples of what women face when discussing their cancer and cancer treatment at work. Macmillan Cancer Support research (Newcombe, 2013) found that 4 in 10 people who return to work following cancer treatment reported discrimination from their employers and were denied time off for medical appointments. In addition, the research found that cancer survivors were passed over for promotion. Ciaran Devane, chief executive at Macmillan Cancer Support, concluded that "Going to work after treatment can be very isolating especially if someone has been off for a while and has lost confidence or contact with colleagues" (cited in Newcombe, 2013, p. 1).

Title I of the Americans with Disabilities Act covers employers with 15 or more employees, in addition to state and local government employers. Furthermore, most states have their own laws prohibiting employment discrimination on the basis of disability. The EEOC is the federal agency enforcing the employment provisions of the Americans with Disabilities Act (EEOC, 2013c). According to the EEOC (2013c):

Despite significant gains in cancer survival rates, people with cancer still experience barriers to equal job opportunities. Often, employees with cancer face discrimination because of their supervisors' and coworkers' misperceptions about their ability to work during and after cancer treatment. Even when the prognosis is excellent, some employers expect that a person diagnosed with cancer will take long absences from work or be unable to focus on job duties. Title I of the Americans with Disabilities Act limits employers' abilities to inquire about cancer as well as other disabilities and to conduct medical examinations pre-job offer, post-job offer and while the individual is employed. This Act also prohibits retaliation against an applicant or employee who has opposed the employers' practices that discriminate based on cancer or for participating in an investigation as a complainant, respondent or witness. (p. 2)

Furthermore, job applicants are not required to disclose that they are cancer patients or survivors unless they are requesting a reasonable accommodation from the employer (e.g., time off to undergo chemotherapy).

The Americans with Disabilities Act also prohibits discrimination against "qualified individuals," individuals who, with or without a reasonable accommodation, can perform "essential functions" of the job. Functions are essential when they are the reason the job exists or because the function is so highly specialized that the individual is hired for his or her expertise in performing the specialized functions.

A modification or adjustment is "reasonable" by law if it "seems reasonable on its face, i.e., ordinarily or in the run of cases." Thus, the request is reasonable if it appears to be plausible or feasible. A reasonable accommodation enables an applicant with a disability such as cancer to have an equal opportunity to participate in the application process and to be considered for hire in an organization. In addition, a reasonable accommodation permits an employee with a disability the equal opportunity to enjoy the benefits and privileges of employment that employees without disabilities enjoy.

Despite the legislation concerning disability discrimination that has existed in the United States since 1992, individuals with disabilities still face enormous discrimination and harassment in the workplace because of stereotyping (e.g., Green, Davis, Karshmer, Marsh, & Straight, 2005). Stereotypes refer to individuals' thoughts/cognitions that typically do not correspond with reality. Stereotypes occur when individuals are classified by others as having something in common because they are members of a particular group or category of people (e.g., employees with cancer). Psychological research has identified that stereotypes have the following characteristics (Fiske, 1993):

1. Groups that are targeted for stereotypes are easily identified and relatively powerless.
2. There is little agreement between the composite picture of the group and the actual characteristics of that group.
3. This misperception is difficult to modify even though individuals who hold stereotypes have interacted with individuals of the group who disconfirm the stereotypes.
4. This misperception is the product of a bias in individuals' information-processing mechanisms.

Disability stereotyping is a psychological process that describes individuals' structured sets of beliefs about the personal attributes of people with disabilities (e.g., incompetent, burdens, incapable of participating fully in all aspects of life, victims, nonsexual, or having an illness that can be contracted by contact at the workplace; Fine & Asch, 1988; Stone-Romero, 2005). Psychologists have identified an emotional component to stereotypic cognitions: prejudice as well as a behavioral component to individuals' cognitions, in other words, discrimination. Thus, individuals' statements and nonverbal gestures toward individuals with disabilities provide insight into their structured sets of beliefs and emotions about people with disabilities (Bruyere, Erickson, & Ferrentino, 2003).

Stereotyping impacts individuals' career development. Doren and Benz (2001) noted in their review of 34 empirical studies dealing with gender, disability, and employment outcomes from 1972 to 1998 that women who have disabilities are less likely to be employed than women without disabilities or men with or without disabilities. In addition, Doren and Benz found that women with disabilities earn less than men with disabilities and that the wage gap increases with time. Women with disabilities are also more likely to be employed in positions rated as having lower status and as part-time employees than are men with disabilities. Finally, Doren and Benz found that women with disabilities do not remain at any one job as long as do men with disabilities.

Thus, stereotypes get expressed behaviorally in discriminatory treatment of employees with disabilities in terms of wages, pay increases, and promotions. In addition, women with disabilities who are of color experience more stereotyping than do white women or men in general, illustrating the concept of "intersectionality," which explains the oppressions faced by people who are simultaneous members of more than one disenfranchised group.

DeBoer (as cited in Rabin, 2009) indicated that cancer survivors have a 37 percent higher rate of joblessness than do individuals without cancer. DeBoer commented that "this issue is so important to patients, because they often regard returning to work as indicative of complete recovery."

Furthermore, women with cancer experience harassment in the workplace on the part of supervisors and coworkers. Such offensive conduct includes mockery, put-downs, making "jokes" about the loss of breasts, and comments about hair loss. Disability harassment is thus any verbal or physical conduct that is directed at a woman (or man) because she has cancer or other disability that is sufficiently severe, pervasive, or persistent so as to have the purpose or effect of creating a hostile work environment. According to the Equal Employment Opportunity Commission (2004):

> The ADA prohibits offensive conduct that is sufficiently severe or pervasive to create a hostile or abusive work environment. Acts of harassment may include verbal abuse, such as name-calling, behavior

such as graphic and written statements, or conduct that is physically threatening, harmful, or humiliating. . . . To be actionable, conduct related to an employee's intellectual disability must be sufficiently severe or pervasive as to be both subjectively hostile and abusive (to the person) and to a reasonable person.

Thus, legally, a hostile work environment may exist with respect to an individual's disability when:

- The employee is a qualified individual with cancer.
- Verbal and/or nonverbal behavior occurs because of an individual being a member of a protected class (e.g., having cancer).
- The harassment is unwanted or unwelcome.
- The harassment is severe or pervasive enough to unreasonably impact the employee's work environment.
- The employer knew or should have known of the harassment and failed to take prompt and remedial action.

Behaviorally, a hostile work environment for disability can include: posters, email, cartoons, or pictures displayed in the work area that create an offensive and intimidating environment for employees with cancer; engaging in threatening, intimidating, or hostile acts toward an employee with cancer; actual denial of a job-related benefit to an employee with cancer; telling jokes pertaining to women with cancer; making suggestive, obscene, or insulting sounds about individuals with cancer. In addition, a hostile work environment for employees with cancer includes inappropriate reference to their cancer, unwelcome discussion of the impact of their cancer and/or cancer treatment, and refusal to work with and exclusion of people with cancer from social events or staff meetings and training programs (Weber, 2007).

Campbell (2001) noted that women with disabilities, including cancer, endure ableism, a type of discrimination defined as:

A network of beliefs, processes and practices that produces a particular kind of self and body (the corporeal standard) that is projected as the perfect, species-typical and therefore essential and fully human. Disability is cast as a diminished state of being human. (a corporeal standard) that is projected as the perfect. (p. 44)

There is thus an intersectionality between gender and disability: women experience harassment and discrimination more than men in general (Emmett & Alant, 2006). However, women with disabilities face compound discrimination or a double jeopardy by being both female and disabled (Banks, 2010). According to Wendell (2009):

> [D]isabled are made "the other" who symbolize failure of control and the threat of pain, limitation, dependency and death. (p. 1527)

Disability microaggressions are subtle verbal, behavioral, or environmental insults that target women with cancer and other disabilities (Nadal, Hamit, & Issa, 2010). Microinsults include verbal and nonverbal behavior that conveys rudeness and demeans a group, such as women with gynecological or breast cancer (Sue, Bucceri, Lin, Nadal, & Torino, 2007). Microinvalidations are actions that negate or exclude the psychological thoughts or feelings of individuals who represent different groups, including women with cancer (Sue, Bucceri, Lin, Nadal, & Torino, 2007). Disability microaggressions are often discounted because they are ambiguous, and individuals who engage in this form of discrimination argue that the slights are unintentional. However, disability microaggressions result in significant impacts for women with cancer. Ignoring or tolerating lower level abuse creates an environment conducive to more serious aggressive behavior, including discrimination/harassment. Thus, when verbal aggression, isolation, and disrespect of individuals are tolerated or go unnoticed by supervisors, teachers, or other administrators, discrimination and harassment will follow.

Employers must prevent discriminatory treatment of women with cancer through exercising "reasonable care" with an effective and enforced antidiscrimination and harassment policy, investigatory procedures, and training programs in disability awareness and the organization's policy and procedures (EEOC, 2013c).

Schingel (2006) noted:

> Until we as a society can take the time to understand the roots of discrimination and take a good look at our own thought patterns, we'll never move forward. (p. 2)

In keeping with Schingel's sentiment, one major goal of this handbook is to provide individuals with the tools necessary to prevent as well as deal with cancer discrimination in the workplace.

REFERENCES

Albino, J., Tedesco, L., & Schenkle, C. (1990). Images of women: Reflection from the medical care system. In M. Paludi & G. Steuernagel (Eds.), *Foundations for a feminist restructuring of the academic disciplines* (pp. 225–253). New York: Haworth.

Americans with Disability Act in the Workplace. Retrieved from http://www.adaintheworkplace.org/settlementagreements.html.

Ayanian, J., Kohler, B., Abe, T., & Epstein, A. (1993). The relation between health insurance coverage and clinical outcomes among women with breast cancer. *New England Journal of Medicine, 329,* 326–331.

Baksh, S. (2011). *Here's how deadly breast cancer is for women of color in the U.S.* Retrieved from http://colorlines.com/archives/2011/11/breast_cancer_awareness.html.

Banks, M. (2010). Special issues for women with disabilities. In M. Paludi (Ed.), *Feminism and women's rights worldwide. Volume 1: Heritage, roles and issues* (pp. 149–160). Westport, CT: Praeger.

Born to rock. (2013, September 2). *People,* p. 82.

Bruyere, S., Erickson, W., & Ferrentino, J. (2003). Identity and disability in the workplace. *William and Mary Law Review, 44,* 1173–1196.

Bury, M. (1982). Chronic illness as biographical disruption. *Sociology of Health and Illness, 4,* 167–182.

Byrne, S. (2013). *Sharon Osbourne, Christina Applegate and other celebrities who had double mastectomies like Angelina Jolie.* Retrieved from http://omg.yahoo.com/blogs/celeb-news/sharon-osbourne-christina-applegate-other-celebrities.

Campbell, F. (2001). Inciting legal fictions: Disability's date with ontology and the ableist body of the law. *Griffith Law Review, 10,* 42–62.

Cancer Research UK. (2013a). *Breast cancer incidence statistics.* Retrieved from www.cancerresearchuk.org/cancer-info/cancerstats/types/breast/incidence/uk-breast/.

Cancer Research UK. (2013b). *Ovarian cancer incidence statistics.* Retrieved from www.cancerresearchuk.org/cancer-info/cancerstats/tpes/ovary/incidence/uk-ovarian.

Clyne, R. (1989). *Cancer: Your life, your choices.* Wellingborough: Thorsons.

Datan, N. (1989). Illness and imaginary feminist cognition, socialization and gender identity. In M. Crawford & M. Gentry (Eds.), *Gender and thought: Psychological perspectives* (pp. 175–187). New York: Springer.

DeLucrezia, N. (2013). *What they didn't tell Angelina Jolie about prophylactic-mastectomy.*

Doren, B., & Benz, M. (2001). Gender equity issues in the vocational and transition services and employment outcomes experienced by young women with disabilities. In H. Rousso & M. Wehmeyer (Eds.), *Double jeopardy: Addressing gender equity in special education* (pp. 289–312). Albany, NY: State University of New York Press.

Ehrenreich, B. (2009). *Not so pretty in pink: The uproar over new breast cancer screening guidelines.* Retrieved from http://ehrenreich.blogs.com/barbaras_blog/2009/12/not-so-pretty-in-pink.html.

Emmett, T., & Alant, E. (2006). Women and disability: Exploring the interface of multiple disadvantage. *Development Southern Africa, 23,* 445–460.

Equal Employment Opportunity Commission. (2004). *Questions & answers about persons with intellectual disabilities in the workplace and the Americans with Disabilities Act.* Retrieved from www.eeoc.gov.

Equal Employment Opportunity Commission. (2013a). *EEOC sues Kyklos Bearing International for disability discrimination.* Retrieved from www.eeoc.gov/ eeoc/newsroom/release/8-1-13.cfm.

Equal Employment Opportunity Commission. (2013b). *EEOC sues Midwest Regional Medical Center for disability discrimination.* Retrieved from www.eeoc .gov/eeoc/newsroom/release/7-30-13.cfm.

Equal Employment Opportunity Commission. (2013c). *Questions and answers about cancer in the workplace and the Americans with Disabilities Act.* Retrieved from www.eeoc.gow/laws/types/cancer.cfm.

Fine, M., & Asch, A. (1988). *Women with disabilities: Essays in psychology, culture and politics.* Philadelphia, PA: Temple University Press.

Fiske, S. (1993). Controlling other people: The impact of power on stereotyping. *American Psychologist, 48,* 621–628.

FORCE. (2011). *Facing our risk of cancer empowered.* Retrieved from http://facingourrisk .wordpress.com/2011/11/08/guest-blogger-reporter-stacey-sager/.

Fulmore, C. (1999). Applying cognitive-social theory of health protective behavior to breast self-examination. *Dissertation Abstracts International, 60 (3-B),* 95–99.

Garrett, J. (2011, September). *Genetics of women's cancers.* Presentation to Hamilton College, Clinton, NY.

Gillette, H. (2013). *New vaccine brings hope for Latinas with ovarian cancer.* Retrieved from http://saludify.com/vaccine-latinas-ovarian-cancer.

Grady, K. (1988). Older women and the practice of breast self-examination. *Psychology of Women Quarterly, 12,* 473–487.

Green, S., Davis, C., Karshmer, E., Marsh, P., & Straight, B. (2005). Living stigma: The impact of labeling, stereotyping, separation, status loss and discrimination in the lives of individuals with disabilities and their families. *Sociological Inquiry, 75,* 197–215.

Guidry, J., Fagan, P., & Walker, V. (1998). Cultural sensitivity and readability of breast and prostate printed cancer education materials targeting African Americans. *Journal of the National Medical Association, 90,* 165–169.

Habermann, E., Abbott, A., Parsons, H., Virnig, B., Al-Refale, W., & Tuttle, T. (2010). Are mastectomy rates really increasing in the United States? *Journal of Clinical Oncology, 28,* 3437–3441.

Hatfield, H. (2012, October). *By the numbers: Breast cancer.* Retrieved from www .webmd.com.

Helgeson, V., Cohen, S., Schultz, R., & Yasko, J. (2000). Group support interventions for women with breast cancer: Who benefits from what? *Health Psychology, 19,* 197–214.

Hollywood Reporter. (2013). *Laura Linney on the poignant value of "The Big C."* Retrieved from http://www.hollywoodreporter.com/live-feed/laura-linney-big -c-finale-448040.

Jolie, A. (2013, May). My medical choice. *New York Times.* Retrieved from www .nytimes.com/2013/05/14/opinion/my-medical-choice.html.

Latteier, C. (1998). *Breasts: The women's perspective on an American obsession*. New York: Taylor and Francis.

Leinster, S., Slade, P., Dewey, M., & Ashcroft, J. (1989). Mastectomy versus conservative surgery: Psychological effects of the patient's choice of treatment. *Journal of Psychological Oncology, 7*, 179–192.

Manderson, L., & Stirling, L. 2007. The absent breast: Speaking of the mastectomied body. *Feminism and Psychology, 17*, 75–92.

Nadal, K., Hamit, S., & Issa, M. (2010). Overcoming gender and sexual orientation microaggressions. In M. Paludi & F. Denmark (Eds.), *Victims of sexual assault and abuse. Volume 2: Cultural, community, educational and advocacy responses* (pp. 21–49). Westport, CT: Praeger.

National Cancer Institute. (2013). www.cancer.gov.

Newcombe, T. (2013). Rise in cancer patients facing discrimination at work. Retrieved from http://www.hrmagazine.co.uk/hro/news/1077127/rise-cancer-patients-facing-discrimination.

Norsigian, J. (2013). *Angelina Jolie, breast cancer, and you: How to make the right decisions for YOUR health*. Retrieved from www.ourbodiesourblog.org/blog/2013/05/the-right-decision-for-breast-cancer-treatment.

O'Connor, M. (2013). *Angelina Jolie: Breasts don't define femininity*. Retrieved from http://nymag.com/thecut/2013/05/angelina-dividing-a-sex-symbol-from-her-breasts.html.

Ovarian Cancer National Alliance. (2013). *Statistics*. Retrieved from www.ovarian-cancer.org/about-ovarian-cancer/statistics.

Pabst, G. (2012). *Breast cancer awareness and women of color*. Retrieved from http://www.jsonline.com/blogs/news/151424355.html.

Paludi, M. (2002). *Psychology of women*. Upper Saddle River, NJ: Prentice Hall.

Paludi, M. (2011, September). *Resilience: Women dealing with the psychological impact of cancer*. Presentation to Hamilton College, Clinton, NY.

Paludi, M. (2013a). Mental health impact of ableism for women with disabilities. In M. Paludi (Ed.), *Psychology for business success* (pp. 115–137). Westport, CT: Praeger.

Paludi, M. (2013b, June). *Inclusive excellence: A strategic process for recruitment, engagement and retention of students and faculty*. Presentation given to the University of Buffalo School of Medicine and Biomedical Sciences, Buffalo, NY.

Parker, W. (2010). Bilateral oophorectomy versus ovarian conservation: Effects on long-term women's health. *Journal of Minimum Invasive Gynecology, 17*, 161–166.

Poran, M. (2002). Denying diversity: Perceptions of beauty and social comparison processes among Latina, Black, and white women. *Sex Roles, 47*, 65–81.

Puvia, E., & Vaes, J. (2013). Being a body: Women's appearance related self-views and their dehumanization of sexually objectified female targets. *Sex Roles, 68*, 484–495.

Rabin, R. (2009). Cancer survivors struggle to find jobs, study finds. *New York Times*. Retrieved from www.nytimes.com/2009/02/18/heath/18 cancer .html.

Richardson, C. (1988). *Mind over cancer*. London: W. Foulasham.

Sacerdoti, R., Lagana, L., & Koopman, C. (2010). Altered sexuality and body image after gynecological cancer treatment: How can psychologists help? *Professional Psychology: Research and Practice, 41*, 533–540.

Saslow, D. (2012). *Can removing fallopian tubes prevent cancer?* Retrieved from http:// www.cancer.org/cancer/news/expertvoices/post/2012/08/28/can-removing -fallopian-tubes-prevent-cancer.aspx.

Schingel, R. (2006). *How the movie "Crash" illustrates race and ethnic relations in America.* Retrieved from www.associatedcontent.com/article/18187/.

Smith, B., & Hutchinson, B. (2004). *Gendering disability.* New Brunswick, NJ: Rutgers University Press.

Sowter, H., & Ashworth, A. (2005). BRCA 1 and BRCA 2 as ovarian cancer susceptibility genes. *Carcinogenesis, 26*, 1651–1656.

Spence, J. (1995). *Putting myself in the picture: A political, personal and photographic autobiography.* London: Camden Press.

Stone-Romero, E. (2005). Personality-based stigmas and unfair discrimination in work organizations. In R. Dipboye & A. Colella (Eds.), *Discrimination at work: The psychological and organizational bases* (pp. 255–280). Mahwah, NJ: Erlbaum.

Sue, D., Bucceri, J., Lin, A., Nadal, K., & Torino, G. (2007). Racial microaggressions and the Asian American experience. *Cultural Diversity and Ethnic Minority Psychology, 13*, 72–81.

Szumacher, E. (2006). The feminist approach to the decision making process for treatment of women with breast cancer. *Annals of Academic Medicine Singapore, 35*, 655–661.

Thomas-MacLean, R. (2005). Beyond dichotomies of health and illness: Life after breast cancer. *Nursing, 12*, 200–209.

Turnbull, B. (2013). *Women with disabilities less likely to be screened for cancer.* Retrieved from http://www.cbcn.ca/index.php?pageaction=content.page&id =7970&lang=enb.

Tuttle, T., Habermann, E., Grund, E., Morris, T., & Virnig, B. (2007). Increasing use of contralateral prophylactic mastectomy for breast cancer patients: A trend toward more aggressive surgical treatment. *Journal of Clinical Oncology, 33*, 5203–5209.

Verbrugge, L. (1984). How physicians treat mentally distressed men and women. *Social Science and Medicine, 18*, 1–9.

Webber, D. (2013). *Angelina Jolie, genetic testing and the ACA.* Retrieved from http:// capsules,laiserhealthnews.org/?p=19480.

Weber, M. (2007). *Disability harassment.* New York: NYU Press.

Wendell, S. (2009). Unhealthy disabled: Treating chronic illnesses as disabilities. *Hypatia, 16*, 17–33.

Wiederman, M., & Hurst, S. (2006). Physical attractiveness, body image, and women's sexual self-schema. *Psychology of Women Quarterly, 21,* 567–580.

Wilkinson, S., & Kitzinger, C. (Eds.). (1994). *Representing the other: A feminism and psychology reader.* Thousand Oaks, CA: SAGE Publications

Young, I. (1992). Breasted experience: The look and feeling. In D. Leder (Ed.), *The body in medical thought and practice* (pp. 215–230). Boston: Kluwer.

Part I

In Women's Own Voices

Chapter 1

My Personal Journey

Stephanie M. Karwan

This can't be happening to me. But it did.

"You need to come in for a consultation," a portentous phrase that I have come to hate and associate with only the worst outcome. It was the tip-off. I knew that it was not going to be good, but you hope against hope. And then your life changes forever—you get the diagnosis that you feared—"You have cancer," three little words that change everything. The most dreaded words that your doctor can ever say to you. It feels like a slap across the face. Your mind races; your heart feels like it is going to jump out of your chest; your hands shake; and your eyes fill with tears. You want to ask all the right questions, but it is hard to focus. You are angry. You are depressed. You are vulnerable. You are afraid. You are sad. You are in denial. And then it finally sinks in—you have "it"; your reality is forever changed.

The cancer diagnosis is very personal on every level. Do I give up and give in to it? Do I fight it? I was hurt—emotionally. I was damaged—physically. I was questioning—spiritually. I was forever changed—psychologically. My mind was spinning, trying to truly comprehend what the doctor was saying.

I am not even sure at that point that I was still listening to the doctor completely. Instantly I made my decision, partly because I still didn't believe it, and partly because I didn't know what else to do. I decided that I was going to fight like hell. After all, as Winston Churchill said, "If you're going through hell, keep going." And I took that to heart. I told the doctor, "Get it out; do it as soon as possible, right now; I want to go to the hospital from here—I don't want to wait." Of course, I had to wait, and it was many surgeries/procedures over three plus months before it was over. But now it is over, and I have been cancer free for 16 years! There is hope; there is healing; there is life after cancer.

Over the days, weeks, and months when it was all unfolding, question after question kept running through my mind. Can it be true? How can this be happening to me? Why me? How did this happen? Was it something that I did? Is it bad karma? What am I going to do? How am I going to tell my mother? How bad is it? Will I die? How long will I live? Will it hurt? Why me, God? I try to be a good person. What did I do to deserve this? What is going to happen now? When will it be over? Are you sure I have cancer?

You see, I had a rare type of cancer that occurs on the outer surface area of the female genitalia—vulvar cancer. There are several types of vulvar cancer, the most common of which is a form of squamous cell cancer that accounts for about 90 percent of all vulvar cancers; then comes melanoma at 5 percent; the remaining 5 percent is made up of less common cancers, including Paget's disease of the vulva, vulvar adenocarcinoma, and basel cell carcinoma. (See www.about.com/cancer.) Squamous cell cancer is the second most common skin cancer in light-skinned people. It is rare in people who have dark skin. I am a very light-skinned person of Eastern European descent. Squamous cell cancer is a type of nonmelanoma skin cancer. Vulvar cancer is very rare. It comprises about 4 percent of gynecologic cancers diagnosed in women.

I had no pain; I had no symptoms—so it couldn't be real. Could it? Cancer hurts. Cancer makes you lose weight. Cancer makes you pale. Cancer makes you gaunt. Cancer makes you tired. Cancer makes you frail. Cancer has some sort of symptom. Doesn't it? Not always.

It was a visual identification from my doctor during a routine yearly gynecological checkup—black and white spots on an area I would never see nor even think of trying to view! And I will thank him forever—it could have been easily missed by another doctor because vulvar cancer is rare in a 44-year-old; it is usually an older woman's disease. It is not common in a woman who is still, albeit late, in her childbearing years. Vulvar cancer can make itself known with lumps or masses, vulvar itching that lasts over a month, tenderness, a cut on the vulva that won't heal, nonmenstrual bleeding, vulvar pain, burning, or a change in a mole on the vulva; early diagnosis and treatment raises the cure rate to more than 90 percent. I had none of the symptoms. What I did have was a very knowledgeable and observant doctor; some others may have dismissed what they were seeing due to my age and the absence of other symptoms. Lucky for me that I had him and that I was eventually found to have carcinoma-in-situ, an early form of cancer that did not invade the surrounding tissue—it was contained.

But at least then I knew—I had cancer—the "other shoe" had dropped, and I could move on; I would fight it with everything I could. It is at that point that you decide to look fear in the face—you need to move forward; you need to deal with it and move on. I told the doctor to do whatever was needed, including chemotherapy and radiation; however, at that time, neither was yet developed for vulvar cancer. So I began the procedures that did exist—I had LEEPs (Loop Electrosurgical Excision Procedure, which uses a thin, low-voltage electrified wire loop to cut out abnormal tissue), excisions to cut out the spots, and oh-so-many biopsies. Biopsies were something I was all too familiar with; I had experienced them too frequently in my life. I had well over 25 biopsies for various issues of the cervix, vulva, endometrium, and breast over those troubling years. And I had LASERs—a focused laser beam that vaporizes (burns off) the layer of vulvar skin containing abnormal cells. Laser surgery is used as a treatment for VIN (vulvar precancer). It is not used to treat invasive cancer.

Nothing was totally successful, so another biopsy, another consultation, another procedure; more tears, more anger, more talks with God. It was at this time that I became extremely discouraged because the spots kept coming back. The doctor informed me that my malignancy was multicentric; he had to keep removing the next spot that popped up, and I kept hoping that each procedure was the last—that it was all gone. Wrong. Finally we reached the point of needing a more invasive approach, a surgery that was going to be more drastic. It turned out to be the final surgery that I needed, and it was very successful. However, not knowing what the outcome would be, I had to be sure that this was the right thing to do for me, so I sought a second opinion from a gynecological oncologist. Surprisingly, getting that second opinion was one of the hardest things that I had to do—but not because I was worried that my doctor was doing the wrong things. I trusted my doctor implicitly; I quite simply did not want to offend him by questioning his approach; I felt that I was betraying him. But this was my body and my fight, and I wanted to be sure that I was doing all the right things. So I gathered my courage, requested copies of all my records, and made an appointment for an exam and consultation with the specialist. Funny, now I wanted a consultation; that consultation could end up being my friend, not my enemy. The new doctor reviewed all my records—no easy task since I had a seriously large file filled with all sorts of tests, procedures, and pictures. The verdict—my doctor was doing, and had done, exactly the right set of things, in the right order, and the specialist agreed that a somewhat more radical surgery was now needed.

Surgery day arrived, and I found myself crying uncontrollably in the patient holding area of the operating suite. I felt so alone, so vulnerable, even though my family was outside, and I certainly had very concerned doctors and nurses consoling me. I was scared. What if this didn't work? What next? After all, chemotherapy and radiation were not options. Would I have to continue to be chopped up until I was some mutilated freak no one wanted to be near? I was feeling my mortality.

The surgery was a hemi-vulvectomy. A hemi-vulvectomy is the removal of not just the skin but also the deep tissue from one side of your vulva. Finally we had a winner! The surgical area was immediately closed satisfactorily by my gynecologist without need for grafting, and I did not need a separate operation by a reconstructive surgeon, which my doctor had predicted and which is often necessary.

Following vulvar surgery (the surgery is called a vulvectomy), recovery requires the normal steps. The area had to be kept very clean and the wound dry in order to heal and avoid infections—not an easy task in the genital area. The doctor provided a peri bottle, which is used to cleanse the surgical wound after urinating, and drying the area is accomplished with a hair dryer and warm air. I had become extremely adept at this and never developed an infection—something that completely surprised my doctor, who remarked that he had never seen anyone without an infection during this recovery. I was determined to do it all right and not jeopardize my recovery in any way—to the point of being obsessive—I just couldn't face a setback; I could not have emotionally handled any more bad news, however minor it may have been.

My first follow-up office visit went well, but the doctor informed me that I would need an exam every three months for the rest of my life. I can only assume that he expected it to spread to the other side and that there was a real possibility that it had spread elsewhere and would need aggressive treatment; perhaps he did not expect me to live long. We did the three-month exams for about four years. Then I graduated to every six months, but I was too afraid to wait that long, so I insisted that I be seen every four months; then we went to five months and eventually to six. And after 10 years he declared me cured, and we are now at regular annual checkups. Woohoo!

Are there complications? There can be. They can range from infections, to blood clots, to physical discomfort, to clothes rubbing, to numbness, to a reduction of sexual desire or pleasure. More radical surgery—a full radical vulvectomy—can remove the clitoris, and there can be a sexual impact. There may be a loss of sensitivity or a narrowing of the opening, making penetration painful, but there are lubricants and therapies that may help.

Does the vulva look different? I guess so, in some respects, but who cares, and who is looking? I am alive, and it is not like it is visible to everyone I pass by! And if a man won't accept me because he feels that I am damaged goods with a funny-looking vulva, then he is not the right one for me. No one is perfect.

Do I have any side effects? Some—I do dribble urine a little bit, and most times I wear a protective "pad" of some sort because it makes me feel fresher, but that is a personal choice, not a requirement. I can predict a change in the weather sometimes by an ache at the surgical site! This does get better over the years and less frequent. The urine stream is altered slightly and directed to the side of the surgery because that side where the tissue was removed is smaller. At night it can be difficult to "hold" my urine. If I turn over—and it is only when turning over—and feel the need to urinate, then I must get up and follow through because in that relaxed state I can't wait, or I will have an accident. During the day, I have no such issue. And I sometimes get "undie wedgies" because one side is smaller. In the grand scheme of things, all these complications are minor, and I have learned to live with them—and the operative word is "LIVE!" I am alive to experience these things—and that is the greatest gift.

In the hospital on the day following the surgery, the doctor turned to my mental state. He sent a social worker to help me cope with the cancer diagnosis and the removal of part of my body that could make me feel less of a woman and less attractive to a man. She found me up, freshly showered, curling my hair, and putting on makeup. She spoke with me for a few minutes, offered any help I wanted, and pointed out support groups—which I refused. She smiled and said, "I think you will be okay emotionally; you have a good attitude, and you are trying to get back to normal much faster than most people"—and I was. I just knew instinctively that this surgery had worked. I felt relieved. I felt rested. I felt alive again. I felt happy. I guess that I did not realize just how much all the stress of the last few months had affected me. My visitors commented on how wonderful I now looked. They also instinctively felt that the cancer was gone. It appears that, after all, I did have one symptom at least—I had not looked healthy, and now I did!

I am generally an optimistic person with strong faith and an incredibly loving and supporting family and priest. I think this combination was very beneficial for me. I remember coming home from the hospital and noticing that the world was so incredibly beautiful in spring. The grass was greener than I could ever remember, the air was fresher, the atmosphere crystal clear, but I must admit, in the weeks at home recuperating, I started to question some things. I knew summer was approaching, and I needed to think about how I wanted to fill my flower gardens, and I remember saying to myself, "Why bother? I am not going to be here." I also needed a new car, and I said the same thing. However, I think these thoughts were products of my eight weeks of recovery hibernation; once I was able to get out and about on my own, I quickly changed my tune and was ready and eager to go.

* * *

My questions then changed to "What caused it?" and "Can I prevent this in the future?" My doctor said, "Bad things happen to good people, and it is not always something that they have done." For me, I will believe to the day I die that my cancer was caused by stress. I was under unbelievable stress at work with a very demanding boss, and my mom had just come through some major life-threatening surgeries. Stress can cause the "fight-or-flight" response and actually be beneficial, but after a certain point it can cause major damage to your health and other areas affecting the quality of your life. That's my lot in life.

My doctor did see white spots on my vulva, so this could point to lichen sclerosus being present in my case; he also saw black spots. Prevention and cure for me starts with faith in three different senses. In the first instance, faith in my doctor—that he was correct, and I am cured. In the second instance, faith in the religious sense—I believe in a higher power, and I have faith that my prayers to my God are heard and answered in a favorable way, in whatever means he feels is beneficial for me. Thirdly, faith that there are, and will continue to be, medical strides every year in the understanding, diagnosis, prevention, and treatment of vulvar cancer.

What I believe is lacking is support for this rare cancer. Over time, I did agree to attend at least one support group meeting for women with cancer, only to find that it was almost solely dedicated to breast cancer. I had nothing in common with those women, except that I was a woman who had cancer; and the social workers and nurses who were there for support had no idea about vulvar cancer and sadly couldn't tell me what I wanted to know. They spent the time talking about Tamoxifen (the prescription drug to fight breast cancer), breast chemotherapy, breast radiation, and other breast cancer issues. All these issues were, and are, very important and need to be discussed and shared with women undergoing the same things, but certainly the session held nothing for me. I wanted to speak with someone who had vulvar cancer, preferably someone younger who could tell me what I could expect to undergo in the future—if I had a future, free or not, of this cancer.

I wanted to know how to deal with the roller coaster of emotions: fear, anger, guilt, anxiousness, insecurity, feeling undesirable and unattractive, being happy, being relieved, being worried, feeling shame, letting in de-pression, being sad, panicking, looking for release, searching for hope, feeling invincible, feeling vulnerable, being empty, feeling alive. Simply put, I just wanted to speak with someone personally knowledgeable and emotionally in tune with me, so I went home. I accepted my journey; I embraced my life and my family and my friends, and I looked forward to the future—even if that future was one day at a time; sometimes it was minute by minute or hour by hour when my emotions took over.

A positive attitude was elusive at times, but I got through it emotionally somehow, largely due to the support of my family, and physically due to my doctor's diligence. One thought I tried to hold in my mind was that cancer happens, and it was not my fault. I also knew that I was extremely lucky that my cancer was found early and that I had no pain. But that was a double-edged sword because then I wondered if it was really gone or was coming back since I had no personal way of knowing what was going on in between doctor's appointments and biopsies. Somehow the frequent appointments and tests became routine and an odd sort of comfort in that I knew anything further, should it come back, would be found sooner rather than later and dealt with before it became too bad.

And before I knew it, the days went by, then a week, then a month, then a year, and here I am 16 years later. My journey is, of course, unique to me, but my goal is to let others know that they are not alone, that there are people who really care, and that there is hope; new strides are being made more often than we know. Get regular checkups—they saved me—and don't give up hope.

Chapter 2

Breast Cancer, My Sister, and Me

Susan Strauss

This chapter is a combination of a review of the scholarly literature on breast cancer, interviews with experts in genetics and in cancer counseling, and information from pertinent websites. I have interspersed an informal conversational tone throughout, using my younger sister Julie's recent breast cancer diagnosis and treatment and its impact on us both as a case study of the disease. It is my hope that Julie's journey will capture the personal element of this devastating disease.

THE LUMP

Julie is a 57-year-old (56 years at the time of her breast cancer diagnosis) petite blue-eyed Caucasian woman. I love her to bits. She and her husband, Michael, are retired, and they live in our hometown in Minnesota.

It was January 2012, and Julie and Michael had just arrived at their new condo in Alabama to escape the Minnesota winter. It was to be their first winter in the condo. On January 11 my phone rang, and it was Julie (otherwise known as Baby Sister, Little Sister, and Squirt) telling me that she had found a lump in her breast and had made an appointment with a health care provider to get it checked out. My heart skipped a beat. I assured her (and me) that it was probably no big deal; most lumps are benign, and I reminded her that I had had a breast biopsy 30 years ago and that it was benign. Because she didn't live in Alabama and knew no physicians, she randomly selected a clinic she found on the Internet that was close to their condo. That scared me; she had no idea how competent the provider would be. She called for an appointment on January 11 and was able to see the nurse practitioner the next day. The nurse practitioner told Julie that the lump was suspicious and sent her for an ultrasound of her breast that same day. When the radiologist viewed the ultrasound, he was concerned and ordered a biopsy for the next day, January 13. When my baby sister called to tell me it wasn't looking good, I wanted to vomit! I couldn't believe it.

She had the biopsy on the 13th, and on visual inspection of the tissue, the doctor told her he was quite sure it was cancer. The tissue was sent to the lab. We waited on pins and needles for the lab results, which didn't come back until January 17. It was not good news. My baby sister had breast cancer!

EPIDEMIOLOGY

Breast cancer is a heterogeneous disease and the most common cancer in women with slightly fewer than 122 of 100,000 women of all races diagnosed per year (Centers for Disease Control and Prevention, 2012). The disease is the second leading cause of death after lung cancer for Caucasian, Black, Asian/Pacific Islander, and American Indian/Alaska Native women and the first cause of death for Hispanic women. Approximately 791,000 women in the United States will be diagnosed with breast cancer, and more than 275,000 women will die from the disease in 2012 (American Cancer Society [ACS], 2012). There are a few less than 3 million breast cancer survivors in the United States (Oz, 2012).

Breast cancer in African American women tends to strike at younger ages and be more deadly than breast cancer in Caucasian women (American Association for Cancer Research [AACR], 2008a). Molecular differences may explain why African American women have a higher breast cancer mortality rate, or it may be because they are often diagnosed at a later stage than Caucasian women (ACS, 2011a).

Breast cancer is predominantly a woman's disease, though it is sometimes found in men as well, with an estimated 2,140 annual cases in men (ACS, 2011c). Variables such as age, socioeconomic level, race, and ethnicity, in addition to the tumor's size, histologic grade, and hormone receptor status, play a critical role in the incidence and mortality of the disease (Henderson, Lee, Seewaldt, & Shen, 2012; Parise, Bauer, Brown, & Caggiano, 2009).

Difficulty in accessing a clinical breast exam (CBE) and mammography, and a lack of health insurance are associated with a diagnosis of advanced breast cancer. Women with lower incomes have a poorer five-year survival rate at every stage of diagnosis than women with higher incomes (Mahon, 2012).

WHAT IS BREAST CANCER?

Anatomy and Physiology of the Breast

In order to understand the complexity of breast cancer, a basic understanding of the breast's anatomy and physiology is required.

The breasts are attached to the chest wall laterally to the sternum (breast bone) by ligaments, and they rest on the pectoralis major muscle of the chest (Mahon, 2012). The breast shape and size are due to adipose tissue (fat) that extends throughout the breasts and surrounds the 15 to 20 milk-producing lobes, which are circular to the nipple. Each of the lobes encompasses numerous lobules, which give rise to very small bulb-shaped glands that produce milk when signaled by the hormones estrogen, progesterone, and specifically prolactin. These glands, lobules, and lobes are connected by ducts that transport milk to the nipple. The darkened area surrounding the nipple is the areola.

Estrogen and progesterone are the hormones responsible for the changes that occur in the breasts and the uterus during the menstrual cycle. As a woman ages, her breasts become less glandular and more fatty, due largely to a decrease in estrogen with menopause (Wood, Muss, Solin, & Olopade, 2005).

Recent Research

Years ago when a woman was screened for breast cancer, she either had it or she didn't. Little else was known about her cancer's receptors and genes. Today's screening is a whole other story. Breast cancer is not a single disease but a multitude of different diseases, each with its own distinct molecular and biological behavior and prognosis (Cancer Genome Atlas Network, 2012; Curtis et al., 2012; Henderson, Lee, Seewalt, & Shen, 2012; Parise, Bauer, Brown, & Caggiano, 2009). It is now believed that cancer is much more complicated and complex than scientists ever imagined.

A 2009 study profiled breast cancer into eight subgroups based on protein expression of the tumor—estrogen, progesterone, and human epidermal growth factor 2 (HER2) receptors (Parise, Bauer, Brown, & Caggiano, 2009). Receptor status will be discussed in more detail later in the chapter.

A large international breast cancer study found 10 different breast cancer subtypes, classified broadly based on their molecular profile/genetic expression, that are associated with survival (Curtis et al., 2012). This research found new genes that had not previously been tied to breast cancer. The study also discovered the relationship between genes and how cells signal cell growth and division. Professor Carlos Caldas, a co-lead author of the study and senior group leader at the United Kingdom's Cambridge Research Institute, said, "Essentially we've moved from knowing what a breast tumour looks like under a microscope to pinpointing its molecular anatomy—and eventually we'll know which drugs it will respond to" (University of British Columbia, 2012).

Yet another large breast cancer study found a prodigious genetic diversity of early-stage breast cancers (Cancer Genome Atlas Network, 2012). Its findings present a comprehensive knowledge of the process behind four breast cancer subtypes involving hormone receptors. This research also found that breast cancer consists of numerous distinct diseases. These three studies and others are exciting because they offer new approaches to successfully treating and curing the disease in the future by aligning treatment with the tumor type to determine the likelihood of metastasis and recurrence.

Types of Breast Cancer

Breast cancer is generally divided into lobular and ductal carcinoma (Mahon, 2012). Lobular carcinoma indicates that the cancer is located in the lobes of the breast, whereas ductal carcinoma indicates that the cancer is found in the milk ducts. These findings are further divided, using microscopic analysis, into in situ (noninvasive) or invasive (Wood, Muss, Solin, & Olopade, 2005). Most breast cancers are, however, invasive (Breastcancer. org, 2012a). In situ cancer indicates that malignant cells have not extended beyond the lobe or duct in which they were found. They are described as ductal carcinoma in situ (DCIS) or lobular carcinoma in situ (LCIS) and could advance as invasive cancer (National Cancer Institute [NCI], 2010). In 2008 roughly 27 percent of newly diagnosed tumors in the United States were DCIS. Very few of these tumors could be felt by palpation, and 80 percent were diagnosed using mammography alone. Additional types of breast cancer include the following:

1. Invasive ductal carcinoma (IDC) begins in the milk ducts and extends to surrounding breast tissue; most common type of breast cancer.
2. Less common subtypes of IDC include tubular, medullary, mucinous, papillary, and cribriform; these cells look and behave a bit differently than IDC cells generally do.
3. Invasive lobular carcinoma (ILC) begins in the lobule and extends to surrounding tissue.
4. Inflammatory breast cancer is a fast-growing cancer, which begins with skin redness and swelling rather than a lump.

5. Male breast cancer is rare and almost always ductal carcinoma.
6. Paget's disease of the nipple is a rare form of cancer around the nipple.
7. Recurrent and/or metastatic cancer returns after treatment or spreads to distant parts of the body.

Normal breast cells have estrogen and progesterone hormone receptors both inside and outside the cell that receive signals from estrogen and progesterone to promote their growth (Breastcancer.org, 2012b; Parise , Bauer, Brown, & Caggiano, 2009). If a cancerous tumor contains these hormone receptors, then it requires estrogen and progesterone to grow. Tumors that contain estrogen or progesterone receptors are referred to as estrogen positive (ER+) or progesterone positive (PR+); those tumors lacking estrogen and progesterone receptors are referred to as estrogen negative (ER-), or progesterone negative (PR-). Approximately 75 percent of invasive breast cancer contain the estrogen receptor, with higher rates seen in postmenopausal women (Harvey, Clark, Osborne, & Allred, 1999); primary breast cancer is also more likely to be positive for the estrogen receptor. About 65 percent of ER+ breast cancers are also PR+ (Breastcancer. org, 2012c). Approximately 13 percent of breast cancers are ER+ and PR-, and roughly 2 percent of breast cancers are ER- and PR+. Very few breast cancers test negative for estrogen receptors but positive for progesterone receptors. About 25 percent of breast cancers are ER- and PR-.

Approximately 20 percent to 30 percent of breast cancers contain a protein on the surface of their cells called human epidermal growth factor receptor-2 (HER2) (Breastcancer.org, 2012d). Normal healthy breast cells contain HER2, which instructs the cell how to grow and develop. But in those women with HER2 cells that overexpress the protein (HER2+) due to a gene mutation, breast cancer results (Pruthi, 2012). HER2+ receptors result in faster cancer cell growth, resulting in the creation of even more HER2+ cancer cells (Pegram & Slamon, 2000). HER2+ breast cancer is more aggressive because it grows and metastasizes more quickly, thereby creating a poorer prognosis and increasing the likelihood of recurrence following treatment (Pruthi, 2012). Fortunately, HER2+ treatments are very effective. Not all HER2+ tumors are alike, and there have been two different types of HER2+ tumors found (Cancer Genome Atlas Network, 2012).

The combination of ER, PR, and HER2 creates eight different subtypes. Examining these eight (ER/PR/HER2) in combination provides physicians with a more accurate indicator for survival (Parise, Bauer, Brown, & Caggiano, 2009). Parise et al.'s study determined that individual tumor markers such as ER or PR or HER2 are not as important to survival as the combination of these markers. "Each subtype appears to be unique and may require individualized clinical management as the concept of a 'one size fits all' strategy slowly vanishes" (p. 600). The eight subtypes and the percentage of relative five-year survival include the following:

1. ER+/PR+/HER2-   96.4%
2. ER+/PR-/HER2-   91.9%
3. ER+/PR+/HER2+   91.3%
4. ER+/PR-/HER2+   88%
5. ER-/PR+/HER2-   82.7%
6. ER-/PR+/HER2+   78.8%
7. ER-/PR-/HER2-   76.2% (referred to as triple negative)
8. ER-/PR-/HER2+   75.9%

Subgroup numbers seven and eight above, which are associated with the worst clinical outcomes, are seen more frequently in African Americans, Hispanics, and low-income women. More clinical and epidemiological information is needed about the other six subgroups.

Women whose cancer markers were ER+ and PR+ had better five-year survival rates than those women with negative markers (Parise et al., 2009). The four breast tumor subgroups with ER- markers had the poorest survival rate. HER2+ cancer equaled a worse prognosis than HER2-. From Parise's study, however, it is the estrogen receptor rather than HER2+ receptor that appears to be the leading factor influencing survival.

Triple negative breast cancer (ER-/PR-/HER2-) is a particularly aggressive form of the disease occurring more frequently in younger women, Hispanic, and African American women (ACS, 2012) and in women with BRCA1 gene mutations (Breastcancer.org, 2012e). Between 10 percent and 20 percent of breast cancers are triple negative (Breastcancer.org, 2012f) and have a high likelihood to reoccur. Triple negative breast cancer was genetically much closer to ovarian cancer than to other breast cancers, raising the question as to whether they share a common cause (Cancer Genome Atlas Network, 2012). The molecular and genetic similarities between triple negative and ovarian cancer suggested that triple negative breast cancer, though located in the breast, is an entirely different disease than other breast cancers. Triple negative breast cancer does not include estrogen and progesterone receptors or HER2 proteins, and therefore it is difficult to treat because it won't respond to current chemotherapy.

Women most likely to have ER- markers were younger than 50, in a low socioeconomic group, were non-Hispanic Black or Hispanic, and had stage III (a more advanced stage that will be discussed later in the chapter) or undifferentiated (abnormal-looking cells under a microscope) tumors (Parise et al., 2009). Women with the highest rate of survival (ER+/PR+/HER2-) were older than 50, non-Hispanic White, in higher socioeconomic levels, presented with stage I tumors or differentiated (cells resembling normal cells) tumors.

Tumor size, stage, and grade were found to be associated with various subtypes and therefore important in diagnosis and prognosis (Parise et al., 2009). ER+/PR+/HER2- were more likely found in small tumors less than 2 centimeters (cm) in size. Tumors 2 cm and larger were more likely to be triple negative, and if the tumors were more than 5 cm, then they were 40 percent more likely to be ER-/PR-/HER2+. Subtypes ER+/PR+/HER2- and ER+/PR+/HER2+ were more prevalent in stage II tumors. Subtype ER-/PR-/HER2+ was more prevalent in stage III and IV tumors; however, triple negative tumors were less likely to occur.

JULIE'S BREAST CANCER

Following the biopsy on Julie's right breast, we were told that she had invasive lobular carcinoma. We had no idea what this meant. As a nonpracticing registered nurse (RN), I was somewhat knowledgeable about breast cancer, but I had never heard of this degree of specificity in a diagnosis. Little did I know that her diagnosis would become even more specific. What in the world does this word *invasive* mean? It didn't sound good; we were alarmed. Julie and I hit the Internet looking for information. We were careful to access only credible Internet sites. Julie was like a bee after honey in her quest to understand the implications of her diagnosis. She spent hours on the Internet learning as much as she could.

After viewing the ultrasound and receiving the pathology results of the tumor in Julie's right breast, the doctor told her not to worry, that at most her cancer was only a stage I (an early-stage breast cancer), that a lumpectomy would be the best treatment, and that she would be just fine. I was livid that he would tell her such a thing. He had no idea of the extent of her cancer because the full lab results had not come back yet, and we had no idea as to how many lymph nodes were involved. Why would a physician make a hopeful statement that he could not support with any medical evidence? Julie, of course, was very relieved to hear such good news. I didn't dare say anything to her to negate the trust she was developing for her physician, and I didn't want her to worry when my concerns might be unfounded. After all, we didn't have the lab results back yet, and my fear was just that—fear. Nonetheless, it was very hard for me to keep my mouth shut. I had a visceral reaction, nausea and lack of appetite, and, thinking a cancer diagnosis equaled death, was fearful that she was going to die. I was premature in my fear, but it was there, nonetheless. I think my nursing background provided me with just enough medical knowledge to capitalize on my fear.

It wasn't until after her lumpectomy that we knew she had not one but two synchronous yet different breast cancers. Can you believe it— two different cancers at the same time in different breasts? Her condition had gone from bad to worse. Then, we found out the most troubling aspect (to this point), which was that the cancer in Julie's right breast, the invasive lobular cancer, was ER+/PR-/HER2+, 4.4 x 3.2 x 2.5 cm in size, and staged at 3C with a grade 3. The cancer cells were also poorly differentiated, with cells that exhibited marked variation in size and shape and occasionally with very large and bizarre forms. She was diagnosed with in situ invasive ductal cancer in her left breast, ER+/PR+/HER2-, with a lesion only 0.6 x 0.6 x 0.5 cm in size, not extensive, and staged at 0 with a grade 1.

Then we learned that she had extensive lymph node involvement. It was as if our world had stopped. I wanted to make the diagnosis go away. I wanted to fix it. I didn't know how I could support her, what I could say, and how I could take care of my little sister. What must she be feeling? What is it like to get this diagnosis?

PREVENTION AND RISK FACTORS

Prevention

Breast cancer prevention and risk factors are intricately linked. Some of the best tactics for preventing the disease deal with avoiding, when possible, the various risk factors, such as obesity and alcohol consumption, to name a couple. An additional preventive practice involves seeking genetic counseling and testing if breast cancer is in the family. If the counseling finds that the risk for acquiring breast cancer is high, choices regarding hormone therapy and prophylactic mastectomy and/or oophorectomy (removal of the ovaries), or chemoprevention such as Tamoxifen, will need to be made (Petrucelli, Daly, & Feldman, 2010).

Exercise, specifically six or more hours a week of strenuous activity, may reduce the risk of invasive breast cancer by 23 percent if there is no family history of the disease (AACR, 2007a). Exercise exerts breast cancer protection throughout a woman's lifetime. It is hypothesized that the strenuous exercise lowers the estrogen exposure, which reduces the risk for the disease.

Obesity in women after the age of 60 increases their risk of developing breast cancer by 55 percent according to a Swedish study (AACR, 2011). The same study found that women with diabetes were at a 37 percent increased risk for breast cancer if they had been diagnosed up to four years prior to their cancer diagnosis.

Women who have borne children may be at a reduced risk of developing breast cancer for a couple of reasons. Pregnancy decreases the amount of time estrogen is circulating in the body because pregnancy decreases estrogen production (Chavez-MacGregor, Elias, Onland-Moret, van der Schouw, Gils, Monninkhof, et al., 2005). Another potential protective effect of pregnancy is that fetal cells are "transplanted" to the mother before birth, a process called microchimerism (AACR, 2007b). The transplanted cells may put the mother's immune system on notice to destroy malignant cells. This research may provide a unique approach for future studies on the prevention of cancer.

The American Cancer Society recommends the following prevention strategies (ACS, 2011c; 2012):

1. Yearly mammogram beginning at age 40
2. Clinical breast exam (CBE) by a health care provider every three years beginning for women in their 20s or 30s and yearly for women age 40 and older
3. Breast self-exam (BSE) beginning during a woman's 20s
4. Magnetic resonance imaging (MRI) and mammography yearly for women at high risk of developing breast cancer (considered greater than a 20% lifetime risk)

Risk Factors

A risk factor refers to a feature or a trait associated with an increased chance to develop the disease (Mahon, 2012). Several types of risks have been identified, including *absolute, relative,* and *attributable* (ACS, 2011c, 2012). An absolute risk refers to the incidence or mortality from breast cancer in the general population. For example, U.S. women have a 1 in 8 risk of developing breast cancer sometime during their lives. Relative risk is a comparison of these incidents or deaths with those women who do not have the specific risk factor. For example, a woman who experiences menarche prior to age 12 has a 1.3 relative risk to (or is 1.3 times more likely to) develop breast cancer compared to a woman who experiences menarche after the age of 12 (ACS, 2011c). And finally, the attributable risk refers to the extent that breast cancer may have been preventable by modifying or minimizing the risk factor.

A number of risks are associated with breast cancer, such as age, weight, alcohol consumption, and reproductive factors, as well as hormone replacement therapy (Anderson, Limacher, Assaf, Bassford, Beresford, Black, et al., 2004), oral contraceptive use (Newcomer, Newcomb, Trentham-Dietz, Longnecker, & Greenberg, 2003), radiation (WebMD, 2012), genetics (Lynch, Snyder, Lynch, Riley, & Rubinstein, 2003), and others. Having a cancer risk factor, or many, does not necessarily result in a diagnosis of cancer according to genetic counselor Shari Baldinger (personal communication, August 24, 2012; WebMD, 2012). Most women who do get breast cancer have no known risk factors, and women with one or more breast cancer risk factors may never develop the disease.

Age

The risk for developing breast cancer increases with age, with an overall lifetime probability of 12.5 percent (1 in 8) (ACS, 2011b). As a woman ages, her risk increases: from age 30 to 39 her risk is .43 percent (1 in 232); age 40 to 49 her risk is 1.45 percent (1 in 69); age 50 to 59 her risk is 2.38 percent (1 in 42); and age 60 to 69 her risk is 3.45 percent (1 in 29). From 2003 to 2007 the median age of death was 68 (Altekruse, Kosary, Krapcho, Neyman, Aminou, & Waldron, et al., n.d.).

Reproductive Factors

Hormonal changes associated with puberty, pregnancy, and menopause cause changes in breast tissue (Chavez-MacGregor et al., 2005). The age of a woman's first menarche; whether she has had children, and if so her age when her first child was born; and finally the age she completed menopause are associated with her exposure to hormones, particularly estrogen. Collectively, menarche, pregnancy, and menopause dictate the number of menstrual cycles a woman experiences throughout her life. The number of menstrual cycles may be the more likely predictor of breast cancer risk. Considering this, a woman with an early menarche before the age of 12, who has never borne a child, and who completed menopause after the age of 50 has experienced more menstrual cycles, resulting in more estrogen. She may, therefore, have an increased risk of breast cancer (Chavez-MacGregor et al., 2005). The more children a woman has, the less risk of breast cancer due to the interruption of estrogen secretion by the ovaries (Collaborative Group on Hormonal Factors in Breast Cancer, 2002). Breastfeeding tends to decrease breast cancer risk as well.

Weight

A woman's weight, specifically her body mass, may be more of a risk factor for postmenopausal women than for premenopausal women (Chavez-MacGregor et al., 2005). Adipose (fat) contains estrogen in postmenopausal women, so the more adipose tissue, the higher the levels of estrogen, adding to the increased risk. One study found that for each point gain of body mass index (BMI), cancer risk increased 4 percent (AACR, 2011). This means that a woman with breast cancer and a BMI of 30 had a 20 percent increased risk of relapse than a woman with a BMI less than 25. (A BMI greater than 30 is considered obese, while a BMI of 25 to 30 is considered overweight.) Overweight or obese pre- and postmenopausal women are also at an increased risk of relapse. Additional research is exploring a correlation of obesity to poverty and breast cancer since poor adults are more likely to be obese.

Oral Contraceptive Use

The use of oral contraceptives and the risk of breast cancer may vary depending on both the type of contraceptive a woman uses and the length of time she uses it (Newcomer et al., 2003). There is an association with a slightly increased breast cancer risk for women who have used contraceptives, which is reduced over time (Marchbanks, McDonald, Wilson, Folger, Mandel, Daling, et al., 2002).

Hormone Replacement Therapy

The Women's Health Initiative study demonstrated that estrogen and progestin, as a combined hormone replacement therapy for women going through menopause, has shown an increased risk of approximately 24 percent for developing breast cancer (Anderson et al., 2004). The risk varied depending on the type of drug and the number of years it was used.

Alcohol Consumption

Two or more drinks of alcohol a day increases breast cancer risk by stimulating the metabolism of carcinogens and interfering with the repair of DNA (AACR, 2008b; Chavez-MacGregor et al., 2005). Studies have demonstrated that alcohol increases the amount of estrogen metabolic by-products circulating in a woman's body. This increase in estrogen then fuels estrogen-sensitive breast cancer. The more a woman drinks, the higher her risk (AACR 2008b). Moderate alcohol consumption was a risk factor for 70 percent of estrogen and progesterone positive tumors. Women who drank three or more alcoholic beverages a day had up to a 51 percent increased risk of developing estrogen and progesterone positive breast tumors.

Radiation Exposure

If women have been exposed to radiation for postpartum mastitis, X-rays for tuberculosis, or radiation prior to the age of 30, then the risk of breast cancer increases (WebMD, 2012).

Genetics

Cancer is caused by damage to DNA that the body is unable to repair. As a result, all cancer is genetic. Fortunately, the body's amazing reparative abilities usually stop the DNA-damaged cells from proliferating. Women can inherit already damaged DNA; however, approximately 80 percent of damaged DNA is due to environmental exposure, such as diet, smoke, and ultraviolet light, to name a few (ACS, 2011c).

Many genes that contribute to breast cancer risk have been identified, and more will be found (S. Baldinger, personal communication, September 6, 2012). One lab has created a 14-multigene breast cancer panel, which includes genes that create high risks for breast cancer as well as some that create a more modest risk. Most of the mutated genes are also associated with some increased risk for other cancers.

BRCA1 and BRCA2

The two gene mutations that are best known and well researched are mutations in the BRCA1 and BRCA2 genes. These two gene mutations are the most common known cause of breast cancer (Petrucelli et al., 2010), yet they account for only about half of inherited breast cancer clusters (S. Baldinger, personal communication, October 3, 2012). Ashkenazi Jewish women have a higher overall prevalence of carrying the BRCA1 and 2 mutations (1 in 40). The overall population of women has a 1 in 400 to 1 in 800 risk of carrying the mutations, depending on ethnicity (Petrucelli et al., 2010). The risk can vary even when the same mutations exist within the same family. The likelihood that a person carries the mutation is dependent on family history and can be determined using various mutation probability models.

Everyone carries the BRCA1 and BRCA2 genes; it is their mutations that cause the problem. The BRCA1 gene's function is to be the "caretaker" in helping to maintain genomic integrity (Petrucelli et al., 2010, p. 246). BRCA2 is active in the repair of DNA and also serves as a caretaker similar to BRCA1. Many mutations have been found in both genes—1,600 mutations in BRCA1 and more than 1,800 in BRCA2. Other cancer risks associated with BRCA1 and 2 include cancers of the fallopian tubes, ovaries, peritoneum, prostate, pancreas, uterus, gallbladder and bile duct, stomach, and skin (melanoma). Interestingly, cancer risks in the BRCA1 and BRCA2 mutations may differ based on where the mutation is found on the gene. BRCA genes are autosomal dominant, meaning that they can be inherited through either the paternal or maternal side of the family (Lynch et al., 2003). The BRCA mutations are most significant with the breast and ovarian cancer known as hereditary breast and ovarian cancer (HBOC). Even one of the following factors in an individual or in a family history suggests hereditary breast/ovarian cancer syndrome requiring additional evaluation:

1. Early-age breast cancer (younger than 50 years old)
2. Two different primary breast tumors, or breast and ovarian/fallopian tube/primary peritoneal tumor in one family member, or two or more different breast tumors, or breast and ovarian/fallopian tube/

primary peritoneal cancers in first, second, or third degree relatives from the same side of the family

3. At-risk population (e.g., Ashkenazi Jewish)
4. BRCA1 or BRCA2 in a family member
5. Any male with breast cancer
6. Ovarian/fallopian tube/primary peritoneal cancer at any age

It is estimated that women with BRCA1 and BRCA2 gene mutations have a 40 percent to 87 percent lifetime risk of developing a minimum of one breast cancer (and 30 percent to 50 percent risk of ovarian cancer), with half of women with the mutations developing the cancer by age 50 compared to 12–13 percent for women overall (Breastcancer.org, 2012g; Easton, Ford, & Bishop, 1995; Hopper et al., 1999; Lynch et al., 2003). Women with a history of significant familial breast cancer (either two or more cases of breast cancer among close relatives younger than age 50, or three breast cancer cases among close relatives of any age), yet without BRCA1 or BRCA2, have a fourfold higher risk of developing cancer than those women without a familial history (AACR, 2008c).This risk indicates gene involvement but without knowledge of what genes are involved.

Breast Density

Genetic influence on breast density is estimated to be 60 percent (AACR, 2007c). Several genes have been discovered that may be associated with dense breast tissue, a breast cancer risk. Women with dense breasts are considered to be three to five times more likely to develop breast cancer than women whose breasts are less dense. Breast density refers to breasts with less fat compared to the connective tissue surrounding the ducts and lobes.

Some states have passed laws requiring that patients be told when a mammogram shows they have dense breast tissue that can hide tumors on their mammograms, thereby increasing the risk of breast cancer (Breast tissue density sparks debate, 2012). There has also been a similar federal law introduced in the House of Representatives. It is estimated that 40 percent of women who have had mammograms have dense breasts, with younger women more likely than older women to have denser breasts. Ultrasounds have detected tumors in women with dense breasts that mammogram failed to detect.

Family History

Family history is one of the strongest risk factors for both breast and ovarian cancer (Lynch et al., 2003), but most women who develop breast cancer have no family history of the disease (Breastcancer.org,

2012g). If one's mother, sister, or daughter (first degree relatives) has breast cancer, then the risk for breast cancer is doubled, and if there are two first degree relatives with breast cancer, then the risk is fivefold. If a woman has a male relative with breast cancer, then she has an increased risk of the disease. There is also a slightly higher risk if aunts, grandmothers, and cousins (second degree relatives) have had the disease (WebMD, 2012). The risk increases if the first degree relative developed breast cancer prior to menopause and had cancer in both breasts.

Approximately 2 percent of Ashkenazi Jews are believed to be carriers of one of three BRCA1 and BRCA2 gene mutations associated with an increased risk of breast, ovarian, and prostate cancers; 20 percent of Ashkenazi Jewish women who developed breast cancer before the age of 40 carry one of these three mutations (Brandt-Rauf, Raveis, Drummond, Conte, & Rothman, 2006).

JULIE'S (AND MY?) RISK FACTORS

Our family's history of breast cancer was one of Julie's biggest risk factors. In the mid-1940s, at about the age of 50, our paternal grandmother had breast cancer in one breast, which was treated with a radical mastectomy, then cancer in the second breast, followed by another radical mastectomy. She died within three years. At about the age of 40, our maternal grandmother had breast cancer in one breast, which was treated with a radical mastectomy, and she appeared to be cancer free. However, the breast cancer recurred in her lungs 35 years later and killed her. We also had a maternal aunt with breast cancer before the age of 50 who had a radical mastectomy and survived the disease, and a cousin who died of breast cancer at around the age of 52.

Is it possible we have a genetic mutation conducive to breast cancer, especially on the maternal side of the family? Could it be the dreaded BRCA1 or BRCA2 gene mutation? If Julie has the mutation, could I have it too? If I have the mutation, could both of my daughters? And, what about my little granddaughter or even my grandson? And if we don't share the BRCA gene mutations, what other gene mutations have been passed on? Does the fact that my sister has breast cancer increase significantly my risk of developing the disease?

Another potential risk factor was that our paternal grandfather had been Jewish and became Christian when he married our grandmother. We do not know if he was ethnically a Jew or whether he merely practiced the Jewish religion. We could, then, be Ashkenazi Jew.

Julie has not had any children, was 11 or 12 at menarche, and experienced menopause at 47. She was on the birth control pill during a portion of her adult years, which minimized normal menstrual cycles. It is unclear what this reproductive history would mean for her risk. She is petite and exercises somewhat.

GENETIC COUNSELING AND TESTING

Genetic counseling is often an appropriate mode for determining breast cancer risk (S. Baldinger, personal communication, August 24, 2012; Mahon, 2012). The counselor will get both an individual and family history for causes of death going back three generations. Gathering family causes of death can be a challenge because it may require reviewing pathology reports from medical records and death certificates. Even if the BRCA gene mutation is found in a family, it doesn't mean that every family member will have inherited it (Breastcancer.org, 2012h; S. Baldinger, personal communication, August 24, 2012). It is possible that family members who did have breast (or ovarian) cancer might test negative for BRCA mutations and contracted the disease from another mutated gene yet to be discovered.

There are three models the genetic counselor may use to determine a woman's breast cancer risk, and six models to determine risk for BRCA1 or BRCA2 mutations (Claus, Schildkraut, Thompson, & Risch, 1996; Couch et al., 1997; Parmigiani et al., 2007). The counselor will determine whether a woman will benefit from genetic testing based on the result of these risk assessments (S. Baldinger, personal communication, August 24, 2012). The tests are expensive ($4,500 was quoted to my sister), so it is important to consider whether one's health insurance will cover the expense. Most insurance covers the cost if the woman displays the required criteria established by the carrier.

The American Society of Clinical Oncology and insurers recommend that genetic counseling be done prior to genetic testing. Counseling prior to testing allows for an informed decision to be made about which genetic tests should be ordered, and the results, positive or negative, can be interpreted correctly (S. Baldinger, personal communication, September 5, 2012; Petrucelli et al., 2010). The counselor examines both the quantitative and qualitative elements of the woman's lineage before making a testing recommendation.

Myriad Genetic Laboratories is the only lab in the United States that tests for BRCA. There are three tests available (Myriad Genetic Laboratories, 2008):

1. *Comprehensive BRAC Analysis* tests for mutations in the BRCA1 and BRCA2 genes associated with hereditary breast and ovarian cancer (HBOC) syndrome.
2. *Single Site BRAC Analysis* examines a small portion of DNA for a specific BRCA gene mutation that has been identified in another family member.

3. *Multisite 3 BRAC Analysis* tests for the three most common BRCA mutations found in people of Ashkenazi or Eastern European Jewish ancestry.

Test results may come back negative, positive, or uncertain. Negative results mean only that the gene mutations tested for were not found; it is important to remember that other mutations that were not tested for may exist. Uncertain results, depending on which test was given, may indicate a gene alteration, but no known cancer risk is confirmed.

There is an initial cancer risk assessment found on the Myriad Genetic Laboratories website (Myriad Genetic Laboratories, 2012) intended to assist in determining one's hereditary risk factors for breast and ovarian cancer. Some question why they should take a breast cancer risk assessment test. It is important to recognize that inherited breast cancer risk is not an inevitable outcome. The knowledge gained from completing the assessment can be used to reduce one's risk, take proactive steps, and make informed choices.

Testing negative for the mutation's presence needs to be interpreted with caution, however, because it may mean that the underlying cause of the breast cancer was not found (Petrucelli et al., 2010). In other words, a negative result may mean that the gene mutation causing the presenting breast cancer was not tested for, or has not yet been found by scientists, or is caused by nonhereditary factors. Testing negative for known breast cancer gene mutations often indicates that the woman has the same risk as the general population. That's not to say, however, that she may not be at risk for developing breast cancer from another gene mutation that hasn't been discovered yet or for which no test has been developed (S. Baldinger, personal communication, August 24, 2012). Those women who test positive for BRCA1 or BRCA2 have a significant risk of developing breast cancer and must make decisions about how to manage that risk.

Deciding which family members should visit a genetic counselor and have genetic testing is sometimes challenging. However, once a family member is found to have the BRCA1 or BRCA2 mutations, the relative most closely related to her (or him) should be tested (Breastcancer.org, 2012i). Let's look at the following scenario. Let's say your mother's sister, your aunt, has the BRCA mutation; then your mother should be tested. If her test results are negative, then you do not need testing because you could not have received the gene mutation from your mother. However, if your mother's results are positive, meaning that she has the BRCA mutation, then you would want to decide whether to be tested. Perhaps your mother is no longer alive; then you might decide to be tested based on your aunt's positive results. If you test positive for the gene mutation, then your siblings and adult children may wish to be tested as well.

JULIE'S GENETIC TESTING AND MY GENETIC COUNSELING

Julie did not have genetic counseling but did have genetic testing for the BRCA1 and BRCA2 gene mutations. Just as I was completing writing this chapter, we found out that Julie's genetic testing showed no signs of the BRCA genetic mutations. This was wonderful news for her, for me, and for my children.

I went through genetic counseling, recognizing that with our family history of breast cancer, and with my sister's diagnosis, my risk was probably high. The counseling session was interesting and took about an hour or so. My lifetime risk of developing breast cancer at my current age is 13 percent, whereas the risk for the general population of women at my age is 4.5 percent. While my risk is a little more than three times that of the general population of women, it is still relatively low. My risk for carrying the BRCA1 gene mutation is 0.023 percent, and for carrying the BRCA2 mutation it is 0.018 percent, both extremely low. I was relieved. The counselor suggested that I have a clinical breast examination (CBE) every six months rather than yearly; otherwise there isn't anything additional she recommended. She said that it was up to me to decide whether to have a magnetic resonance imaging (MRI) of my breasts. I haven't decided if I will do so or not.

BREAST CANCER SCREENING AND DIAGNOSTIC TESTS

Breast Cancer Screening

Breast cancer screening is credited with reducing the mortality and morbidity of breast cancer, and is usually associated with women who have no signs or symptoms of breast cancer. Screening includes breast self-examination (BSE), clinical breast examination (CBE), mammography, and perhaps a magnetic resonance imaging (MRI) (Mahon, 2012).

Breast Exams

Both BSE and CBE have detected breast lesions that were not detected by mammography (Mahon, 2012). BSE has historically been considered the best preventive screening technique for women to detect an abnormal lump or mass in their breasts. It is not considered necessary for women to do a monthly BSE. Often women discover breast changes while showering or dressing. However, BSE is a useful technique in discerning a mass in the length of time between CBE and mammography.

CBE is conducted by the health care clinician. Though CBEs are recommended for all women, particularly those women at increased risk for breast cancer and/or who carry the BRCA1 or BRCA2 genetic mutations, research studies are ambiguous in demonstrating that they actually reduce the incidence of breast cancer or the mortality rate (United Nations Population Fund, 2002).

Mammography

Mammography, an X-ray of the breasts, has been credited as the most effective screening method to detect breast cancer often many years before a lump can be palpated (ACS, n.d.). A mammogram can detect cysts, calcifications, and masses while enabling a physician to view the overall breast tissue due to the compression of the breast. A woman should begin having mammograms at the age of 40 and continue for as long as she is still at any risk for breast cancer (ACS, 2011b). Mammograms reveal 80 percent to 90 percent of breast cancers in asymptomatic women. The screening is a bit more accurate for postmenopausal women, probably due to less breast density. The mammogram is not foolproof, however, and false negative findings may occur if there is increased density, a faster tumor growth rate, poor positioning of the breast, or an overlooked abnormality during clinical examination of the mammogram (Mahon, 2012). Anywhere from 5 percent to 10 percent of mammograms detect either abnormal or inconclusive results requiring further testing, such as mammogram imaging studies or a biopsy.

Yearly mammograms may not be adequate for high-risk women with known BRCA1 or BRCA2 genetic mutations. These women should begin mammography by 25 years of age and also have an MRI of the breasts (Saslow et al., 2007). Women who have other risk factors and no known BRCA gene mutations are encouraged to have a mammogram at a younger age and to undergo a breast MRI (National Comprehensive Cancer Network [NCCN], 2010).

Breast MRI

Breast MRIs are done in conjunction with mammograms for women who are at a high risk for developing breast cancer (Mayo Clinic Staff, 2011a). A high risk is defined as a 20–25 percent or greater risk as calculated by a genetic counselor using tools that include examining the family's history of breast or ovarian cancer. Other indicators for a breast MRI may include a prior breast cancer diagnosis, a suspicious area on the mammogram, palpation of a lump that isn't detectable on a mammogram or ultrasound, suspected rupture of a breast implant, dense breast tissue, and a history of precancerous breast changes. One of the problems with breast MRIs is the risk of a false positive, which may result in additional testing such as a biopsy, increased cost, overestimation of tumor size, and undue anxiety (Onesti, Mangus, Helmer, & Osland, 2008).

DIAGNOSING BREAST CANCER

Women who display questionable signs of breast cancer require a diagnostic evaluation. There are numerous signs and symptoms that should signal a visit to a health care provider (ACS, 2011c, 2012):

Lump or mass felt in the breast
Lump or mass felt under the arm
Swelling of the breast
Dimpling of the breast
Pain in the breast or in the nipple
Nipple turning inward
Nipple discharge (other than milk)
Skin irritation of the breast
Redness, scaliness, or thickening of the nipple or breast skin

If when conducting a BSE a suspicious lump is found, a visit to one's health care provider for evaluation is essential. The provider will do a CBE and order a mammography and a biopsy (Mahon, 2012). Additional diagnostic tests may include a positron emission tomography (PET), computerized tomography (CT) scan, and if it is suspected that the cancer has metastasized, then bone, liver, and lung scans may be required.

Biopsy

A biopsy may be one of the first examinations done if a woman has found a mass in her breast. This may be a surgical procedure in which the surgeon makes an incision and removes, often, the entire area of cells to be examined microscopically to determine if there is cancer (Mayo Clinic Staff, 2011b). A microscopic exam is the only way to differentiate the types of cells in the tumor for diagnosis. Sometimes the biopsy is done using a needle that extracts cells from the mass. There are several types of needle biopsy procedures that may be used, including: a) a fine-needle aspiration (a syringe draws out the cells or fluid from the mass), b) core needle biopsy (a larger needle draws out a column of tissue), c) vacuum-assisted biopsy (use of suction to extract cells or fluid via a needle), or d) image-guided biopsy (use of imaging procedures such as X-rays or ultrasound with a needle biopsy).

Staging

One of the aspects of diagnosing breast cancer is determining the *stage* of the disease, thereby assessing the amount of cancer in the body and its location (Mahon, 2012). Staging refers to the tumor's size; the degree, if at all, that the cancer cells have invaded the lymph nodes; and whether the cancer has spread to any *distant* parts of the body. Staging is determined using the physical exam, radiologic studies of the lymph nodes, and surgical techniques. A TNM system categorizes each cancer and is used as a means for staging (Susan G. Komen for the Cure, 2011). The cancer is assigned a T category, which describes the measured primary tumor. The N category denotes whether the cancer has metastasized into the nodes, and M refers to whether there is distant metastasis to other parts of the body. This TNM system then is used to create the staging of breast cancer as 0, I, II, III, or IV, with additional detail allocated to each stage and identified as A, B, and C. The following list describes the stages of breast cancer (Cancer Treatment Centers of America, n.d.):

1. Stage 0, referred to as carcinoma in situ or sometimes as a precancerous condition, indicates that the cancer cells are located only in that part of the breast in which they began and have not invaded any other breast tissue.
2. Stage 1 indicates a tumor no more than 2 cm in size and with no lymph nodes showing cancer cells.
3. Stage II is descriptive of an invasive cancer in which the tumor is 2–5 cm or has spread into the axillary lymph nodes on the side where the breast cancer was located. Stage II also includes two subcategories, 2A and 2B. 2A indicates any of these: a) cancer is found in the axillary lymph nodes but not in the breast; b) the breast cancer is 2 cm and is also in the lymph nodes; or c) the breast tumor is larger than 2 cm but smaller than 50 cm, and is not found in the lymph nodes. Stage 2B may indicate either of these: a) the size of the tumor is 2–5 cm and has also spread to the axillary lymph nodes; or b) the tumor is larger than 5 cm, but there is no cancer in the lymph nodes.
4. Stage III involves a tumor more than 2 inches in diameter and extensive axillary lymph node involvement, or indicates that the cancer has spread to lymph nodes or other tissue near the breast. There are three subcategories with stage III breast cancer. Stage 3A is characterized by a tumor larger than 5 cm or by significant lymph node involvement, in which the nodes lump together or stick to surrounding tissue. Stage 3C cancer may have spread to the skin or chest wall, clavicle, or the nodes surrounding the sternum, and may or may not be in the breast.
5. Stage IV, also referred to as metastatic breast cancer, means that the cancer has spread beyond the breast, surrounding tissue, and all surrounding lymph nodes (mammary and axillary) to other lymph nodes, the brain, bones, lungs, liver, or skin.

In addition to staging breast cancer (which details the extent and severity of cancer) is the grading of the tumor on a scale of 1 to 4 (National Cancer Institute, 2004). Grading, based on the structure and growth pattern of cells, refers to how the tumor's cells compare to normal cells, with higher graded tumors suggesting a poorer prognosis and perhaps a different type of treatment. Grade 1 cells are usually considered to be the least aggressive, while grades 3 and 4, which do not resemble normal cells, grow rapidly and tend to spread faster.

JULIE'S SCREENING AND DIAGNOSTIC TESTING

Along with the ultrasound on January 13, which showed a right breast lesion measuring 19 x 16 millimeters (mm), and the initial biopsy, Julie's surgeon ordered a mammogram of both breasts. She had always been compliant in having a mammogram every year because of our family history of breast cancer, but she had lost track of time, and it had been two years since her last mammogram. The mammogram of her right breast on January 12 found a hyper-dense lesion in the upper outer quadrant. There was also an area of density, which was initially seen as benign, in the upper outer quadrant of her left breast.

Fortunately the surgeon felt that a more extensive examination of her left breast should be done, considering the diagnosis of the right breast. As a result, Julie underwent bilateral MRIs of both breasts on January 20, 2012. The right breast showed a mass at the 9:00 position measuring 2.4 x 2.1 cm. (The ultrasound, mammogram, and MRIs each showed a different sized tumor based on the type of test and its limitations.) The left breast showed a 0.4 cm abnormal lesion at the 9:00 position with an unclear diagnosis.

As a result of the right breast MRI, an ultrasound-guided vacuum-assisted core biopsy was done on both breasts. The right breast biopsy results showed that Julie had lobular breast cancer. The left breast biopsy came back as highly suspicious for carcinoma. Her surgeon stated that the left breast biopsy results really didn't tell him anything and that he believed the lesion was probably not breast cancer. However, he rightly decided that she required a lumpectomy of lesions in both breasts, which took place on February 7, 2012. As a result, the pathology report clearly stated that she had different cancers in her left and right breasts.

In less than a month, Julie had gone from a seemingly healthy middle-aged woman enjoying the warmer winter in the South to a woman with bilateral breast cancer; she had experienced two breast biopsies, two lumpectomies, mammography, breast MRIs, and an echocardiogram to ensure that her heart was healthy enough to withstand chemotherapy.

It was overwhelming. It consumed our thinking. We were afraid.

BREAST CANCER TREATMENT

Even though all breast cancers share the trait of pathological cell division due to the damage in their DNA, each breast cancer is different, and one therapy does not fit all types of breast cancers. Breast cancers may have many mutations of the genes causing the disease, often occurring in different combinations, which causes the cancer to differ from one patient to the next. As a result, different women may respond differently to various treatments. What compounds the problem is that the cancer cells can adapt under treatment and can adapt differently in different people (Slear, 2012).

Breast cancer treatment most often comprises one or more of the following options: surgery, radiation, hormone therapy, monoclonal antibodies, and chemotherapy, though not all of these treatments are used with the same diagnosis (Mahon, 2012). Surgical procedures are pivotal in diagnosing, staging, and treating breast cancer. Surgery may play several different roles in treating cancer, including removal of the cancer, treatment of advanced cancer, restoration or reconstruction of the breast, and prophylactic or preventative use.

Lumpectomy

A lumpectomy involves the removal of the tumor and the tissue surrounding the tumor to minimize recurrence. Removal of the surrounding tissue, referred to as *margins*, is an important element of the procedure to ensure that the entire cancerous mass has been removed and no cancer cells remain in the surrounding tissue (Mayo Clinic Staff, 2011c). Wider margins that are clear of cancer are not an assurance that the cancer will not recur, however (Oz, 2012). A lumpectomy may be done as a diagnostic procedure to determine if the mass is cancerous, or it may be a treatment for early stage breast cancer (Mayo Clinic Staff, 2011c). Studies have confirmed that a lumpectomy followed by radiation is as effective a treatment for early stage breast cancer as is a mastectomy. Up to 75 percent of women choose a lumpectomy or breast-conserving surgery (Oz, 2012). Oz reported on a new British study showing that 20 percent of women who opted for a lumpectomy, however, required a mastectomy within three months. A U.S. study found considerable differences in reoperation rates depending on the surgeon and the hospital in which the initial surgery was performed (McCahill et al., 2012). These data are concerning for patients who are unable to assess the competence, accountability, and transparency of their surgeons and the hospitals in which the surgery is performed.

Lumpectomy is not for everyone, however, including women who have scleroderma, systemic lupus erythematosus, two or more tumors in different quadrants of the breast, previous radiation to the breast, cancer that has spread throughout the breast, a large tumor, small breasts, or no access to radiation (Susan G. Komen for the Cure, 2012). In addition to the lumpectomy, axillary lymph nodes may be removed, as well as the lining of the chest muscles lying under the mass (Mahon, 2012).

Sentinel Lymph Node Biopsy

Sentinel lymph node biopsy is a technique in which specific (sentinel) lymph nodes are observed for a radioactive substance that was injected near the tumor prior to a lumpectomy or mastectomy (Mahon, 2012; Mayo Clinic Staff, 2011c). The radioactive contrast flows into the lymphatic system to the first lymph nodes where the cancer is likely to have spread, thus the name "sentinel." Using a scanner to detect which nodes contain cancerous cells, the surgeon then removes those nodes in which radioactivity is present (Gawlick, Mone, Hansen, Connors, & Nelson, 2008). If cancer cells are found in one to three axillary nodes, in more than three nodes, or if the breast tumor is large, then the physician will recommend radiation following a mastectomy.

The examination of lymph nodes during surgery is a best practice in determining whether the cancer has metastasized to the nodes (Breastcancer. org, 2012j). Nodes are small organs that filter lymph as it leaves the breast and heads into the blood, catching and trapping cancer cells before they metastasize to other body parts. The more axillary lymph nodes that show cancer, the more serious the diagnosis. Cancer cells found in the lymph nodes denote an increased likelihood of metastasis.

Researchers at the ACS found that 11 percent of women did not have their nodes examined (AACR, 2007d). These women were more likely to be African American, elderly, have no health insurance, or live in neighborhoods where there were low levels of education. These disparities are cause for concern because it suggests that breast cancer decisions may be made differently for marginalized patients. Failure to examine the nodes negatively impacts the staging of a woman's cancer and therefore her treatment.

It is estimated that 70 percent of women with early-stage breast cancer have no lymph node involvement, which indicates less likelihood of metastasis (Mahon, 2012). Sentinel node biopsy with accompanying lymph node dissection provides accurate diagnostic data to aid in the prognosis of the cancer (Gawlick et al., 2008).

Mastectomy

The most extensive breast cancer surgery is a mastectomy or removal of the breast. There are several types of mastectomies, including the following (Mayo Clinic Staff, 2011d):

1. Modified radical mastectomy is recommended for women whose cancer has metastasized to the lymph nodes or if she has large

tumors. The procedure is the most extensive because it removes the breast, skin, areola, nipple, lining of the chest muscles, and axillary lymph nodes. In some cases part of the chest wall is also removed.

2. Simple or total mastectomy removes the breast, including the skin, areola, and nipple and may include a sentinel node biopsy.

3. Skin-sparing mastectomy is the removal of the breast, areola, and nipple but not the skin. The skin remains for breast reconstruction surgery.

4. Nipple-sparing (subcutaneous) mastectomy spares the skin, nipple, areola, and chest-wall muscles and removes only the breast tissue. This type of mastectomy is another option for women who will be having breast reconstruction surgery.

Radiation

Radiation therapy utilizes X-rays, gamma rays, electrons, or protons to destroy or damage cancer cells (Breastcancer.org, 2012k; Mayo Clinic Staff, 2011e). The high energy radiation particles break the DNA strand, thereby preventing the cancer from growing. Some normal cells are affected, but most recover. Even though the surgeon removes the cancerous breast, there is no guarantee that every cancer cell is removed; therefore radiation kills whatever cancer cells may be hiding in the tissue (Breastcancer.org, 2012k). Women who did not get radiation following a lumpectomy were at 60 percent greater risk of cancer recurrence in the same breast.

Women may receive external radiation therapy following a lumpectomy or a mastectomy (Mahon, 2012), with treatments typically five days a week for six or more weeks. Some women require brachytherapy, which is radiation delivered within the breast. One technique involves a thin catheter with a balloon inserted into the portion of the breast where the lump was removed. Twice a day radioactive material is placed into the balloon via the catheter and then removed. As with external radiation, this is done as an outpatient procedure but usually for only five days. A second form is referred to as interstitial brachytherapy. This form of radiation involves numerous small catheters inserted into the area of the breast where the lump was removed, and radioactive pellets are introduced into the breast through the catheters for short periods of time and then removed. Radiation and lumpectomy have shown to be as effective a breast cancer treatment, with fewer complications, as a mastectomy (Nesvold, Dahl, Lokkevik, Marit Mengshoel, & Fossa, 2008).

Radiation may be performed at different times during a woman's breast cancer treatment and for different reasons (Mayo Clinic Staff, 2011e). It may be administered with other treatments such as chemotherapy to kill cancer cells, prior to a mastectomy to shrink the cancer (neoadjuvant therapy), after surgery to kill any remaining cancer cells (adjuvant therapy), or to alleviate symptoms caused by advanced cancer.

Some breast cancer radiation treatment requires the use of a bolus, which enhances the amount of radiation directed to the identified area (Cooney, Irani, Stalnecker, & Johnston, 2006). A bolus is a material that provides an adequate radiation buildup in the skin and superficial chest wall, and is commonly used during postmastectomy radiotherapy, particularly for locally advanced breast cancer. The most frequent site of breast cancer recurrence is the chest wall, so delivering adequate radiation doses to the chest wall is crucial to reducing the risk of treatment failure.

Chemotherapy

Chemotherapy (chemo) refers to the use of chemicals (drugs) as a therapeutic agent to kill any cancer cells that have metastasized to the nodes or distant body parts (Mahon, 2012). Chemotherapy is a systemic treatment administered before surgery or after surgery, and is intended to augment surgery and radiation therapy to treat cancer that has metastasized. Chemo usually consists of a cocktail of drugs rather than a single drug because combinations of drugs are often more effective (Gullatte, 2007). The medications may be administered intravenously or orally.

When the cancerous tumor is large or difficult to remove, physicians may suggest neoadjuvant chemo to shrink the tumor by destroying the cancer cells, thereby easing the surgical removal of the tumor (Mahon, 2012). Adjuvant chemo is seen with women whose cancers tend to be stage II and stage III and is administered to enhance their prognosis of a cure.

Hormone (Endocrine) Therapy

These medications treat hormone receptor positive breast cancer (only) by either lowering the amount of estrogen (most of which is produced in women's ovaries) or blocking estrogen's action on breast cancer cells (Breastcancer.org, 2012l). The treatment reduces the recurrence of early-stage hormone receptor positive breast cancer and slows the growth of advanced or metastatic hormone positive breast cancers.

Women whose breast cancer shows positive estrogen or progesterone receptors, or who do not know whether they are ER+ or PR+, benefit from hormone therapy, particularly those women who are postmenopausal or have metastasis (Mahon, 2012). Hormone therapy works by reducing the amount of estrogen that stimulates breast cancer, resulting, in many cases, in preventing breast cancer recurrence. Sixty percent of patients who are ER+ respond to endocrine therapy, while less than 10 percent of ER- patients respond (Harvey et al., 1999). Patients who are both ER+ and PR+ benefit the most from endocrine therapy. If only one of the hormone receptors is expressed, then endocrine therapy may decrease by up to half (Bardou, Arpino, Elledge, Osborne, & Clark, 2003).

Numerous hormonal drugs are used, including Herceptin and Tykerb (biologic response modifiers), which prevent breast cancer cells' growth (Mahon, 2012). Aromasin, Femara, Arimidex, and Megace (referred to as aromatase inhibitors) prevent the production of estrogen in the adrenal glands (which sit on top of each kidney and produce a variety of hormones). And finally, Tamoxifen, Evista, and Fareston (selective estrogen-receptor modulators) bind to the estrogen receptors in the cancer cells and block their growth.

Immunotherapy

Monoclonal antibodies drugs are relatively new in treating cancer (Mayo Clinic Staff, 2011f). These drugs are produced in the laboratory and are carefully created to attach to specific defective proteins (antigens) on the cancer cell. These drugs mimic the body's own naturally occurring antibodies (which attack antigens) that comprise the immune system. When the monoclonal antibodies attach to the cancer cell, they enhance the ability of the immune system to find the cancer cells and destroy them. The drug also blocks cancer cell receptors that promote growth and overexpression of cancer-causing genes.

Herceptin (Trastuzumab), one of the most common of these innovative drugs, is used to treat HER2+ breast cancer. It is often infused via a port that has been surgically implanted under a woman's clavicle. A port is a small plastic or metal round disc attached to a catheter and inserted into the subclavian vein, which leads to the superior vena cava and into the heart for distribution throughout the body via the bloodstream (Breastcancer.org, 2012m). The drug is administered into the port through a needle. The use of a port prevents having to experience the stress of a venipuncture every time the drug is administered. Because the drug is administered roughly every three weeks for a year, the use of a port, allowing the drug to be infused into the larger vessel, minimizes the potential irritation that the drug may cause to the lining of a smaller vein in the arm. The drug may be given in conjunction with chemotherapy or hormonal therapy, or administered alone (Mahon, 2012; Mayo Clinic Staff, 2011f).

Some HER2+ breast cancers do not respond as well to Herceptin as to other drugs (AACR, 2007e). These Herceptin-resistant tumors continue to overexpress the HER2 protein. Scientists have studied these tumors looking for specific genes that may be the culprit. The discovery of pertinent genes opens options for additional drug treatment.

Breast Reconstruction

One of the many decisions a woman with breast cancer must make is whether she will have a mastectomy and, if so, whether she will have breast reconstruction surgery. The surgery is a procedure to create a new breast in place of the breast that was removed. The procedure may be done at the same time as the mastectomy or at a later date (Mahon, 2012). Reconstructive surgery is done by a plastic surgeon, and there are two options—implanting a silicone breast implant or using a transverse rectus abdominis myocutaneous (TRAM) flap approach (Mayo Clinic, n.d.). The TRAM approach uses abdominal muscle, fat, and skin to create a breast shape. It often appears more natural looking because it uses the patient's own tissue. An added benefit is that the procedure involves a "tummy tuck," which makes the patient's abdomen look flatter.

For those women who choose to forgo breast reconstruction, several breast prostheses are available. They are made from various substances and can either be adhered to the chest or fit into pockets of postmastectomy bras (Mahon, 2012). The prosthesis is often weighted to match the weight of the remaining breast.

Women with stage IV breast cancer often have chemotherapy with hormone therapy, and some have biological therapy as well (Mahon, 2012). These therapies, along with radiation and surgery, will not cure them but may help manage the disease and enhance their possibility for survival.

Complementary or Alternative Medicine

Complementary or alternative medicine (CAM) breast cancer therapies have been effective in decreasing depression and anxiety, minimizing pain, and boosting immune function (Aghabati, Mohammadi, & Esmaiel, 2008). There are numerous safe, complementary cancer treatments that may provide symptomatic relief and promote healing, though they do not cure cancer (Mayo Clinic Staff, 2011f). The following healing modalities have shown various levels of effectiveness in those with cancer:

1. Music therapy
2. Biofeedback
3. Tai chi
4. Hypnosis
5. Massage
6. Meditation
7. Relaxation techniques
8. Exercise
9. Yoga
10. Acupuncture

11. Aromatherapy
12. Therapeutic Touch

JULIE'S BREAST CANCER TREATMENT

Julie and her Alabama oncologist and surgeon discussed treatment options prior to knowing that there was cancer in the left breast. (She had two oncologists, one in Alabama and the other in Minnesota.) Should she begin her chemo prior to a lumpectomy, or after? Should she consider a mastectomy? She discussed the pros and cons of neoadjuvant chemotherapy followed by a lumpectomy, or the reverse—having the lumpectomy prior to chemotherapy. She decided that she would have the lumpectomy first. She wanted the cancer out of her body; psychologically, she needed the actual physical removal of the cancerous tumor, then the chemo. She was informed that the size of the lesion could result in a deformity of her breast contour, but that was not important to her. In retrospect, it probably would have been better for her to have had the chemo prior to the lumpectomy.

At this point, neither Julie's physicians nor Julie were even thinking about a mastectomy. That thinking changed when: a) the results of the lumpectomies of both breasts revealed that she had cancer in the left breast as well as the right, and b) the surgeon failed to remove enough margins in her right breast during the lumpectomy. The failure to remove the margins meant she still had cancer in the right breast—a mastectomy was needed to remove the remaining cancerous breast tissue. Then, there was the news of the lymph nodes.

Alarmingly, after finding that two sentinel nodes were positive for cancer during the lumpectomies, the pathology report showed that Julie had cancer in 20 out of 21 lymph nodes. She also had extracapsular extension in several nodes, meaning that the cancer had spread outside the lymph node itself (Breastcancer.org, 2012j). In addition, she had both lymphovascular and perineural invasion, meaning that the cancer cells were also found in the lymph, blood vessels, and tissue surrounding the nerves.

We wondered—could it get any worse? I had never heard of anyone having two different cancers at the same time, let alone metastasis into 20 lymph nodes. The extensive metastasis in her nodes and surrounding tissue, the HER2+ diagnosis, and two different kinds of breast cancer—well, it was just too much, way too much. It was like being punched in the gut and not being able to breathe. It was overwhelming. It felt insurmountable.

Due to her concerning pathology report, doctors were anxious to start Julie on chemotherapy (Taxotere and Carboplatin) and Herceptin. Since she needed Herceptin for one year, she decided to have a port implanted for ease of infusion. This involved a surgical procedure, yet another invasion of her little body. By February 22 she had her first chemo and Herceptin infusion. Following her first chemo, she e-mailed her family saying, "I feel so good knowing that those drugs are now circulating in my body killing off those f*** cancer cells. . . . I'm gonna kick this cancer's ass! I'm ticked!" With each chemo, she received a steroid infusion as well, which gave her quite a bit of energy for the first 24 hours. She would often go home and cook and clean. She said it felt like how she would imagine a hit of speed would feel. She finished her chemo treatments (six infusions of chemo, one infusion every three weeks) on June 8, 2012, and continued with the Herceptin into February 2013.

Because Herceptin can damage the heart, Julie had an echocardiogram, an imaging test to examine the anatomy and physiology of the heart, to ensure that her heart was healthy enough to withstand the rigors of Herceptin. When a patient is on Herceptin, an echocardiogram should be done every six months.

Much to our family's dismay, midway through Julie's chemo treatment, her husband, Michael, was diagnosed with colon cancer! Talk about life not being fair! It was just more than we thought we could handle. Somehow, though, we all reached into our reserves, which we didn't even know we had, and supported both Julie and Michael upon this terrible news. Fortunately, the colon cancer was encapsulated and had not metastasized to any lymph nodes or other organs. He had surgery to remove the cancerous tumor, and that was it—he needed no chemo and no radiation. Thank goodness for small favors.

Julie came back to Minnesota for the mastectomies. I was so glad to have her home, with Minnesota health care. The bilateral mastectomy took about two and a half hours, a long two and a half hours. Julie wanted to see her breasts after they were removed—and so did I. This may seem pretty weird, but Julie is also very interested in the human body, anatomy, and physiology, and had attended a year of nursing school. My nursing background also spurred my interest. I wanted to see if any of the cancer was visible. We knew that we shouldn't be able to see it since she had had the chemo, but nonetheless we both wanted to see her breast. We needed reassurance that no cancer was observable. It was reassuring to see what appeared to be normal breast tissue.

Seeing her in that hospital bed was awful. She was bald from the chemo, was missing both breasts, had a large hematoma (pocket of blood under the skin) on her surgical wound on her left chest, and was wearing what had to be absolutely the ugliest hospital gown I'd ever seen. The colors of the gown were tan and green print; can you imagine? Why in the world would any manufacturer make hospital gowns with those ugly colors, which do nothing but make a patient look more pale and sick? The nurses came in with pretty bright blue scrubs; you would think some pretty bright colors could be used for patient gowns. The gown was also huge on her, hanging on her small frame.

The surgeon angered me when, after her modified radical bilateral mastectomies, he told me that he had removed another lymph node, positive that it was cancerous. This news devastated me. He claimed that, with his experience, he could tell by visual inspection whether the node was cancerous. HA! Who did he think he was to make a comment like that? I felt like the wind had been knocked out of me. Why would he say such a thing, when he could not possibly know whether the node was cancerous until the lab results came back? I asked him how in the world there could be a cancerous lymph node after all the chemo she had received. He erroneously told me that chemotherapy doesn't kill localized (within the breast tissue) cancer, that it only kills cancer cells that had metastasized throughout the body. His comment contradicted the common medical practice of using chemotherapy prior to surgery, which is frequently done to reduce the size of the tumor by killing cancer cells, thereby making the surgical removal of the tumor easier.

We had to wait over the weekend to get the lab results from the node. Julie's Facebook post on July 24 said:

My pathology report was back, and it shows NO CANCER in any of the breast tissue that was removed. So chemo destroyed leftover breast cancer in my right breast and hopefully has destroyed breast cancer cells elsewhere in my body. Now I will pray that it will be a helluva long time before any cancer returns (it took my grandmother's cancer 35 years to resurface!). Feeling good!

Julie's surgery wounds needed to heal before she could start radiation. Her mastectomies took place on July 18; her radiation began on August 30 and ended on October 24. She needed 37 radiation treatments, with the first 28 radiating her entire right chest, right axilla, and clavicle, and the final 9 radiating her scar from her right mastectomy only. Her radiation oncologist told her that most recurrences of breast cancer occur at the scar. Julie's radiation involved the use of a bolus every other treatment. A bolus is an 8 x 8 square inches of opaque, pliable material that, according to Julie, feels like rubbery skin; it is about a fourth of an inch thick and is placed over the affected area to enhance the radiation's effectiveness on the skin. The radiologist said that he used the bolus in all mastectomy patients. The radiation didn't give her the sensation of burning, but rather she said her skin's itching drove her nuts. She used a hydrocortisone cream, aloe vera gel (which she kept in the refrigerator), and emu oil, which helped minimize the severe itching.

Following the radiation Julie began taking Arimidex on October 25, 2012, two days after completing her radiation. She will be on Arimidex for five years. The drug decreases the amount of estrogen in the body, thereby minimizing ER+ cancer growth (AstraZeneca, 2012). The side effects from the drug include hot flashes, nausea, pain, back pain, headache, bone pain, coughing and shortness of breath, swelling of arms and legs, decreased energy, and weakness.

COMPLICATIONS OF BREAST CANCER TREATMENT

Considering the intensity, the numerous types, and the length of treatment, it would be unrealistic to expect that a woman would not experience any complications. The complications are from the chemical, surgical, and radiation attack on her body's systems. It is often the complications that cause the breast cancer patient to feel sick, rather than the cancer itself.

Radiation Complications

Radiation complications include red, dry, itchy, and tender skin with some desquamation toward the end of therapy (Mahon, 2012). Though the effects of radiation on the skin disappear, the skin may have permanent discoloration. Another radiation side effect is fatigue.

Chemotherapy

Chemotherapy complications vary depending on the drugs used and include the following (Gullatte, 2007):

1. Decrease in white blood cells, resulting in increased risk of infection
2. Decrease in blood platelets, with increased risk of bleeding
3. Anorexia (loss of appetite)
4. Alopecia (hair loss)
5. Nausea and vomiting
6. Mouth sores
7. Darkening of nail beds and skin creases of hands
8. Edema (swelling due to accumulation of fluid)
9. Allergic reactions
10. Diarrhea
11. Cessation of menstruation

Hormonal Therapy Complications

Hormonal therapy complications may include symptoms similar to menopause: hot flashes, vaginal discharge, vaginal dryness, itching, irritation of the skin around the vagina, headaches, irregular menstruation, nausea and vomiting, rash, and fatigue (Mahon, 2012).

Herceptin Complications

Herceptin complications, though rare, include fever, chills, weakness, nausea, vomiting, diarrhea, headaches, rash, dyspnea, fatigue, and cardiac toxicity, which may lead to heart failure. Other side effects may include a drop in red blood cells, which carry oxygen, and a drop in platelets, which play a pivotal role in blood clotting (Genetech, n.d.). Because of the potential damage to the heart, most physicians order an echocardiogram prior to beginning Herceptin to ensure that the woman's heart is healthy.

Fatigue

Approximately 33 percent of breast cancer survivors experience fatigue that can persist for years following treatment (AACR, 2006). The fatigue appears to be the immune system's response to inflammation.

Lymphedema

Lymphedema is a complication from the surgical removal (or the radiation) of axillary lymph nodes in which the arm on the affected side swells (Mayo Clinic Staff, 2011g). There is significantly less lymphedema following breast-conserving surgery than when a modified radical mastectomy is performed (Nesvold et al., 2008). Twenty percent of women developed lymphedema following a modified radical mastectomy, whereas only 8 percent developed it following breast-conserving surgery. When the nodes are removed, it minimizes the ability of the remaining nodes to drain the lymph fluid from the breast, causing the swelling. The swelling may be mild to severe and may occur shortly after the removal of the nodes, or years later. In addition to swelling of the arm, there may be a feeling of heaviness, restricted ability to move the arm, achiness or discomfort, risk of infection, and a hardening or thickening of the skin.

There is no cure for lymphedema, but there are a number of effective treatments that can minimize swelling and discomfort (Mayo Clinic Staff, 2011g):

1. Gentle exercises of the arm stimulate muscle contractions and therefore circulation of lymph fluid out of the arm. A physical therapist teaches these exercises.
2. A compression stocking or wrapping of the arm compresses the arm, thereby minimizing swelling and encouraging lymph fluid to flow from the arm toward the axillary nodes. Sometimes a pneumatic pump is attached to the compression stocking and intermittently presses on the arm, forcing the fluid out toward the remaining nodes.

3. Massage, again taught by a physical therapist, uses a particular technique of hand strokes on the chest and arm. Referred to as *manual lymph drainage*, this technique pushes lymph fluid to the nodes, where it can drain into the lymphatic system.

Surgical Complications

Complications from lumpectomies and mastectomies may include bleeding, infection, poor cosmetic scarring, chronic pain, numbness, seroma (a pocket of clear fluid), hematoma, adverse reaction to anesthesia, and even death.

Recurrent Breast Cancer

A recurrence of breast cancer is a common fear. The American Society of Clinical Oncology (ASCO) recommends that a breast cancer survivor should have a history and physical examination and mammography every 3–6 months for the first three years following her treatment, every 6–13 months for years four and five, and annually thereafter (Khatcheressian et al., 2006). Women who chose breast-conserving surgery should have a mammogram six months after completing radiation. Other monitoring tests such as chemistry panels, bone scans, chest X-rays, ultrasounds, MRIs, CT scans, PET scans, or checking for tumor markers in the blood are not recommended follow-up courses of action in women with no symptoms or no findings on physical exam. It is only after a woman becomes symptomatic or a physical exam demonstrates possible metastasis that additional surveillance tests should be considered.

Despite five years of adjuvant therapy, 20 percent of women are plagued by a recurrence within 10 years following treatment, with higher risk for higher staged cancers (Brewster et al., 2008). More than half of breast cancer recurrences present symptoms and are therefore found between scheduled follow-up visits (de Bock, Bonnema, van Der Hage, Kievit, & van de Velde, 2004). Breast cancer may occur many years after treatment; however, most recurrences appear within the first two or three years following treatment (Cancer Treatment Centers of America, n.d.). The recurrent cancer may be found back in the breast or in the chest wall, or it may have metastasized to other parts of the body.

The treatment options for recurrent breast cancer vary based on the location, the scope of recurrence, and the type of the original cancer (Mahon, 2012). All of the same treatments offered for the original breast cancer are once again available, though in all likelihood with some variation. If the recurrence is in a distant organ, then treatment is ineffective in curing the cancer but rather becomes a treatment to manage the metastasis.

JULIE'S COMPLICATIONS

Julie has had no known complications so far from the Herceptin. Complications from her chemotherapy caused mild nausea for the first two or three days following the infusion of the drugs and fatigue that became extreme toward the end of the first week, then gradually dissipated. Her nausea responded well to antiemetic drugs. The fatigue worsened throughout the months of chemo. She lost all hair from her body. She laughed about how loss of her nose hair made her sniff more, and losing pubic hair even made a difference in the stream of her urine. She was delighted that she no longer had to pluck her chin hairs. She looked forward to buying cute little hats and opted not to use a wig. With the loss of all her hair, including eyebrows and eyelashes, she looked just like our Dad, which we laughed about.

The first chemo reduced Julie's white blood cell count (the cells that fight infection) down to a little more than 1,000 cells per microliter. Normal white cell count is 5,000 to 10,000 per microliter. Consequently, she was at an increased risk of infection and was required to wear a facial mask, stay away from people, and take a small dose of antibiotics for a few weeks until she received an injection of Neulasta following the remainder of each chemo infusion. Neulasta, given the day after chemo, works on the bone marrow, where white blood cells are created, increasing the rate at which the cells are produced and therefore increasing the amount of white blood cells circulating in the blood (Neulasta, 2012). The drug is expensive, costing up to $5,000 an injection, Julie was told.

Before her mastectomies, Julie's hemoglobin had dropped down to 7 grams per deciliter, which caused her doctors to be concerned about the possibility of internal bleeding. One of the most common sites of bleeding is the gastrointestinal tract; consequently, her surgeon wanted her to have a colonoscopy prior to the mastectomy. Poor little Squirt just didn't have the emotional wherewithal to deal with that, so she bargained with the surgeon that if she could get her hemoglobin up to 10 grams by five days prior to surgery, then he would hold off on the colonoscopy. Well, bless her little heart, between taking iron pills and eating iron-enriched food, she got it up to 10, and so talked him out of the colonoscopy, at least temporarily.

Following her mastectomies, she developed a hematoma along the mastectomy incision of her left breast. Between the blood drainage from her wounds and the hematoma, there was enough blood loss to cause her hemoglobin (the part of the red blood cell that carries oxygen) to drop from a normal of 12–16 grams to 7 grams, which is extremely low. The blood loss also caused her blood pressure to drop down to 85/56, which was low. I wasn't happy. I said to the surgeon, "It looks like you missed a bleeder, huh?" He denied it. But as a result of the hematoma and blood loss, she required two units of blood and had to go back to surgery two days after her mastectomy to remove the hematoma. She had her mastectomy on Wednesday, had the hematoma removal on Friday morning at 7:00 a.m., and walked out of the hospital by noon, feeling good and full of energy. She is amazing.

When she had her postoperative appointment with the surgeon and exclaimed how wonderful it felt to be cancer free, his response was something to the effect of "well, at least in your breasts." Now why would her surgeon take the wind out of her sails by insinuating that the cancer was elsewhere, when she was feeling so good about the cancerous breasts and nodes being out of her body? I thought it was cruel and insensitive. This man had absolutely no idea whether she had cancer elsewhere in her body, so why make that comment?

Because of the extensive involvement of cancer in her nodes and the subsequent removal of 20 nodes, she has lymphedema in her right arm. She wears a compression sleeve and massages her arm several times a day to keep the swelling and discomfort to a minimum. She will likely need to do so for the rest of her life.

The radiation has really taken a toll on her little body. By the beginning of October, the skin over her clavicle was so badly burned that the radiation oncologist gave her a day of reprieve. She said that the radiation treatment itself actually hurt. Her skin had split and was blistered. However, what really bothered her was her skin's itching. She used anti-itch cream and another cream to sooth her burns. One evening she and Michael were going out for dinner, and she just smeared the burn cream on quite thick. At the restaurant, she noticed a little girl staring at her from a nearby table. Julie thought it was probably because she had not worn her little hat out to eat, and little tufts of hair were growing back on her head. However, when she went into the bathroom and looked at the skin visible under her tank top, she noticed that her skin had turned black. She had no idea the cream turned her skin black and now knew what the little girl was staring at.

Julie decided not to have reconstructive surgery. It was a fairly easy decision for her to make. She didn't want to experience additional surgery, Michael didn't mind one way or the other, and it wasn't an important issue for Julie whether or not she had breasts. Her surgeon gave her a prescription for prosthetic bras and breast prostheses, but so far she's been wearing bras with heavy padding and it works fine for her because she is so petite. She's not sure if she will ever get the prosthetic bras and breast prostheses.

EMOTIONAL ASPECTS OF BREAST CANCER

A study comparing women who were diagnosed with early-stage breast cancer compared to women who had benign tumors found that women with breast cancer demonstrated more emotional control than did women with benign breast disease (Watson et al., 1991). Additionally, there was a poorer prognosis if a breast cancer survivor displayed a helpless attitude toward the disease. The results of this study suggested an association between controlling one's anger and a helpless or fatalistic attitude about a diagnosis and prognosis of breast cancer.

A diagnosis of breast cancer brings on a myriad of emotional and psychological challenges, as well as sexual concerns, according to healing coach Nancy Cox, RN (N. Cox, personal communication, October 1, 2010). Cox describes cancer as a *noisy* disease because cancer patients and their families are always thinking about the disease and struggling to quiet their minds and reduce their anxiety. The breast cancer patient and her family experience a number of emotions: fear, sadness, uncertainty, anxiety, anticipatory grief, shock, anger, and worry over body image and sexuality. Each emotion is not felt in isolation but rather within a tapestry of all the other emotions, all interwoven and convoluted. In addition, all patients come into the cancer experience with the personal histories, issues, and concerns that existed prior to their diagnosis. The patient's life prior to the diagnosis doesn't just stop at the cancer diagnosis door, according to Nancy.

Women must also deal with their sense of self as a sexual being if their breasts have been removed and with how the various treatments impact their sexuality. Approximately 70 percent of early-stage breast cancer survivors in one study experienced a loss of libido and vaginal dryness (Panjari, Bell, & Davis, 2010). Potential causes of these physical responses may be hormonal or a changed sense of body image, or being postmenopausal. Women taking aromatase inhibitors, which mimic menopausal symptoms such as vaginal dryness, were more likely to experience these physical changes.

Fear is perhaps one of the most pressing emotions that Cox helps the breast cancer patient and her family express and deal with. They are afraid that the cancer diagnosis is equivalent to a death march. Additionally, women fear losing their breasts, jobs, and money, as well as the pain, sickness, and complications from chemotherapy and radiation. Sadness about the loss of their health, and potentially their lives, is tied into uncertainty and the anxiety of what will happen to them and their families. The patient is often angry, which is part of the grief process, and may be depressed and anxious. There may be even more anger at a physician if she or he missed diagnosing the disease when she first went in for a visit after finding a lump.

Every patient is so different in her or his response to a breast cancer diagnosis, according to Cox. The responses can vary depending on the patients' age; partnership status; support network; degree of illness; faith; philosophy about life, health, and disease; and whether they have young children, among other considerations. Cox meets people where they are— she has no agenda other than to guide them through their journey with breast cancer and perhaps death and dying.

Sometimes Cox's work is less about helping the woman deal with the diagnosis and treatment to heal and more about helping her deal with impending death. Cox views this work as sacred and powerful—she is helping her patient to live freely and honestly, truly making the most of the time she has left.

Cox also counsels family members of breast cancer patients. She has often found that the patient is doing "better" with the diagnosis than is the family member. Family members often feel helpless, and they struggle with seeing their loved ones in emotional and physical pain. One of the things she helps the family members deal with is their own self-care because they are so focused on the one with cancer. Family members often withhold talking about their emotions, particularly their fear, with their loved ones with breast cancer. Cox describes it as a dance that goes on—what to say, what not to say. Family members often discount their own emotional turmoil, thinking that they are not the one going through the diagnosis. But, as Cox points out, the family is going through the diagnosis as well. It may be from a different perspective than the patient, but it is a family diagnosis. The breast cancer patient is busy with doctors' appointments, infusions, radiation, and surgery. The family members are involved in those activities but more as observers and supporters; they are not experiencing the treatment so sometimes feel helpless.

JULIE AND ME

When Julie was first diagnosed, and for many months thereafter, I felt disbelief and denial. That old saying that you don't expect it to happen in your family hit me across the face. I was weepy and disengaged, and life's little trials and tribulations weren't important. I didn't want to talk about it with my friends because then I had to feel it all the more. I'm usually quite a talker, an extrovert, and share my feelings, but during those first months I just couldn't do it. I felt so raw, depressed, empty, and on automatic, going through the exercise of life. I cried easily and frequently at seemingly little, inconsequential things. I've cried writing this book chapter and have had to take many breaks from my writing. My stomach aches with the fear of losing her, which is so very painful. I have to keep reminding myself a) that she is a survivor of breast cancer; b) that she is not dying from the disease; c) to enjoy her and love her; d) to keep things in perspective; and e) to live life to the fullest (such a common phrase that takes on new meaning in these times).

There were so many times when Julie and I would talk about her cancer and her treatment. At times she would gently (usually) remind me, "I am more than my cancer. . . . I don't just want to talk about my cancer." It was such a healthy reminder. Yet, it was her cancer that was foremost on my mind.

Reading Julie's pathology and surgical reports was painful. This wasn't just medical information about a patient that I would read as a former RN—it was about my little sister. It was agonizing to read such physicians' notations as:

1. "The fact that the cancer is invasive lobular in type is concerning regarding the possibility that it might be more extensive than originally appreciated."
2. "[H]er advanced disease will also require radiation therapy."
3. "Impression: Right-sided breast cancer unfortunately of invasive lobular type."

I know that a breast cancer diagnosis is not an automatic death sentence. But her diagnosis is a pretty severe one. I'm scared for her. I hate that she is experiencing this awful monster attacking her precious little body. We recognize how the medical treatment, wonderful as it is, is also ravaging her body with the poison and radiation required to kill those cancer cells, and knowing the potential adverse long-term impact on her future health is devastating.

Her oncologist had initially suggested that she have a CT/PET scan to determine the extent of the disease, which she refused to do. In April 2012 she said her emotions just couldn't handle it; if the scans showed that the cancer had spread, then she would give up, and she doesn't want to do that. At that point she still had many months of treatment ahead of her. She needed to keep her energy high and to hang on to hope. She sees metastasis as a death sentence. She e-mailed me, "I can't imagine that there isn't some mets [metastasis], given all the positive nodes. I can only hope the chemo is killing whatever is there." She went on to say,

> There is ZERO cure for stage IV; they just do chemo to keep it at bay to keep you alive as long as they can. I do not want to know that I am going to die. I will be going through what I have to do right now, and take things one step at a time. That is how I feel right now. I may be stage IV right now and don't know it cuz I haven't been scanned, but I DO NOT WANT TO KNOW; there is NOTHING that can be done about it, and if other cancer was found, all of my hope would disappear. I'm not saying that I might not change my mind down the road: right now I only have the strength to deal with the breast aspect. My emotions just could not handle it if had spread. . . . Honey, you'll definitely be outliving me.

Every day she lives with the fear that the cancer either is not gone or will return. She said when she gets a pain in her hip, she automatically wonders if the cancer is in her bone; or when she coughs, if it has metastasized to her lungs; or when she has a headache, if it is in her brain. She said she feels as though her cancer will always be "simmering in the background, just waiting to boil up again."

When our dad died, we cremated him with several items that had personal significance in his life. One day Julie left a voice mail for me, and as she was crying she told me the things she wanted cremated with her. I cried. I've saved the voice mail.

I find it difficult to know what to say to my baby sister when she speaks about dying, that the breast cancer will be her demise. She speaks about it being gone from her body now, but the fear is that it will come back and kill her. It is my fear as well. What do I say to her? I want to tell her not to worry and that it won't come back, but I'm afraid it might. I feel inadequate in those moments—how can I best support her, be honest and real, and provide hope for a long life? I struggle with it.

Despite her poor prognosis and her intermittent but rare days of depression, anger, and as she terms it, "the pity-pot" over how the disease has changed her life, Julie's positive attitude and physical strength are amazing. She has courage, resilience, and determination. I am in awe of her. Her daily routine has not changed—she cooks, cleans, walks her dogs, and does the grocery shopping, and at their new condo she has painted every room, shampooed the carpet, and overseen the installation of new wood floors. Her life continues; her cancer is not her life.

Julie and I have butted heads as sisters; we are both strong-willed and like to control our own destinies and sometimes each other's destinies too. There were times when she had to tell me to back off. My sense of helplessness in trying to advocate for her and to try to minimize what she was experiencing felt to her on occasion like I was usurping her decision making. I should have known better; she is such a well-informed patient.

Her cancer diagnosis has brought us much closer. We talk on the phone much more. Right after her diagnosis, and for many months following, we talked every day. It was like I wanted to get as much of her as I could. I realized how very much I loved her when I feared she would be taken from me. Her diagnosis hit me between the eyes, and those things she does that bug me to no end, somehow don't bug me anymore. Well, almost.

I periodically read the obituaries, looking to see the age and cause of death. Now when I see that someone has died of breast cancer, it hits me in my gut in a way it didn't before. Or, I will see that someone died of damage to their heart and lungs after radiation to their chest, and it scares me.

I'm a fan of the television show *Dancing with the Stars*. On the show that aired October 29, 2012, a couple danced to a song about a woman having been diagnosed with cancer. I wasn't expecting a moving song on cancer, with dancers interpreting the emotion of such a diagnosis. It came out of nowhere, and I sobbed and sobbed some more. The emotions of cancer are always on the surface for the family too. Sometimes family members can be caught off guard when going through the routine of life.

THE FUTURE OF BREAST CANCER TREATMENT

The future of breast cancer treatment looks exciting and hopeful, with much of it focusing on a complicated approach to treatment called *personalized medicine* (Cantlupe, 2012). Personalized medicine focuses on customizing medications for each individual patient to attack that person's specific type of cancer. The new drugs and other treatments will be specific to the patient's tumor and genomes.

According to Maurie Markman, MD, with the Cancer Treatment Centers of America (CTCA), "Within the next year, it will be possible to sequence the entire genome of a tumor and the corresponding normal genome of an individual cancer patient for $3,000. Twelve to fifteen years ago, it would have cost about $6 million" (CTCA, n.d., p. 48). CTCA is partnering with a biopharmaceutical company to begin researching molecular-targeted drugs to treat breast cancer. Fortunately the timeframe and the cost for research to conduct gene sequencing have decreased considerably. Several years ago it took one year and cost $75,000; today it takes a day and costs $1,000.

One significant clinical trial for breast cancer is known as the I-SPY 2 trial through the Knight Cancer Institute in Portland, Oregon. The trial involves women with newly diagnosed advanced breast cancer, using genetic markers from their tumors to screen for effective treatment (Cantlupe, 2012). Other cancer care programs are partnering with hospitals and research agencies to collect cancer tumors and profile them to categorize the tumors' genetic and genomic portraits for effective treatment. One example of such a partnership is the Personalized Medicine Institute, through its subsidiary M2Gen, which has collected 32,500 tumors and genetically profiled 16,000 of them. The Mayo Clinic's efforts in personalized medicine include its Breast Cancer Genome Guided Therapy Study. This study examines the breast tumor genetic mutations of 200 women to determine why some cancers actually adapt and thrive during chemotherapy.

FINAL REMARKS

I am absolutely in awe of my little sister's responsibility in staying on top of breast cancer. She is a role model for other women experiencing the trauma of the diagnosis and the treatment. While the worst of her treatment is over, her next step is to meet with her gynecologist to decide whether the removal of her fallopian tubes, ovaries, and perhaps uterus is a necessary next step. Removal of some or all of these organs requires

careful consideration as a viable preventative measure. If she does not require the surgery, then her remaining treatment is to receive Herceptin
through February 2013 and to stay on Arimidex through 2017. Hopefully
she will never require any additional cancer treatment, the disease is out
of her body forever, and she will live a long life.

This chapter is written in tribute to my little sister, Julie, and in memory of my two grandmothers, my aunt, my cousin, my many friends, and
women worldwide who have both survived or died from this awful
disease.

RESOURCES

Aghabati, N., Mohammadi, E., & Esmaiel, Z. P. (2008). The effect of therapeutic
    touch on pain and fatigue of cancer patients undergoing chemotherapy.
    eCAM, 7, 375–381. doi:10.1093/ecam/nen006.
Altekruse, S. F., Kosary, C. L., Krapcho, M., Neyman, N., Aminou, R., Waldron,
    W., et al., (Eds.). (n.d.). *SEER cancer statistics review, 1975–2007.* Bethesda,
    MD: National Cancer Institute. Retrieved from http://www.stanford.edu/
    group/ecampus/cgi-bin/cancerpen/node/21.
American Association for Cancer Research. (2006). Inflammation markers identify
    fatigue in breast cancer survivors. Retrieved from http://www.aacr.org/
    home/public--media/aacr-press-releases/press-releases-2006.aspx?d=852.
American Association for Cancer Research. (2007a). Active lifestyle reduces risk of
    invasive breast cancer. Retrieved from http://www.aacr.org/home/public
    --media/aacr-press-releases.aspx?d=708.
American Association for Cancer Research. (2007b). The benefits of motherhood:
    Fetal cell "transplant" could be a hidden link between childbirth and re-
    duced risk of breast cancer. Retrieved from http://www.aacr.org/home/
    public--media/aacr-press-releases.aspx?d=904.
American Association for Cancer Research. (2007c). Discovery suggests location of
    genes for breast density, a strong risk factor for breast cancer. Retrieved from
    http://www.aacr.org/home/public--media/aacr-press-releases.aspx?d=815.
American Association for Cancer Research. (2007d). New perspectives on health
    disparities in breast cancer research. Retrieved from http://www.aacr.org/
    home/public--media/aacr-press-releases/press-releases-2007.aspx?d=927.
American Association for Cancer Research. (2007e). Gene profiling predicts resist-
    ance to breast cancer drug Herceptin. Retrieved from http://www.aacr.org/
    home/public--media/aacr-press-releases/press-releases-2006.aspx?d=710.
American Association for Cancer Research. (2008a). Health disparities: Genetics
    plays an important role in cancer detection, prognosis among minorities. Re-
    trieved from http://www.aacr.org/home/public--media/aacr-press-releases/
    press-releases-2008.aspx?d=1049.
American Association for Cancer Research. (2008b). How what and how much we
    eat (and drink) affects our risk of cancer. Retrieved on July 23, 2013 from

http://www.aacr.org/home/public--media/aacr-press-releases/press
-releases-2008.aspx?d=1055.

American Association for Cancer Research. (2008c). Breast cancer common among women with family history but without BRCA1 or BRCA2. Retrieved from http://www.aacr.org/home/public--media/aacr-press-releases/press-releases -2008.aspx?d=1205.

American Association for Cancer Research. (2010). AACR in the news: Clue found in aggressive breast cancer (CNN.com). Retrieved from http://www/aacr .org/home/public--media/aacr-in-the-news.aspx?d=2133.

American Association for Cancer Research. (2011). Diabetes and obesity increase risk for breast cancer development. Retrieved from http://www.aacr.org/ home/public--media/aacr-press-releases/press-releases-2011.aspx?d=2657.

American Cancer Society. (n.d.). Mammograms and other breast imaging proce-dures. Retrieved from http://www.cancer.org/Healthy/FindCancerEarly/ ExamandTestDescriptions/MammogramsandOtherBreastImagingProcedures/ mammograms-and-other-breast-imaging-procedures-toc.

American Cancer Society. (2011a). Cancer facts and figures for African Americans, 2011–2012. Atlanta, GA: American Cancer Society. Retrieved from http:// www.cancer.org/acs/groups/content/@epidemiologysurveilance/documents/ document/acspc-027765.pdf.

American Cancer Society. (2011b). Breast cancer facts & figures, 2011–2012. Atlanta, GA: American Cancer Society. Retrieved from http://www.cancer.org/acs/ groups/content/@epidemiologysurveilance/documents/document/ acspc-030975.pdf.

American Cancer Society. (2011c). Breast cancer: Early detection. Retrieved from http://www.cancer.org/Cancer/BreastCancer/MoreInformation/BreastCancer EarlyDetection/breast-cancer-early-detection-acs-recs.

American Cancer Society. (2012). Cancer facts & figures, 2012. Atlanta, GA: American Cancer Society. Retrieved from http://www.cancer.org/acs/groups/content/ @epidemiologysurveilance/documents/document/acspc-031941.pdf.

Anderson, G. L., Limacher, M., Assaf, A. R., Bassford, T., Beresford, S. A., Black, H., et al. (2004). Effects of conjugated equine estrogen in post-menopausal women with hysterectomy: The Women's Health Initiative randomized controlled trial. *Journal of the American Medical Association, 291*, 1701–1712. doi:10.1001/jama.291.14.1701.

Andic, F., Ors, Y., Davutoglu, R., Cifci, S. B., Ispir, E. B., & Erturk, M. E. (2009, March 24). Evaluation of skin dose associated with different frequencies of bolus applications in post-mastectomy three-dimensional conformal radio-therapy. *Journal of Experimental and Clinical Research Online, 28.* doi: 10.11.86/ 1756-9966-28-41.

AstraZeneca. (2012). Arimidex Direct. Retrieved from http://www.arimidex.com/.

Bardou, V., Arpino, G., Elledge, R. M., Osborne, C. K., & Clark, G. M. (2003). Pro-gesterone receptor status significantly improves outcome prediction over estrogen receptor status alone for adjuvant endocrine theory in two large breast cancer databases. *Journal of Clinical Oncology, 21,* 1973–1979. doi: 10.1200/JCO.2003.09.099.

BRACAnalysis. (n.d.). A quiz for HBOC testing. Retrieved from http://www.bracnow .com/considering-testing/check-inherited-cancer-risk.php.

BRACAnalysis. (n.d.). Why take a breast cancer/ovarian cancer risk assessment test? Retrieved from http://www.bracnow.com/considering-testing/why -take-a-breast-ovarian-cancer-risk-test.php.

Brandt-Rauf, S. I., Raveis, V. H., Drummond, N. F., Conte, J. A., & Rothman, S. M. (2006). Ashkenazi Jews and breast cancer: The consequences of linking ethnic identity to genetic disease. *American Journal of Public Health, 96,* 1988–1989. doi/pdfplus/10.2105/AJPH.2005.083014.

Breastcancer.org. (2012a). Non-invasive or invasive breast cancer. Retrieved from http://www.breastcancer.org/symptoms/diagnosis/invasive.jsp.

Breastcancer.org. (2012b). Triple-negative breast cancer. Retrieved from http:// www.breastcancer.org/symptoms/diagnosis/trip_neg/.

Breastcancer.org. (2012c). How to read hormone receptor test results. Retrieved from http://www.breastcancer.org/symptoms/diagnosis/hormone_status/ read_results.

Breastcancer.org. (2012d). HER2 status. Retrieved from http://www.breastcancer .org/symptoms/diagnosis/her2.

Breastcancer.org. (2012e). Who gets triple-negative breast cancer? Retrieved from http://www.breastcancer.org/symptoms/diagnosis/trip_neg/who_gets.jsp.

Breastcancer.org. (2012f). Triple-negative breast cancer. Retrieved from http:// www.breastcancer.org/symptoms/diagnosis/trip_neg/.

Breastcancer.org. (2012g). BRCA1 and BRCA2 testing. Retrieved from http://www .breastcancer.org/symptoms/diagnosis/brca.jsp.

Breastcancer.org. (2012h). Deciding who in the family should get tested. Retrieved from http://www.breastcancer.org/symptoms/testing/genetic/who_to_test .jsp.

Breastcancer.org. (2012i). Scientists re-write rulebook on breast cancer in landmark global study. Retrieved from http://www.publicaffairs.ubc.ca/2012/04/18/ scientists-re-write-rulebook-on-breast-cancer-in-landmark-global-study/.

Breastcancer.org. (2012j). Lymph node involvement. Retrieved from http://www .breastcancer.org/symptoms/diagnosis/lymph_nodes.

Breastcancer.org. (2012k). How radiation works. Retrieved from http://www .breastcancer.org/treatment/radiation/how_works.jsp.

Breastcancer.org. (2012l). Hormonal therapy. Retrieved from http://www.breastcancer .org/treatment/hormonal/.

Breastcancer.org. (2012m). How is chemotherapy given? Retrieved from http:// www.breastcancer.org/treatment/chemotherapy/process/how.jsp.

Breastcancer.org. (2012n). Lymph node involvement. Retrieved from http://www .breastcancer.org/symptoms/diagnosis/lymph_nodes.jsp.

Breast tissue density sparks debate. (2012, October 28). *Star Tribune.* Retrieved from http://www.startribune.com/lifestyle/health/176111231.html.

Brewster, A. M., Hortobagyi, G. N., Broglio, K. R., Kau, S., Santa-Maria, C. A., Arun, B., et al. (2008). Residual risk of breast cancer recurrence 5 years after adjuvant therapy. *Journal of the National Cancer Institute, 100,* 1179–1183. doi: 10.1093/jnci/djn323.

Cancer Genome Atlas Network, The. (2012, September 23). Comprehensive molecular portraits of human breast tumours. *Nature Online.* doi:10.1038/ nature11412.

Cancer Treatment Centers of America. (n.d.). Breast cancer stages/staging. Retrieved from http://www.cancercenter.com/breast-cancer/breast-cancer-taging.cfm? source=GOOGLPPC&channel=paid%20search&c=paid%20search:Google: National%20Search:Broad:breast+cancer+staging:Broad&OVMTC=Broad&sit e=&creative=8469525561&OVKEY=breast%20cancer%20staging&url _id=129085313&adpos=1t 3&gclid=CKyxjP_-gLMCFcxcMgodpiQAKg.

Cantlupe, J. (2012). Tailoring treatment for cancer. *HealthLeaders, 15,* 46–53.

Chavez-MacGregor, M., Elias, S. G., Onland-Moret, N. C., van der Schouw, Y. T., Van Gils, C. H., Monninkhof, E., et al. (2005). Postmenopausal breast cancer risk and cumulative number of menstrual cycles. *Cancer Epidemiology, Biomarkers & Prevention, 14,* 799–804. doi:10.1158/1055-9965.EPI-04-0465.

Centers for Disease Control and Prevention. (2012). Cancer among women. Retrieved from http://www.cdd.gov/cancer/dcpc/data/women.html.

Claus, E. B., Schildkraut, J. M., Thompson, W. D., & Risch, N. (1996). The genetic attributable risk of breast and ovarian cancer. *Cancer, 77,* 2318–2324.

Collaborative Group on Hormonal Factors in Breast Cancer. (2002). Breast cancer and breastfeeding: Collaborative reanalysis of individual data from 47 epidemiological studies in 30 countries, including 50,302 women with breast cancer and 96,973 women without the disease. *Lancet, 360,* 187–195. doi: 10.1016/S0140-6736(02)09454-0.

Collado-Hidalo, A., Bower, J. E., Ganz, P. A., Cole, S. W., & Irwin, M. R. (2006). Inflammatory biomarkers for persistent fatigue in breast cancer survivors. *Clinical Cancer Research, 12,* 2759–2766.

Cooney, T., Irani, F., Stalnecker, A., & Johnston, S. (2006). Development of a novel bolus material for radiation therapy. Duke University. Retrieved from http://bme227.pratt.duke.edu/downloads/S06/Bolus_Proposal.pdf.

Couch, F. J., DeShano, M. L., Blackwood, M. A., Calzone, K., Stopfer, J., Campeau, L., et al. (1997). BRCA1 mutations in women attending clinics that evaluate the risk of breast cancer. *New England Journal of Medicine, 336,* 1409–1415.

Curtis, C., Shah, S. P., Chin, S.-F., Turashvili, G., Rueda, O. M., Dunning, M. J., et al. (2012). The genomic and transcriptomic architecture of 2,000 breast tumours reveals novel subgroups. *Nature, 486,* 346–352. doi:10.1038/nature10983.

de Bock, G. H., Bonnema, J., van Der Hage, J., Kievit, J., & van de Velde, C. J. H. (2004). Effectiveness of routine visits and routine tests in detecting isolated locoregional recurrences after treatment for early-stage invasive breast cancer: A meta-analysis and systematic review. *Journal of Clinical Oncology, 22,* 4010–4018. doi: 10.1200/JCO.2004.06.080.

Decarli, A., Calza, S., Masala, G., Specchia, C., Palli, D., & Gail, M. H. (2006). Model for prediction of absolute risk of invasive breast cancer: Independent evaluation in the Florence-European Prospective Investigation into cancer and nutrition cohort. *Journal of the National Cancer Institute, 98,* 1686–1693. doi:10.1093/jnci/djj463.

Easton, D. F., Ford, D., & Bishop, D. T. (1995). Breast and ovarian cancer incidence in BRCA1-mutation carriers: Breast Cancer Linkage Consortium. *American Journal of Human Genetics, 56,* 265–271.

Evans, D. G., Eccles, D. M., Rahman, N., Young, K., Bulman, M., Amir, E., et al. (2004). A new scoring system for the chances of identifying a BRCA1/2 mutation outperforms existing models including BRCAPRO. *Journal of Medical Genetics, 41,* 474–480.

Frank, T. S., Deffenbaugh, A. M., Reid, J. E., Hulick, M., Ward, B. E., Lingenfelter, B., et al. (2002). Clinical characteristics of individuals with germline mutations in BRCA1 and BRCA2: Analysis of 10,000 individuals. *Journal of Clinical Oncology, 20,* 1480–1490. doi:10.1200/JCO.20.6.1480.

Gawlick, U., Mone, M. C., Hansen, H. J., Connors, R. C., & Nelson, E. W. (2008). Selective use of intraoperative sentinel lymph node pathological evaluation in breast cancer. *American Journal of Surgery, 196,* 851–855.

Genetech. (n.d.). Adjuvant breast cancer treatment. Retrieved from http://www .herceptin.com/breast/adjuvant.

Gullatte, M. M. (2007). *Clinical guide to antineoplastic therapy: A chemotherapy handbook* (2nd ed.). Pittsburgh, PA: Oncology Nursing Society.

Harvey, J. M., Clark, G. M., Osborne, C. K., & Allred, D. C. (1999). Estrogen receptor status by immunohistochemistry is superior to the Ligand-Binding Assay for predicting response to adjuvant endocrine therapy in breast cancer. *Journal of Clinical Oncology, 17,* 1474–1481.

Henderson, B. E., Lee, N. H., Seewaldt, V., & Shen, H. (2012, September). The influence of race and ethnicity on the biology of cancer. *Nature Reviews: Cancer, 12,* 648–653. doi:10.1038/nrc3341.

Hopper, J. L., Southey, M. C., Dite, G. S., Jolley, D. J., Giles, G. G., McCredie, M. R. E., et al. (1999). Population-based estimate of the average age-specific cumulative risk of breast cancer for a defined set of protein-truncating mutations in BRCA1 and BRCA2: Australian Breast Cancer Family Study. *Cancer Epidemiology Biomarkers and Prevention, 8,* 741–747. Retrieved from http:// cebp.aacrjournals.org/content/8/9/741.full.

Hoskins, K. F., Zwaagstra, A., & Ranz, M. (2006). Validation of a tool for identifying women at high risk for hereditary breast cancer in population-based screening. *Cancer, 107,* 1769–1776. doi: 10.1002/cncr.22202.

Khatcheressian, J. L., Wolff, A. C., Smith, T. J., Grunfeld, E., Muss, H. B., Vogel, V. G., et al. (2006). American society of clinical oncology 2006 update of the breast cancer follow-up and management guidelines in the adjuvant setting. *Journal of Clinical Oncology, 24,* 5091–5097. doi: 10.1200/JCO.2006. 08.8575.

Krieger, D. (1997). *Therapeutic touch inner workbook*. Santa Fe, NM: Bear and Company.

Lynch, H. T., Snyder, C. L., Lynch, J. F., Riley, B. D., & Rubinstein, W. S. (2003). Hereditary breast-ovarian cancer at the bedside: Role of the medical oncologist. *Journal of Clinical Oncology, 21*, 740–753. doi:10.1200/JCO.2003.05.096.

Mahon, S. M. (2012). *Trends in selected cancers affecting women: Updated edition*. CE Express Home Study. Brockton, MA: Western Schools.

Marchbanks, P. A., McDonald, J. A., Wilson, H. G., Folger, S. G., Mandel, M. G., Daling, J. R., et al. (2002). Oral contraceptives and the risk of breast cancer. *New England Journal of Medicine, 346*, 2025–2032. Retrieved from ProQuest database.

Mayo Clinic. (n.d.). Breast cancer: TRAM surgery. Retrieved from http://www .mayoclinic.org/breast-cancer/tramsurgery.html.

Mayo Clinic Staff. (2011a). Breast MRI. Retrieved from http://www.mayoclinic .com/health/breast-mri/MY00300.

Mayo Clinic Staff. (2011b). Biopsy: Types of biopsy procedures used to diagnose cancer. Retrieved from http://www.mayoclinic.com/health/biopsy/CA00083.

Mayo Clinic Staff. (2011c). Lumpectomy. Retrieved from http://www.mayoclinic .com/health/lumpectomy/MY00833.

Mayo Clinic Staff. (2011d). Mastectomy. Retrieved from http://www.mayoclinic .com/health/mastectomy/MY00943.

Mayo Clinic Staff. (2011e). Radiation therapy. Retrieved from http://www.mayoclinic .com/health/radiation-therapy/MY00299.

Mayo Clinic Staff. (2011f). Monoclonal antibody drugs for cancer treatment: How they work. Retrieved from http://www.mayoclinic.com/health/monoclonal -antibody/CA00082.

Mayo Clinic Staff. (2011g). Lymphedema. Retrieved from http://www.mayoclinic .com/health/lymphedema/DS00609.

Mayo Clinic Staff. (2012). Alternative cancer treatments: 11 options to consider. Retrieved from http://www.mayoclinic.com/health/cancer-treatment/CM00002.

McCahill, L. E., Single, R. M., Bowles, E. J. A., Feigelson, H. S., James, T. A., & Barney, T. (2012). Variability in reexcision following breast conservation surgery. *Journal of the American Medical Association, 307*, 467–475. doi:10.1001/jama.2012.43.

Myriad Genetic Laboratories. (2008). Understanding and managing your risk. Retrieved from http://www.inheritedrisk.com/inherit-risk-cancer/managing -your-risk.htm.

Myriad Genetic Laboratories. (2012). A quiz for HBOC testing. Retrieved from http://www.bracnow.com/considering-testing/check-inherited-cancer-risk .php.

National Cancer Institute. (2004). Fact sheet: Tumor grade. Retrieved from http:// www.cancer.gov/cancertopics/factsheet/detection/tumor-grade.

National Cancer Institute. (2010). Breast cancer treatment PDQ. Retrieved from http:// www.cancer.gov/cancertopics/pdq/treatment/breast/healthprofessional/ page3.

National Cancer Institute. (2012). Fact sheet: Mammograms. Retrieved from http://www.cancer.gov/cancertopics/factsheet/detection/mammograms.

National Comprehensive Cancer Network. (2012). *NCCN guidelines.* Retrieved from http://www.nccn.org/professionals/physician_gls/f_guidelines.asp.

Nesvold, I. L., Dahl, A. A., Lokkevik, E., Marit Mengshoel, A., & Fossa, S. D. (2008). Arm and shoulder morbidity in breast cancer patients after breast-conserving therapy versus mastectomy. *Acta Oncologica, 47,* 835–842. doi:10.1080/02841 860801961257.

Neulasta. (2012). White blood cell counts: How Neulasta works. Retrieved from http://www.neulasta.com/starting-chemo-with-neulasta/white-blood-cell -counts.html?src=ppc&WT.srch=1&SRC=2.

Newcomer, L. M., Newcomb, P. A., Trentham-Dietz, A., Longnecker, Mp. P., & Greenberg, E. R. (2003). Oral contraceptive use and risk of breast cancer by histologic type. *International Journal of Cancer, 106,* 961–964. doi: 10.1002/ ijc.11307.

Onesti, J. K., Mangus, B. E., Helmer, S. D., & Osland, J. S. (2008). Breast cancer tumor size: Correlation between magnetic resonance imaging and pathology measurements. *The American Journal of Surgery, 196,* 844–850. doi:10.1016/j .amjsurg.2008.07.028.

Oz, M. (2012, October/November). Save or sacrifice your breasts. *AARP: The Magazine,* 18.

Panjari, M., Bell, R. J., & Davis, S. R. (2010). Sexual function after breast cancer. *Journal of Sexual Medicine, 8,* 294–301.

Parise, C.A., Bauer, K. R., Brown, M. M., & Caggiano, V. (2009). Breast cancer subtypes as defined by the estrogen receptor (ER), progesterone receptor (PR), and the human epidermal growth factor receptor 2 (HER2) among women with invasive breast cancer in California. *Breast Journal, 16,* 593–602.

Parmigiani, G., Sining, C., Iversen, E. S., Friebel, T. M., Finkelstein, D. M., Anton-Culver, H., et al. (2007). Validity of models for predicting BRCA1 and BRCA2 mutations. *Annals of Internal Medicine, 147,* 441–450.

Pegram, M., & Slamon, D. (2000). Biological rationale for HER2/neu (c-erbB2) as a target for monoclonal antibody therapy. *Seminars in Oncology, 27,* 13–19.

Petrucelli, N., Daly, M. B., & Feldman, G. L. (2010). Hereditary breast and ovarian cancer due to mutations in BRCA1 and BRCA2. *Genetics in Medicine, 12,* 245–259. doi:10.1097/GIM.0b013e3181d38f2f.

Pruthi, S. (2012, April 11). HER2-positive breast cancer: What is it? *Mayo Clinic.* Retrieved from http://www.mayoclinic.com/health/breast-cancer/AN00495.

Saslow, D., Boetes, C., Burke, W., Harms, S., Leach, M. O., Lehman, C. D., et al. (2007). American Cancer Society guidelines for breast screening with MRI as an adjunct to mammography. *CA: A Cancer Journal for Clinicians, 57,* 75–90. doi: 10.3322/canjclin.57.2.75.

Shattuck-Eidens, D., Oliphant, A., McClure, M., McBride, C., Gupte, J., Rubano, T., et al. (1997). BRCA1 sequence analysis in women at high risk for susceptibility mutations. Risk factor analysis and implications for genetic testing. *Journal of* the *American Medical Association, 278,* 1242–1250. doi:10.1001/jama.1997 .03550150046034.

Slear, T. (2012, May). Cancer: More Americans are surviving, here's why. *AARP: The Magazine,* 50–54.

Susan G. Komen for the Cure. (2011). Staging of breast cancer. Retrieved from http://ww5.komen.org/BreastCancer/StagingofBreastCancer.html.

Susan G. Komen for the Cure. (2012). Lumpectomy. Retrieved from http://ww5 .komen.org/BreastCancer/Lumpectomy.html.

United Nations Population Fund. (2002). Breast cancer: Increasing incidence, limited options. Retrieved from http://screening.iarc.fr/doc/eol19_4-rev.pdf.

University of British Columbia. (2012, April 18). Scientists re-write rulebook on breast cancer in landmark global study. *Public Affairs Online.* Retrieved from http://www.publicaffairs.ubc.ca/2012/04/18/scientists-re-write-rulebook -on-breast-cancer-in-landmark-global-study/.

Watson, M., Greer, S., Rowden, L., Gorman, C., Robertson, B., Bliss, J. M., & Tunmore, R. (1991). Relationships between emotional control, adjustment to cancer and depression and anxiety in breast cancer patients. *Psychological Medicine, 21,* 51–57. doi: 10.017/SOO33291700014641.

WebMD. (2012, May 16). Breast cancer health center: Risk factors for breast cancer. Retrieved from http://www.webmd.com/breast-cancer/guide/overview-risks -breast-cancer.

Wood, W. C., Muss, H. B., Solin, L. J., & Olopade, O. I. (2005). Malignant tumors of the breast. In V. T. DeVita Jr., S. Hellman, & S. A. Rosenberg (Eds.), *Cancer: Principles and practice of oncology* (7th ed., pp. 1415–1477). Philadelphia: Lippincott Williams & Wilkins.

Chapter 3

HERA Women's Cancer Foundation

Meg Steitz, HERA Women's Cancer Foundation

HERA Women's Cancer Foundation is a nationally recognized nonprofit organization whose mission is to stop the loss of women from ovarian cancer by promoting Health, Empowerment, Research, and Awareness. In doing so, HERA promotes cross-disciplinary science and seeks to attract young researchers to expand the scientific understanding of ovarian cancer while improving the lives of those battling the disease. HERA provides funding for cutting-edge research grants to scientists at respected medical institutions around the country, including the Johns Hopkins University, the MD Anderson Cancer Center, the University of Colorado, and others. The projects funded by HERA focus on mechanisms of ovarian cancer development, growth, and treatment.

HERA also embraces projects related to raising awareness about ovarian cancer and its symptoms in different communities around the country. By stressing the concept of "community," HERA supports and empowers those undergoing treatment for ovarian cancer, as well as women who are healthy.

Through its signature Climb4Life[SM] and auxiliary events, along with proceeds from multiple other sources, HERA invests at least 85 percent of the funds raised each year into programs that provide research, awareness, education, and community support for ovarian cancer patients and their families.

OVARIAN CANCER: THE SILENT KILLER

While progress has been made diagnosing other forms of female cancers, the survival statistics for women diagnosed with ovarian cancer are grim. According to the American Cancer Society in 2013, 1 in 72 women will be diagnosed with ovarian cancer in her lifetime. With early detection about 94 percent will survive longer than five years; however, only 20 percent of ovarian cancer is caught early.

Currently, there is *no* early detection test for ovarian cancer. Pap smears test only for cervical cancer. More than 78 percent of the women diagnosed in 2013 will be diagnosed after the disease has spread, when the chance for survival is less than 20 percent.

To improve early detection of ovarian cancer, researchers are actively working to develop effective screening tests, and advocates are working to educate women about symptoms. Research studies have identified four common symptoms experienced by women with a new diagnosis of ovarian cancer:

- Bloating
- Pelvic or abdominal pain
- Difficulty eating or feeling full quickly
- Urinary symptoms (urgency or frequency)

Although these symptoms may be vague and can be associated with other conditions, women are advised to report them to their doctor if they persist for more than two weeks. Also, women with a family history of breast, ovarian, colon, or other gastrointestinal cancers should consider a consultation with a genetic counselor to determine whether they carry genetic mutations that increase their risk of ovarian cancer.

OUR ROOTS

The HERA Women's Cancer Foundation was established in 2002 by Sean Patrick of Carbondale, Colorado. Patrick, who had been diagnosed with ovarian cancer in 1997, was frustrated that the prognosis for women with ovarian cancer had not changed in decades and by the disproportionate amount of government funds that went to other cancers. To make a change, she founded HERA and its signature fund-raising series, the Climb4Life^SM weekends.

Patrick, an avid skier, mountain biker, and hiker, learned to rock climb. She saw the correlation between the skills needed for rock climbing (confidence, refined decision making, and a sharp eye for assessing a situation quickly) and the skills needed for coping with health issues. In 2001 she began the first HERA Climb4Life^SM weekend in Salt Lake City, Utah. These events are truly unique, providing climbing, hiking, yoga, outdoor photography, and many more activities in beautiful settings with professional athletes and guides, as well as others who support ovarian cancer research and awareness initiatives. These two- to three-day events now take place annually in Boston, Massachusetts; Boulder, Colorado; and Washington, D.C., in addition to Salt Lake City.

In January 2009 Patrick succumbed to ovarian cancer after a 12-year battle. In the whirlwind that characterized her life as an advocate for women, she passed on a valuable lesson: "We all have the power within us to change the world in a positive way. It just takes one idea, one individual, one scientist, one company, or one community to make a difference in the world. That's the power of one."

KUED-TV, the PBS affiliate in Salt Lake City, created a documentary called *Climb for Life: A Legacy*, which can be viewed at www.herafoundation .org/newsletters/celebrate-hera/. The documentary originally aired in 2012 to commemorate HERA's 10th anniversary. It received a 2012 Emmy Award for Public/Current/Community Affairs—Program/Special and a Gold Award from the Utah Broadcasters Association for Best Lifestyle Program.

HERA'S IMPACT

Since its founding in 2002, HERA has awarded nearly $875,000 for scientific research and community grants. HERA awards the following grants annually after an intensive application and review process:

- OSB (Outside the Box) Grants to scientists with "outside the box" ideas regarding the research of new directions in the treatment, early detection, and prevention of ovarian cancer. Over the last 10 years, HERA has raised and awarded Johns Hopkins Medicine with nearly $525,000 in grant funding through 26 awards made to 23 scientists focused on early detection and targeted therapy for ovarian cancer. These HERA-funded scientists are spread all over the world in Japan, France, China, Thailand, Taiwan, and throughout the United States, training other young scientists to fight ovarian cancer at their new institutions.

- The Sean Patrick Multidisciplinary Collaborative Grant was established in 2011 to provide $50,000 for a cross-disciplinary research project that is collaborative in nature. Projects must identify two (or more) scientists with different yet complementary skills and explain how these skills will be synergistic in addressing the ovarian cancer problem. The first grant was awarded to the University of Colorado; the 2012 grant was awarded to a joint project between the University of Chicago and the University of Texas, and the University of Minnesota was recently selected as the 2013 recipient.

HERA also awards community grants each year to five nonprofit organizations around the country that are working to improve quality of life for women with ovarian cancer or to raise awareness of the disease in novel and unusual ways. Through its Community Grants Program, HERA has awarded more than $48,000 and supported more than 35 programs, which have included the development of advertising campaigns, promotional materials, support groups, educational conferences and events, and therapeutic and outreach services for women with ovarian cancer.

GET INVOLVED

Each year HERA presents its signature Climb4Life^{SM} series as the primary fund-raiser for its research and community grants. The Climb4Life^{SM} events are rock climbing and hiking weekends, some held in indoor gyms and some held at outdoor crags in four cities across the country. People of all ages and skill levels participate—beginning climbers, experienced mountaineers, courageous cancer survivors, people whose lives have been affected by cancer, and people who just love the outdoors.

HERA's outreach activities also include a series of "women's only" 8K runs, called Run Like a Girl, held annually on the East Coast, as well as the Mother's Day 5K run in Denver's beautiful City Park.

Ovarian cancer is a very serious yet underrecognized threat to women's health. HERA's Climb4Life^{SM} weekends and community events empower women and their families to challenge themselves. These events raise awareness about the signs and symptoms of ovarian cancer while raising money that goes directly to much-needed scientific research and unique awareness programs. Through awareness and research, HERA is fighting this deadly disease and encouraging women to pay attention to their bodies, speak up when something isn't right, and be their own advocates when it comes to their health.

In 2013 alone, HERA's Climb4Life^{SM} events raised more than $100,000 to fund ovarian cancer research grants and community grants. For more information about HERA Climb4Life^{SM}, or to donate, visit HERA's website (www.herafoundation.org).

Part II

Sexism and Racism in Women's Cancer Diagnosis and Treatment

Chapter 4

Women's Health: Biological and Social Systems

Cheryl Brown Travis and Andrea L. Meltzer[1]

BACKGROUND

One might begin analysis of the women's health movement in Greek antiquity with Hypatia, said to be one of the first women physicians, who disguised herself as a man in order to practice. The story may be apocryphal, but it is the case that from the time of Hippocrates, women were increasingly and systematically excluded from the practice of medicine of any sort and legally prohibited in many instances. The exclusion of women from the practice of medicine probably arose from a variety of factors, such as a general fear of and mystery regarding women's biology. Economic competition undoubtedly played a role in the diminution of women in medicine, especially as male physicians sought to enter the field of birth and family planning, and midwifery was made illegal in many countries (Marieskind, 1980). Nursing gained some increased professional status under the activism of Florence Nightingale during the Crimean War of 1854. One is reminded that all the nurses were volunteers and that the Charge of the Light Brigade took place prior to morphine, antibiotics, or analgesics.

Margaret Sanger must be noted as one of the stellar figures to presage a women's health movement. She and her sister, Ethel Byrne, and another woman, Fania Mindell, opened a birth control clinic in Brooklyn, New York, in 1916, a time when it was illegal to provide even information on birth control, let alone birth control devices. Sanger and her coworkers were arrested at various times for publicly speaking and imparting information on birth control. To get a sense of the times in which she braved this monolithic opposition, it may help to recall that in 1916 women did not have the right to vote.

The contemporary women's health movement, as it emerged in the 1960s and 1970s in the United States, was situated in a sociopolitical context that saw the birth, or rebirth, of a number of social and political movements: the civil rights movement, feminist movement, and antiwar movement, along with the farm workers movement and a centralization of the labor organizations in general. The first modern nationally inclusive meeting of feminists occurred in 1977, partially in response to a United Nations initiative, the Decade of Women.

Early scholars and activists in the women's health movement included Gena Corea (1977), Mary Daly (1978), Claudia Dreifus (1977), Sheryle Ruzek (1978), Helen Marieskind (1980), Diana Scully (1980), and Peggy Sandelowski (1981).

A central feature of the women's health movement has been to offer practical information and guidance directly to women regarding their own bodies. *Our Bodies, Ourselves*, first published by the Boston Women's Health Book Collective in 1970, has been one of the most widely distributed resources. Regularly updated and revised, the most recent edition (Boston Women's Health Book Collective, 2005) continues to be highly regarded.

Feminism and feminist principles favor the political, economic, and social equality of women and men and therefore favor legal and social change necessary to secure this equality (Hyde, 2006). Collectively, feminist principles serve as a framework for conceptualizing health care issues (Travis & Compton, 2001). They support work that illuminates health outcomes for girls and women and other oppressed groups, medical planning and decision making that is consensual, and exposure of the hidden power and privilege within health care systems that benefit some while excluding others. Although feminism is not a homogeneous philosophy, there are some general principles that seem to hold whether one assumes a liberal, socialist, or cultural standpoint or a postmodern perspective.

The women's health movement has centered on four broad issues. A primary issue is that traditional approaches to medicine have promoted a social construction of women, women's bodies, and women's roles that undermines the human rights of women, the safety and health of women, and the general political and social status of women. That is, the institution of medicine has actively contributed to the oppression of women.

A related issue is that the traditional physician-patient relationship reflects a traditional hierarchy and subordination of the patient and is especially onerous for women. This has been particularly grievous in the areas of gynecology, contraception, pregnancy, and birth.

A third, and related, concern is that women's voices have been trivialized and discounted in such settings, with the result that women often do not receive appropriate or timely care. In particular, women's biomedical symptoms may be discounted or reinterpreted as emotional or psychosomatic. Accounts are not rare of delayed and ponderous diagnostic processes for women with life-threatening heart conditions, painful ovarian cysts, or chronic diseases such as hypothyroidism. Conditions such as hypothyroidism (even if seemingly subclinical) may contribute to higher levels of cholesterol and subsequently to increased risk of heart disease (Michalopoulou et al., 1998). Underdiagnosis or prolonged delays in diagnosis may preclude the most effective medical interventions and necessitate more invasive procedures that are both more risky and more costly. To the extent that biomedical problems are misattributed to women's emotions or psychological distress, women also may be overmedicated with psychotropes. The problems of underdiagnosis and overmedication are compounded by the fact that many randomized clinical trials to assess diagnostic techniques or primary interventions have been developed and tested on men. The historic assumption has been that safety and effectiveness for women can be assumed if results were favorable among men.

A fourth and continuing concern of the women's health movement has been the professional standing and opportunities for women as health care providers and administrators. Some notable improvements have evolved since the 1970s, and the Health Resources and Services Administration reports that as of 2000, slightly more than 40 percent of students entering medical schools are women.

GENERAL FEMINIST PRINCIPLES

Historically, American society has been patriarchal, and feminist theory has had one main goal: gender equality for women and men as well as other oppressed groups. In the health care system, giving women access to the rights and privileges they have been denied could break down this patriarchal system (Miller & Kuszelewicz, 1995). This may be achieved by providing women with additional skills and knowledge so they may further understand their rights.

Basic feminist principles may help to explain our thinking on women's health. These principles—including societal expectations and cultural context, bringing an end to patriarchal power, unity and diversity, and women's movement and activism—all play a role in reaching egalitarianism between the sexes.

Societal Expectations and Cultural Context

Our patriarchal world is shaped by societal actions and expectations. Beginning at their day of birth, boys and girls are taught how to act "masculine" and "feminine," respectively. In our society, as well as in most other societies worldwide, strength, control, and domination are all associated with males (Johnson, 1997), while quietness, gentleness, and subordination are associated with females. Historically and evolutionarily, men have had power and control because they were physically stronger and bigger and were needed to protect pregnant women, in order to carry on their genes. This view may have once held strong, but it no longer is relevant to our history and advances in biology and genetics. Women are not a weaker sex and should not be treated as one.

Bringing an End to Patriarchal Power

The health care system is a male-dominated institution of social control, and there must be an end to the patriarchal power in order to gain equality between the sexes (Hercus, 2005). Women should become educated regarding their rights and privileges to ensure they receive accurate and timely care. As women empower themselves through voicing their opinion to their health care providers, this inequality begins to break down. It is also important for women to share their feelings and to build a support system (Miller & Kuszelewicz, 1995). By doing so, the minority may begin to feel less invisible and more powerful.

Unity and Diversity

Women are frequently isolated from men in many aspects of Westernized culture, including the health care system. A goal of feminism is to reduce this inequality (White, Russo, & Travis, 2001). However, one's status is marked by more than just one's sex. Other factors include race, religion, ethnicity, and sexual orientation. To create true unity for women and incorporate these other factors regarding their health, feminist theory must include multiculturalism. Progress is starting to be made in this area. For example, the American Psychological Association created multicultural guidelines in 2002. Unfortunately, feminist theory is only now beginning to incorporate multiculturalism (Silverstein, 2006).

Women's Movement and Activism

Feminists are ideally attempting to break down the sex inequality in the health care system in hopes of gaining more opportunities for women. Women must become empowered and take action to gain this equality (White et al., 2001). However, it is important to remember that feminist activists should be represented by more than just middle-class, white women (Hutchison, 1986). Multiculturalism is an important aspect of feminism and must be incorporated to reach true equality between the sexes.

HUMAN RIGHTS AND WOMEN'S BODIES

Women's health is a political as well as biomedical phenomenon, shaped by social, political, and economic contexts. These contexts make women's health simultaneously an aspect of human rights. In this respect, security of person and quite literally the boundaries of one's body are essential rights. As Margaret Sanger so eloquently expressed it, "No woman can call herself free who does not own and control her own body" (see Rossi, 1973, p. 533). Slavery, torture, forced marriage, genital mutilation, rape as military or political policy, sexual trafficking, forced sterilization, or forced pregnancy are all anathema to human rights. A declaration on these points is provided by the United Nations' 1948 Universal Declaration of Human Rights (UDHR), which, among its 30 articles, prohibits slavery and regulates against human cruelty and torture (United Nations, 1948).

It took nearly 30 years for a focus to emerge specifically on the status and rights of women in the first World Conference on Women, held in 1975. Simultaneously the UN created the United Nations Development Fund for Women (UNIFEM) with the goal of fostering women's empowerment and gender equality. In 1979 the UN General Assembly adopted the Convention on the Elimination of All Forms of Discrimination against Women (CEDAW), sometimes referred to as the International Bill of Rights for Women. This document defines discrimination against women and national aims to end the discrimination. The basic thesis of CEDAW is that "the full and complete development of a country, the welfare of the world and the cause of peace require the maximum participation of women on equal terms with men in all fields" (United Nations, 1979).

In an ongoing monitoring of human rights and welfare, the United Nations publishes the annual Human Development Report (HDR). The HDR puts forth goals that are based on three main ideas: equality for all people, the continuation of equality from one generation to the next, and the empowerment of people so that they may be included in the development process. In 1995 this report had an expanded focus on the disparity of equality between men and women (United Nations, 1995b). The UN acknowledged that men and women are unequal in every society and that strong action needs to be taken to obtain and maintain equal gender opportunities worldwide.

The 1995 HDR introduced the Gender-related Development Index (GDI). The GDI is a measurement of gender disparity, based on items such as life expectancy, literacy, educational attainment, and income. The UN ranked 130 countries on this scale and found that the 4 top-ranked countries were Sweden, Finland, Norway, and Denmark. Each of these countries has adopted gender equality as a national policy, perhaps leading to less disparity. Nevertheless, the report stated that even though these four countries in the Nordic Belt are high on the GDI, no one society is free of gender disparity.

Also in 1995 the Beijing Declaration was promulgated at the UN Fourth World Conference on Women. This document, like the HDR, recognized gender inequalities everywhere and affirmed a commitment that would "ensure the full implementation of the human rights of women and of the girl child as an inalienable, integral, and indivisible part of all human rights and fundamental freedoms" (United Nations, 1995a).

The quality of women's physical and psychological health is very much shaped by these human rights of women. Despite various centers and institutes that affirm the inclusion of women's rights as fundamental to human rights, most human rights policies leave females vulnerable, especially when women's bodies are concerned. The egregious oppression and control of women by the Taliban government of Afghanistan is just one example.

Battery against women's bodies is one example of violation against human rights (Momoh, 2006). Unfortunately, in countries where customs, rituals, and tradition are highly valued, violence against women in this context is still permitted; female genital mutilation (FGM) is one example of this. It is estimated that between 100 million and 140 million women and girls worldwide have undergone FGM, and each year another 2 million females are at risk (World Health Organization, 2000). The prevalence remains high in approximately 28 African countries, as well as in some areas of Asia and the Middle East. In addition, increasing instances are found in Europe, Australia, Canada, and the United States.

There are several deleterious health consequences of FGM, including, but not limited to, severe pain, hemorrhaging, ulceration of the genital region, possible transmission of HIV, cysts, damage to the urethra, difficulties in childbirth, and even death (Momoh, 2006). This procedure is a violation of women's physical and psychological integrity, but it used to be viewed as a matter of cultural values. In such patriarchal cultures where women have relatively few resources and fewer alternatives, accepted cultural wisdom may even create meanings for such acts that seem to protect or exalt women. In a totalizing environment, some women may themselves endorse such practices. We suggest that it be viewed as oppression.

It may appear as though gender policies in distant lands are most in violation of human rights. However, many of the same issues remain problematic in the United States. For example, access to a means of safe and reliable birth control, to privacy in medical decision making, and to abortion without harassment remain areas of fatal violence in the United States. It is ironic that U.S. lawmakers might vehemently resist compulsory human papillomavirus vaccination of young girls to prevent cervical cancer as a governmental invasion of personal integrity but at the same time feel little compunction about effectively forcing a woman to maintain a pregnancy and give birth.

It is clear that internationally human rights are protected in the home, in the workplace, in the government, and elsewhere. But when it comes to the rights of women's bodies, these principles are regularly ignored, with profound impact on women's health.

Equity and Health Care

Health care spending in the United States is currently measured in the trillions of dollars and will account for 17 percent of the gross domestic product by 2011 (Heffler, Smith, Won, Clemens, Keehan, & Zezza, 2002). How the delivery of health care is organized is therefore a national priority. Policy within the U.S. Department of Health and Human Services has organized health care goals for the nation in terms of prevention, protection, and promotion. Prevention typically deals with efforts to minimize the impact of disease and to reduce the number of individuals having impaired health. It encompasses areas such as high blood pressure control, infant health, immunizations, and sexually transmitted diseases. Protection goals focus on topics such as injury prevention, the control of toxic agents, and occupational health and safety. Health promotion is a relatively recent concept and is directed toward increasing the number of individuals who adhere to healthy lifestyles. Goals of health promotion focus on areas such as smoking cessation, the reduced misuse of alcohol and drugs, improved nutrition, physical fitness, managing stress, and reduction of violence.

In addition to the areas of prevention, protection, and promotion (the "three P's"), one might conceptualize health and medical issues in terms of three E's: efficacy, efficiency, and equity. Efficacy and efficiency would seem to be obvious and extremely salient features of health decision making, and researchers have been addressing these questions for more than 20 years. Efficacy and efficiency prompt researchers to ask the questions, "Does it work safely?" and "Do the benefits outweigh the costs?"

In contrast to the long-standing recognition of the relevance of efficacy and efficiency, formal policy regarding equity has only recently begun to receive the attention it deserves. Equity addresses the questions of barriers to individual access to care and the availability of care as a function of the organization and distribution of resources; it also pertains to variation in the quality of care across recipients. For example, studies on heart disease have found that black patients with coronary artery disease were less likely to receive revascularization than were white patients (Leatherman & McCarthy, 2002).

Equity in access and quality of care has come increasingly to the forefront of attention, and in 1999 the U.S. Congress directed the Institute of Medicine (a component of the National Academy of Sciences) to conduct a study of health care disparities. The study was designed to evaluate potential sources of racial and ethnic disparities in health care, including the role of bias, discrimination, and stereotyping at the individual (provider and patient), institutional, and health-system levels. As part of this initiative, in November 2000 President Bill Clinton signed into law an act that created a National Center on Minority Health and Health Disparities at the National Institutes of Health (NIH). However, this center gives primary focus to ethnicity as the critical distinction relevant to health care delivery and outcomes; gender is not particularly salient in the rhetoric associated with this work.

Access to Insurance and Care

Access to care and the potential effect of limited access on the national costs of health care have become major focal points for current policy and planning. Despite general economic growth over two decades, a housing boom, international trade agreements, and a stock market that has broken successive records, health care coverage was worse in 2006 than it was 20 years earlier. Results from the 2006 National Health Information Survey (Cohen & Martinez, 2006) indicate that 67 percent of the population were covered by private health insurance.

There is an assumption that some government program or another safety net will provide for individuals without private insurance. Among individuals without private health insurance, Medicaid covers roughly 11 percent, and about 2 percent are covered by Medicare or military provisions (National Center for Health Statistics, 1996).[2]

Current estimates by the U.S. Bureau of the Census are that approximately 15.9 percent of the U.S. population, or roughly 47 million people, lack health insurance of any sort, and another sizable percentage is under-insured (DeNavas-Walt, Proctor, & Lee, 2006). However, in 1987 only 12.9 percent of the population was uninsured (U.S. Census Bureau, 2006b). Thus, a strong argument can be made that improvements in state-of-the-art interventions and pharmaceutical breakthroughs are less available today than 20 years ago.

This increase in the percentage of uninsured cannot be dismissed as deadbeat drifters or welfare artists, because many full-time workers lack insurance. Health care for indigent and homeless individuals is only a small part of the trouble, and it cannot be solved simply by putting people to work, because most individuals below the poverty level already have one or more jobs (Travis & Compton, 2001). Those who work full time may not escape the conundrum of how to get health care insurance. Among people ages 18–64 (and therefore not eligible for Medicare coverage) who worked full time in 2005, 17.7 percent were uninsured (U.S. Census Bureau, 2006a).

Among those without any health coverage, more than 70 percent are people of color, even though people of color represent only about 15 percent of the general population. Asian, Black, and Hispanic individuals are much more likely to be without insurance of any kind (U.S. Census Bureau, 2006a). Women in these groups are disproportionately disadvantaged. Hispanic women, especially poor Hispanic women, consistently have the worst access to health care. These women have no regular health care providers, even for routine preventive care. They are less likely to know their blood pressure or cholesterol levels and may be more likely to have high blood pressure that is not effectively controlled by medication.

Approximately 36 percent of poor women are uninsured (National Center for Health Statistics, 1996), and this figure is even higher among Hispanic women in poverty, with approximately 45 percent having no health insurance (Pamuk, Makuc, Heck, Reuben, & Lochner, 1998).

Problems of insurance coverage and access to care are magnified for older women not yet eligible for Medicare. Women are likely to have problems in maintaining health insurance because gender roles and sexism influence individual work histories. Women are more likely to work part time, to have interrupted work histories, and to work in settings without benefit plans. Since only about 10–15 percent of women collect pensions or annuities from private plans, their ability to maintain health insurance or to remediate problems is limited (Kirschstein & Merritt, 1985).

Medicare coverage for those over age 65 does not solve these problems. Out-of-pocket expenses (those expenses not covered by the main insurance program) are often higher for events experienced by older women in comparison to events common among older men.

UNDERSTANDING BREAST CANCER

Cancer is the second leading cause of death in the United States, and approximately half a million deaths are attributed to cancer each year (Minino, Heron, & Smith, 2006). However, many more people live with cancer or have had a diagnosis of cancer at some time in their lives, about 15 million in any given year, or roughly 7 percent of the entire U.S. population (Lethbridgeejku, Rose, & Vickerie, 2004). Over the course of a lifetime, a little more than a third of all women will have a diagnosis of some form of cancer (Ries et al., 2006). There is a great dread of breast cancer, partly because any diagnosis of cancer is seen as a death sentence, but in fact a high percentage of women live quite full lives despite having a diagnosis. About 88 percent of women will survive five or more years, and if the cancer is in situ at the time of diagnosis, 100 percent of the women will survive five or more years (Ries et al., 2006). Treatments for breast cancer are continually developing and will not be described here. Instead we concentrate on understanding cancer biology and some of the risks.

Cancer Biology

Although one might commonly think of cancer as a single entity, such as a tumor, it is better understood as a process involving the actions of many different types of cells and messenger substances, that is, a constellation of genes, cells, and the communication pathways between them. The development of cancer (carcinogenesis) typically requires genetic changes that affect cell function. These errors may occur at several points in the genes and communication pathways. Errors early in the process might have the effect of "initiating" a cell, but these errors must accumulate before a cell becomes transformed to frankly cancerous. Changes throughout the cancer process might involve the increased frequency of cell division (proliferation), an impaired ability to repair errors, or the failure of immature (stem) cells to develop into functioning mature cells that can perform functions in an organ. Later errors in the cancer process might involve a reduced likelihood that a flawed cell will have the ability to shrink, fragment, or otherwise deactivate itself (apoptosis).

The cancer process ultimately will involve genetic mutations (mutagenesis); this is true even for individuals with no family history or genetic precursors for cancer. Genes are part of the DNA residing in the nucleus of a cell; they influence not only appearance (e.g., eye color) but also such functions as cell growth. Some gene mutations are heritable and passed from parent to child, that is, germ-line mutations. These germ-line mutations appear in special cells involved in reproduction (i.e., egg or sperm germ-line cells) and occur during a special type of cell division called meiosis. These germ-line mutations appear in every cell of the bodies of offspring. Many other mutations occur in general cells of the body and take place during general cell division, or mitosis. These general errors occur hither and thither in individual cells. Every time any cell divides, there is a window of opportunity for genetic alterations.

Mutations can take several forms (e.g., deletions, breakages, insertions of extra components or adducts, amplifications of existing genes, or the translocation crossovers of genetic material between chromosomes). Some genes act to suppress cell growth, while others contribute to DNA repair; changes in the function of these genes can easily contribute to cancer. Changes or errors may impair cell function or communication pathways external to the cell (e.g., hormones). Errors in a communication pathway include a cell not being able to receive needed messages, messages not being sent at all, or the wrong messages being sent. The communication pathway may be impaired because something needed to activate a gene (phosphorylate) has been blocked and can no longer attach or communicate with the cell.

One hypothesis suggests that individuals with an inherited (germ-line) mutation that is present in every cell of the body may have initiated cancer cells after only one additional mutation to any cell (Knudson, 1971). This partially explains why individuals with inherited mutations are more likely to develop cancer at a younger age: They are born with one strike against them and thus start life further along a cancer pathway. Cancers without inherited germ-line mutations are likely to be based on a number of alterations in several different genes. It is unlikely that a single error, or even two or three errors, will produce cancer.

To a certain degree, the body has the capacity to repair or otherwise cope with errors. Some errors may be repaired through the immune system (e.g., macrophages), by removal of the sources of harmful messages (e.g., losing fat), or by deactivation of the affected cells themselves (apoptosis). However, virtually all cells divide and multiply on a regular basis, and as they do so, they replicate any errors so that new cells are also flawed. In fact, with each cell division, there is an increasing chance for initial errors to have cascading effects so that additional alterations may occur. This replication of existing errors is the second major component of the cancer process and is commonly termed cell proliferation or cancer promotion. Thus, anything that tends to increase or accelerate cell division beyond normal rates is typically correlated positively with cancer and often is termed a cancer promoter.

Since changes in communication pathways, in genes, and in cell activity are multifaceted and occur over time in a cascading manner, the single largest risk factor for cancer is time, that is, age. According to the Surveillance, Epidemiology, and End Results (SEER) review of cancer statistics, the majority of cancers occur in people over 50 years of age (Ries et al., 2006). Age is a major risk factor for cancer primarily because it reflects the opportunity for thousands of cell divisions and the accumulation of various glitches or errors in genes and communication pathways. In general, the types of cells that divide most frequently as part of normal bodily functions are also the cells most vulnerable to cancer. For example, cells that line the colon (a type of epithelial cell) need to be replaced frequently, and cells in the colon divide and multiply accordingly.

BREAST CANCER RISKS

Genetic

As with almost all fatal diseases in the United States, age is the greatest risk factor for breast cancer. In addition to age, a family history that includes an inherited genetic germ-line mutation adds significantly to the risk. Typically a "family history" of cancer is given more weight if it involves first-degree relatives, for example, mother or sisters. More than 70 genes have been associated with the prognosis (outcome) of breast cancer. Research to assess the information value of this complex gene profile has been conducted in the Netherlands (Buyse et al., 2006) and is reported to offer a better prediction about survival without recurrence than is possible with basic clinical factors. Prognosis based solely on gross clinical factors looks at patient age, tumor size, lymph system involvement, and estrogen receptor status (Ravdin et al., 2001). The Adjuvant! computerized software tool is based on these and other clinical factors for estimating prognosis and is available online (www.adjuvantonline.com). However, most genetic research on cancer has involved research on the risk of getting cancer in the first place.

Genes associated with breast cancer susceptibility include BRCA1 (located on chromosome 17) and BRCA2 (chromosome 13).The general function of these genes is still being researched, but it is thought to influence DNA repair, gene stability, and overall orderly development and transition of breast stem cells to functioning cells in the breast (Foulkes, 2004; Reynolds, 2001; Starita & Parvin, 2003). The normal function of BRCA1 may be as a tumor suppressor gene that detects and promotes repair of damaged DNA (Tan, Zheng, Lee, & Boyer, 2004). Thus, having a healthy BRCA1 gene is a good thing.

Problems arise when mutations to this gene interfere with its normal function. Mutations to these genes may be inherited but more rarely may occur by any of the random errors that occur during any cell division. Only 5–10 percent of breast cancer cases are found to have an inherited (germ-line) mutation in BRCA1 or BRCA2, and if one has an inherited mutation to this gene, then the risk of breast cancer is more than double the risk for an average person (Antoniou et al., 2003; Malone, Daling, Thompson, O'Brien, Francisco, & Ostrander, 1998; Newman, Mu, Butler, Millikan, Moorman, & King, 1998). Women who have inherited mutations in these genes are likely to have a number of close relatives who have breast or ovarian cancer. A review of studies assessing the risk of breast cancer among women with a BRCA1 mutation suggests roughly a 65 percent risk of a breast cancer diagnosis by age 70. The risk is elevated, but not quite as high, if there is a BRCA2 mutation (Antoniou et al., 2003). In contrast, the lifetime risk of breast cancer for all women is approximately 1 in 8 women, or about 13 percent.

Age is the key to understanding the implications of "family history" as an indication of an inherited genetic mutation (Newman et al., 1998). Typically, when there is an inherited genetic mutation, it is more likely that cancer will have developed prior to menopause among relatives (Malone et al., 1998). Thus, family history alone is not good evidence of an inherited genetic risk of cancer. For example, if Aunt Em develops breast cancer at age 75, that has little implication for the risk of other relatives. On the other hand, if she develops breast cancer at age 35, there is more reason for concern.

Estrogen

The natural history of breast cancer is firmly linked with exposure to estrogen; this may be in the form of endogenous estrogens produced in the body, exogenous estrogens in pharmaceutical treatments, or estrogen-like substances associated with environmental toxins. The initial links between the lifetime dose of estrogen and risk of breast cancer can be seen most simply in the fact that women with early menarche (prior to age 11; Trichopoulos, MacMahon, & Cole, 1972) or those with late menopause (after age 55; Trichopoulos, MacMahon, & Cole, 1972) have a greater exposure to estrogen over the course of their lifetimes and also have a higher incidence of breast cancer. Additionally, large-scale prospective longitudinal studies conducted through the Nurses' Health Study[3] have found that women with higher levels of estrogen in the blood are over time more likely to develop breast cancer; this is true for both postmenopausal (Missmer, Eliassen, Barbieri, & Hankinson, 2004) and premenopausal women (Eliassen, Colditz, Rosner, Willett, & Hankinson, 2006). Women with the highest quartile of circulating sex steroids had two to three times the risk of breast cancer in comparison to women in the lowest quartile. Cancers among those women with higher levels of circulating estrogen also were more likely to be invasive rather than in situ.

Exogenous estrogens supplied through hormone replacement therapy among menopausal women correspond to similar increased risks for breast cancer. This general association was documented a generation ago by Jick and colleagues (1980) in an epidemiological study. More recent research has continued to document exogenous estrogens with an increased risk of breast cancer. A national study known as the Women's Health Initiative and developed by the National Institutes of Health followed 16,000 women over the age of 50 for five years. Those who received replacement hormones had approximately a 25 percent greater likeli-hood of developing breast cancer in comparison to randomly assigned women who received only placebos (Chlebowski et al., 2003). Other recent studies have supported the increased risk (Barlow et al., 2006; Million Women Study Collaborators, 2003; Writing Group for the Women's Health Initiative Investigators, 2002).

The biological mechanisms by which extra estrogen might induce cancer are closely related to the general biology of carcinogenesis discussed earlier. The natural role of estrogen in the body is to promote cell division and growth. This necessary component of human reproduction is part of the monthly menstrual cycle and affects breast as well as uterine tissue. Unfortunately, tissues that go through frequent cell division and growth have a greater baseline risk of incurring a series of errors in cell genes and gene-to-gene communication pathways.

The risk of uterine cancer due to replacement estrogens can be reduced to some extent by the inclusion of progestins that induce a menstrual cycle. The progestins induce menstruation, when flawed cells of the endometrium lining are sloughed off, but there is no similar sloughing process of flawed cells in breast tissue. Since replacement estrogen increases cell division and proliferation, it technically falls in the category of a cancer promoter. Estrogen does not necessarily cause errors or mutations, but it does result in an increased number of any cells that happen to have mutations.

Despite the historical and contemporary research documenting the role of estrogen in carcinogenesis, there are benefits and uses of estrogen supplements. The ostensible benefits of estrogen supplements for other health conditions, such as Alzheimer's disease, migraines, and osteoporosis, are based on mixed and conflicting studies and are seldom based on clinical trials with random assignment of participants to treatment or control groups. The touting of estrogen benefits for these other health conditions often ignores other more effective treatments that do not include estrogen. Yet, newspaper stories continue to appear with suggestions as to the potential benefits of estrogen, and general medical practitioners continue to discuss with women "safe" approaches to estrogen replacement. Typical recommendations are to use the smallest effective dose for the particular woman in order to transition through menopause and to take supplements for a "short" period of time as a way to control hot flashes and other menopausal symptoms. What women may not understand is that estrogen supplements may delay menopausal symptoms, but going off estrogen supplements is likely to provoke a return to the very symptoms they hoped to avoid. Hot flashes, sweats, flushes, and sleep disturbance are not pleasant and, if very frequent, can be disruptive. On the other hand, it would be so much more disruptive to be scheduling one's next chemotherapy or radiation treatment.

NOTES

1. Portions of this chapter were published in Denmark & Paludi (Eds.). (2008). *Psychology of women: A handbook of issues and theories.* New York: Praeger.

2. Medicaid is available to individuals in poverty who are younger than age 65, while Medicare is available nationally to all individuals over age 65.

3. The Nurses' Health Study II, established in 1989, recruited 116,609 female registered nurses, ages 25–42. This group has been followed biennially by the members answering a questionnaire and in some cases giving blood samples.

REFERENCES

Antoniou, A., Pharoah, P. D. P., Narod, S., Risch, H. A., Eyfjord, J. E., Hopper, J. L., et al. (2003). Average risks of breast and ovarian cancer associated with BRCAl or BRCA2 mutations detected in case series unselected for family history: A combined analysis of 22 studies. *American Journal of Human Genetics, 72,* 1117–1130.

Barlow, W. E., White, E., Ballard-Barbash, R., Vacek, P. M., Titus-Ernstoff, L., Carney, P. A., et al. (2006). Prospective breast cancer risk prediction model for women undergoing screening mammography. *Journal of the National Cancer Institute, 98,* 1204–1214.

Boston Women's Health Book Collective. (2005). *Our bodies, ourselves.* New York: Simon & Schuster.

Buyse, M., Loi, S., Veer, L. V., Viale, G., Delorenzi, M., Glas, A. M., et al. (2006). Validation and clinical utility of a 70-gene prognostic signature for women with node-negative breast cancer. *Journal of the National Cancer Institute, 98,* 1183–1192.

Centers for Disease Control and Prevention. (2004). *The burden of chronic diseases and their risk factors: National and state perspectives, 2004.* Atlanta: U.S. Department of Health and Human Services. Retrieved from http://www .cdc.gov Inccdphp/burdenbook2004.

Chlebowski, R. T., Hendrix, S. L., Langer, R. D., Stefanick, M. L., Gass, M., Lane, D., et al. (2003). Influence of estrogen plus progestin on breast cancer and mammography in healthy postmenopausal women: The Women's Health Initiative randomized. *Journal of the American Medical Association, 289,* 3243–3253.

Cohen, R. A., & Martinez, M. E. (2006). *Health insurance coverage: Early release of estimates from the National Health Interview Survey, January–June 2006.* Retrieved from http://www.cdc.gov /nchs/nhis.htm.

Corea, G. (1977). *The hidden malpractice.* New York: Jove.

Daly, M. (1978). *Gyn/ecology.* Boston: Beacon Press.

DeNavas-Walt, C., Proctor, B. D., & Lee, C. H. (2006). *Income, poverty, and health insurance coverage in the United States: 2005.* Current Population Reports, P60-231. Washington, DC: U.S. Census Bureau.

Dreifus, C. (Ed.). (1977). *Seizing our bodies.* New York: Random House.

Eliassen, A. H., Colditz, G. A., Rosner, B., Willett, W. C., & Hankinson, S. E. (2006). Adult weight change and risk of postmenopausal breast cancer. *Journal of the American Medical Association, 296,* 193–201.

Foulkes, W. D. (2004). BRCAl functions as a breast stem cell regulator. *Journal of Medical Genetics, 41,* 1–5.

Heffler, S., Smith, S., Won, G., Clemens, M. K., Keehan, S., & Zezza, M. (2002). Health spending projections for 2001–2011: The latest outlook. *Health Affairs, 21,* 207–218.

Hercus, C. (2005). *Stepping out of line: Becoming and being feminist.* New York: Routledge.

Hutchison, L. (1986). A radical feminist perspective. In M. Bricker-Jenkins & N. R. Hooyman (Eds.), *Not for women only: Social work practice for a feminist future* (pp. 53–57). Silver Spring, MD: National Association of Social Workers.

Hyde, J. (2006). *Half the human experience.* New York: Houghton Mifflin.

Jick, H., Walker, A. M., Watkins, R. N., D'Ewart, D. C., Hunter, J. R., Danford, A., et al. (1980). Replacement estrogens and breast cancer. *American Journal of Epidemiology, 112,* 586–594.

Johnson, A. G. (1997). *The gender knot: Unraveling our patriarchal legacy.* Philadelphia: Temple University Press.

Kirschstein, R. L., & Merritt, D. H. (1985). *Women's health: Report of the Public Health Service Task Force on Women's Health Issues.* Washington, DC: Public Health Service.

Knudson, A. G. (1971). Mutation and cancer: Statistical study of retinoblastoma. *Proceedings of the National Academy of Sciences, 68,* 820–823.

Leatherman, S., & McCarthy, D. (2002). *Quality of care in the United States: A chartbook.* No. 520. New York: Commonwealth Fund.

Lethbridgeejku, M., Rose, D., & Vickerie, J. (2004). Summary health statistics for U.S. adults: National Health Interview Survey, 2004. *Vital Health Statistics, 10*(228).

Malone, K. E., Daling, J. R., Thompson, J. D., O'Brien, C. A., Francisco, L. V., & Ostrander, E. A. (1998). BRCAl mutations and breast cancer in the general population: Analyses in women before age 35 years and in women before age 45 years with first-degree family history. *Journal of the American Medical Association, 279,* 922–929.

Marieskind, H. (1980). *Women in the health system.* St. Louis: C. V. Mosby.

Michalopoulou, G., Alevizaki, M., Piperingos, G., Mitsibounas, D., Mantzos, E., Adamopoulos, P., et al. (1998). High serum cholesterol levels in persons with "high-normal" TSH levels: Should one extend the definition of subclinical hypothyroidism? *European Journal of Endocrinology, 138,* 141–145.

Miller, J., & Kuszelewicz, M. A. (1995). Women and AIDS: Feminist principles in practice. In N. Van Den Bergh (Ed.), *Feminist practice in the 21st century* (pp. 295–311). Washington, DC: NASW Press.

Million Women Study Collaborators. (2003). Breast cancer and hormonereplacement therapy in the Million Women Study. *Lancet, 362,* 419–427.

Minino, A. M., Heron, M. P., & Smith, B. L. (2006). *Deaths: Preliminary data for 2004. National Vital Statistics Report, 154*(19).

Missmer, S. A., Eliassen, A. H., Barbieri, R. L., & Hankinson, S. E. (2004). Endogenous estrogen, androgen, and progesterone concentrations and breast cancer risk among postmenopausal women. *Journal of the National Cancer Institute, 96,* 1856–1865.

Momoh, C. (2006). *Female genital mutilation.* Oxford, England: Radcliffe.

National Center for Health Statistics. (1996). *Health, United States, 1995.* Hyattsville, MD: National Center for Health Statistics.

Newman, B., Mu, H., Butler, L. M., Millikan, R. C., Moorman, P. G., & King, M. C. (1998). Frequency of breast cancer attributable to BRCAl in a population-based series of American women. *Journal of the American Medical Association, 279,* 915–921.

Pamuk, E., Makuc, D., Heck, K., Reuben, C., & Lochner, K. (1998). Socioeconomic status and health chartbook. In *National Center for Health Statistics, Health, United States, 1998.* Hyattsville, MD: National Center for Health Statistics.

Ravdin, P. M., Siminoff, L. A., Davis, G. J., Mercer, M. B., Hewlett, J., Gerson, N., et al. (2001). Computer program to assist in making decisions about adjuvant therapy for women with early breast cancer. *Journal of Clinical Oncology, 19,* 980–991.

Reynolds, T. (2001). BRCAl: Lessons learned from the breast cancer gene. *Journal of the National Cancer Institute, 93,* 1200–1202.

Ries, L. A. G., Harkins, D., Krapcho, M., Mariotto, A., Miller, B. A., Feuer, E. J., et al. (Eds.). (2006). *SEER cancer statistics review, 1975–2003.* Bethesda, MD: National Cancer Institute. Retrieved from http://seer.cancer.gov/csr/1975_2003/.

Rossi, Alice S. (Ed.). (1973). *The feminist papers: From Adams to de Beauvoir.* New York: Columbia University Press.

Ruzek, S. (1978). *The women's health movement.* New York: Praeger.

Sandelowski, M. (1981). *Women, health, and choice.* Englewood Cliffs, NJ: Prentice-Hall.

Scully, D. (1980). *Men who control women's health.* Boston: Houghton Mifflin.

Silverstein, L. B. (2006). Integrating feminism and multiculturalism: Scientific fact or science fiction? *Professional Psychology: Research and Practice, 37,* 21–28.

Starita, L. M, & Parvin, J. D. (2003). The multiple nuclear functions of BRCA1: Transcription, ubiquitination and DNA repair. *Current Opinion in Cell Biology, 15,* 345–350.

Tan, W., Zheng, L., Lee, W. H., & Boyer, T. G. (2004). Functional dissection of transcription factor ZBRKl reveals zinc fingers with dual roles in DNA-binding and BRCAl-dependent transcriptional repression. *Journal of Biological Chemistry, 279,* 6576–6587.

Travis, C. B., & Compton, J. D. (2001). Feminism and health in the decade of behavior. *Psychology of Women Quarterly, 25,* 312–323.

Trichopoulos, D., MacMahon, B., & Cole, P. (1972). Menopause and breast cancer risk. *Journal of the National Cancer Institute, 48,* 605.

United Nations. (1948). *Universal declaration of human rights.* General Assembly Resolution 217 A (III), December 10, 1948. Retrieved from http://www.un .org/Overview/rights.html.

United Nations. (1979). *Convention on the elimination of all forms of discrimination against women.* Retrieved from http://www.un.org/womenwatch/daw/ cedaw/cedaw.htm.

United Nations. (1995a). *Fourth World Conference on Women: Beijing Declaration.* Retrieved from http://www.un.org/womenwatch/daw/beijing/platform/ declar.htm.

United Nations. (1995b). *Human development report, 1995.* New York: Oxford University Press.

U.S. Census Bureau. (2006a). Table HIOl. Health insurance coverage status and type of coverage by selected characteristics: 2005 all races. Annual demographic survey, March supplement.

U.S. Census Bureau. (2006b). Table HI-1. Health insurance coverage status and type of coverage by sex, race and Hispanic origin: 1987 to 2005. Historical health insurance tables. Retrieved from http://www.census.gov/hhes/www/ hlthins/historic/hihisttl.html.

White, J. W., Russo, N. F., & Travis, C. B. (2001). Feminism and the decade of behavior. *Psychology of Women Quarterly, 25,* 267–279.

World Health Organization. (2000). *Factsheet 241.* Geneva: World Health Organization.

Writing Group for the Women's Health Initiative Investigators. (2002). Risks and benefits of estrogen and progestin in healthy postmenopausal women: Principal results from the women's health initiative randomized trial. *Journal of the American Medical Association, 22,* 2819–2820.

Chapter 5

Cultural Consideration for Mental Health Treatment with Women of Color

Silvia L. Mazzula and Rebecca Rangel[1]

INTRODUCTION

Racial and ethnic differences in the prevalence of mental and physical illnesses have been widely noted. Racial/ethnic minority populations[2] (African Americans, Asian Americans and Pacific Islanders, and Native Americans) tend to have higher prevalence of psychiatric disorders and physical illnesses, such as cancer, compared to non-Hispanic Whites[3] (Breslau, Kendler, Sue, Gaxiolaaguilar, & Kessler, 2004). For example, the National Survey of American Life shows that African Americans and Caribbean Blacks are more likely to have a chronic major depressive episode (Williams et al., 2007). African Americans are also more likely than non-Hispanic Whites to be victims of violent crimes and to experience trauma as a result of these aggressions (U.S. Department of Health and Human Services [DHHS], 2001). Similarly, Asian Americans have higher prevalence of depression compared to non-Hispanic Whites (Davey & Watson, 2008), and Asian American women have higher rates of suicide compared to both Whites and African Americans (Suicide

Prevention Resource Center, 2010). However, despite service need, racial/ethnic minorities with mental and physical illnesses have less access to care and are less likely to obtain professional treatment[4] (DHHS, 2001; Shim, Compton, Rust, Druss, & Kaslow, 2009). For example, Asian Americans underutilize mental health services more than any racial group, Whites or other people of color (David, 2010; Uba, 1994). Both African Americans and Hispanics receive about half the outpatient mental health services that Whites do (Lasser, Himmelstein, Woolhandler, McCormick, & Bor, 2002).

Moreover, intragroup ethnic factors (e.g., ethnicity, immigration status, language) also show differences in access to services. For example, data from the Collaborative Psychiatric Epidemiology Surveys Initiative of the National Institute of Mental Health (NIMH) show that while Puerto Ricans receive approximately the same amount of services as non-Hispanic Whites (54 percent and 50 percent, respectively), Mexican Americans (34%) are the least likely to receive services or service consistent with established guidelines for adequate treatment (González et al., 2010). Similarly, while fewer than 1 in 11 Hispanics with mental illness receive conventional services, the ratio decreases significantly among Hispanic immigrants to less than 1 in 20 (DHHS, 2001).

It is also acknowledged that when racial/ethnic minorities do receive treatment, they tend to receive poorer quality of services (DHHS, 2001). Treatment services devoid of contextual and cultural factors have also explained poorer engagement in treatment (Chow, Jaffee, & Snowden, 2003), higher rates of premature termination, and higher number of failed appointments by some racial/ethnic minorities in treatment (Atdjian & Vega, 2005). Therefore, this chapter focuses on ethnocultural considerations to improve quality of services and delivery of culturally competent and relevant treatment for racial/ethnic minorities, specifically women.

CULTURAL COMPETENCE

Developing culturally sensitive services has become a national priority (DHHS, 2001). Demonstrating such competence has also become a central aspect in both health organizations and psychology training programs, which are now held accountable by ethical standards, guidelines, and professional governing boards (American Psychiatric Association, 1994; DHHS, 2001). Cultural competence can appear both overwhelming and challenging to master (Ecklund & Johnson, 2007). At times, the mere thought of demonstrating cultural competence can engender diverse and conflicting feelings in practitioners,[5] supervisors, educators, and trainees. However, most conflict may arise from viewing cultural competence as a set of prescribed skills or interventions that practitioners can incorporate into their theoretical framework. Therefore, this chapter supports the notion that providing culturally competent services is neither a particular set of skills nor something to be feared. Culturally competent practices can be integrated within any theoretical framework so long as the practitioner is open and willing to conceptualize clinical presentations more broadly—that is, to expand his or her worldview beyond conventional (i.e., Western) teachings of therapy, human behavior, and normal vs. deviant presentations.

CULTURAL COMPETENCE FRAMEWORK

While numerous and diverse cultural competency domains have been identified, cultural competence can be summarized as practitioners' ability to (1) understand their own biases, assumptions, and worldviews; (2) integrate social and cultural factors in treatment; and (3) deliver appropriate and relevant interventions (Ecklund & Johnson, 2007). These domains call attention to knowledge of the client and practitioner's worldview as well as the thoughts, feelings, and behaviors associated with being members of their respective racial/cultural groups. Therefore, this chapter is grounded in systems theory, which provides a useful way to understand "the context in which a behavior occurs and the sociopolitical factors that may influence an individual's behavior" (McRae & Short, 2010, pp. 2).

From a systems perspective we believe that (a) clients are part of multiple systems (e.g., cultural group, ethnic group, family, racial group) and are therefore multidimensional beings; (b) as members of these various systems, clients endorse values, ideas, assumptions, and beliefs about themselves, their physical or mental illness, and their well-being on both a conscious and unconscious level; and (c) a client's worldview plays an integral part in seeking professional services, remaining in treatment, and completing recovery. Therefore, ethnocultural considerations for treatment are provided in the context of the following assumptions. First, that illness and symptom manifestations are not determined solely by intrapsychic or individual characteristics but are also shaped and informed by their context. Second, that therapy with women of color, who are members of marginalized communities based on race, gender, or cultural heritage, can be most effective when racial and cultural factors are acknowledged and understood by practitioners and integrated in treatment. Lastly, that practitioners themselves are part of multiple systems and therefore their clinical formulations and interventions are grounded in the context of their own worldviews.

Due to the dearth of literature on treatment for women of color, this chapter highlights what we believe to be salient ethnocultural considerations based on the extant literature on racial/ethnic minority issues in general and on women of color in particular. Throughout the chapter, the term "women of color" is used broadly to include women from racial/ethnic minority groups and subgroups (Hispanic [of any racial group], Asian

American and Pacific Islander, and African American). Considering the distinct history of each racial/ethnic group and the unique cultural considerations within those groups is beyond the scope of this chapter. Therefore, readers are cautioned from overgeneralizing the discussion to all racial/ethnic minorities or to all women of color. This chapter is meant to be used as a starting point to explore what *may* be important and critical ethnocultural issues in treatment. The chapter is divided into two sections: structural barriers (including issues of discrimination and racism) and cultural values (including preference for interpersonal relationships, gender roles, religiosity, and cultural expressions of symptomontology). The importance of the practitioner's understanding of her/his own worldview, assumptions, and biases are woven throughout the aforementioned sections.

STRUCTURAL BARRIERS TO ACCESS AND ENGAGEMENT

Structural barriers such as unequal access to quality care, language barriers, and discrimination, and socioeconomic factors such as poverty or lack of insurance (DHHS, 2001) have been the main focus in explaining racial/ ethnic disparities in access and utilization of mental and physical health services. Therefore, treatment with women of color requires special consideration of these barriers.

Language

Language has been a central factor in explaining several treatment barriers. For example, although almost half of Hispanics and Asian Americans are foreign born and non-English speakers (DHHS, 2001), the shortage of practitioners who can communicate in these groups' native languages impacts both access and utilization of services. Language difficulties can be a significant barrier to discussing presenting problems, building rapport, and establishing a therapeutic alliance. In addition, it can be very difficult, and can often rise to the level of stress reactions, for recent immigrants to navigate a new culture, a difficulty that can be exacerbated when the individual does not know the primary language or the language of the service provider.

Ramos-Sánchez, Atkinson, and Fraga (1999) found that clinicians' "preoccupation of English subordinate clients on producing grammatically correct speech may interfere with the clients' emotional expression" (p. 126). For non-English-speaking clients, it can be challenging to both explore their emotional state and search for words in a second language to explain their experience. This can be very taxing for any client, which may cause further distress as a result of misinterpretation by practitioners, particularly during initial evaluation sessions, when clients "may be seen as uncooperative, sullen, negative, nonverbal, or repressed on the basis of language expression alone" (Sue & Sue, 2008, p. 153). Thus, practitioners may perceive what is expressed in body language as stress from the psychological, and sometimes physical exertion, of speaking in a second language as symptoms of anxiety or other forms of pathology. Sue and Sue (2008) caution practitioners that the problem may be linguistic and not psychological when working with minorities by saying that "Euro-American society places such high premium of one's use of English, it is a short step to conclude that minorities are inferior, lack awareness, or lack conceptual thinking powers" (p. 153). Therefore, non-English speakers or those with limited English proficiency may worry about being understood verbally and/or experience fear of being misdiagnosed as a result of language barriers.

Studies have shown that a practitioner's ability to converse in the client's preferred language may demonstrate greater cultural sensitivity and thus she/he may be perceived as more credible by minority clients (Ramos-Sánchez et al., 1999). However, for bilingual practitioners trained in the English language, providing linguistically relevant treatment can be challenging. For example, Biever, Castaño, de las Fuentes, González, Servín-López, and Sprowls (2002) note that "psychologists with conversational proficiency in Spanish have very few resources or guidance in making the transition from social to professional levels of Spanish proficiency" (p. 330). The need for linguistically relevant training when working with Asian American women can become even more challenging, considering that Asian Americans speak more than 100 different languages and dialects (Kramer, Kwong, Lee, & Chung, 2002). Currently, training for bilingual practitioners is significantly limited. For example, while Hispanics are the largest ethnic minority group in the United States, a review of the literature shows the existence of only one program, which was launched in the spring of 1997 at Our Lady of the Lake University in Texas, where psychology courses are conducted in Spanish (Biever et al., 2002). The lack of training programs for bilingual therapists can be somewhat alarming. The lack of training can also create undue stress in many bilingual practitioners, who would benefit from specialized training in psychological terminology and conceptualization in the language spoken in treatment, bilingual supervision that emphasizes the cultural context, and training in adequate translation of documentations to present to their monolingual clients.

In instances when a bilingual practitioner is not available, English-speaking practitioners are left with the ethical dilemma of how best to treat a non-English speaker, and interpreters are often used when a referral is unavailable (Hays, 2001). However, the role of the interpreter is to act as an oral translator of the conversation between the client and the practitioner, adding no additional side remarks or questions during a therapy session. Sue and Sue (2008) question whether interpreters really give accurate translations. For the monolingual English-speaking practitioner, there is no way to know whether the translations are accurate, which highlights the importance of having certified interpreters available. Moreover, there are very few training programs that properly train interpreters in the delicate intricacies of therapy (Bradford & Muñoz, 1993). Therefore, even when interpreters are certified to accurately translate the client's verbal communication, the practitioner is bound to miss the idiosyncrasies and meaning behind the spoken words. Overreliance on verbal expression of feelings and experiences may also be inappropriate for some women of color, such as Asian American women, who value emotional regulation and constriction of affect as a sign of strength (Marcella, 2010).

On some occasions, practitioners may be tempted to utilize family members. While using family members as interpreters appears to be a good solution where interpreters are not available, practitioners must exercise great caution, especially in the context of the confidential therapeutic relationship. Furthermore, children of non-English-speaking parents (or other adults in their extended family network) are often used as interpreters or "language brokers," which has significant consequences on both the non-English-speaking adult and the child. For example, the use of children may "undermine the authority" of the parental figure, disrupting the hierarchical structure in the family (Sue & Sue, 2008). This becomes a salient issue for some racial/ethnic minority groups whose cultural values and heritage emphasize strict family roles and structures. In addition, some clients may feel embarrassed or shame and consider it inappropriate to discuss certain matters in front of children or spouses, especially to practitioners who may be considered as outsiders due to their race or ethnic background. Similarly, in instances when a perpetrator, unbeknownst to the practitioner, serves as an interpreter, the client can undergo undue emotional and psychological stress and retraumatization. These issues have broadly been addressed by ethical codes and guidelines, while others remain to be thoroughly examined. Thus, practitioners should avoid using family members as interpreters whenever possible; referring clients to practitioners competent in the clients' language appears the most effective solution.

Racism and Discrimination

Racism and discrimination are additional structural barriers to service utilization and perceived comfort with treatment providers. The United States has been marked by notions of inferior and superior peoples based on the social construction of race. Therefore, power differentials between minority and majority groups are embedded in all institutions, and mental health systems are no exception. Psychological theories have also been largely grounded on Western- and male-dominated notions of healing, which at times are in stark contrast to non-Western healing practices used by many individuals in the United States. Practitioners also continue to be majority non-Hispanic Whites for various reasons, such as glass ceilings, racism, discrimination, and socioeconomic barriers. Therefore, it is important for practitioners to acknowledge that they represent a system that may be perceived as oppressive and that lacks understanding of racial/ethnic minority issues. Furthermore, both historical and current events laced with discrimination may engender feelings of mistrust and discomfort (Shim et al., 2009) in women of color entering health settings characterized by those who have oppressed their group (whether male or racial majority group). For example, in a study of perceptions of psychotherapists, Sanders Thompson and her colleagues (2004) found that African Americans tended to describe therapists as older White males who were impersonal, uncaring, unavailable, and not in touch with the African American community in order to provide adequate support. Therefore, issues of discrimination, racism, or stressors related to being a member of a racial/ethnic minority group or a woman of color may not be disclosed by clients who perceive that White practitioners may not understand (Sanders Thompson, Bazile, & Akbar, 2004).

This is not to say that practitioners actually endorse those discriminatory or racist beliefs or that they are impersonal, but that providers and physicians must be willing to discuss these critical issues in treatment, as they relate to the woman of color's presenting problem and her engagement in treatment (Dana, 2000). Although discussing racism and discrimination may create feelings of discomfort in the practitioner, incorporating these issues in treatment is essential for women of color who have a history of experiences with racism and may continue to encounter these experiences on a daily basis (Carter, Forsyth, Mazzula, & Williams, 2005; Nadal, 2011). Acknowledging "what" practitioners may represent to a particular woman of color (i.e., a system that has often been oppressive to women and racial minorities) is the first step toward effective and culturally competent treatment. In addition, examining how she may feel about seeking services will allow women of color to feel understood and respected (Nunez & Robertson, 2006), will assist in building a healthy client-therapist alliance, and will begin to break down cultural mistrust of the mental health system.

Racial Identity

Theories of racial identity also suggest that both the client's and therapist's level of racial identity may implicate engagement in treatment, progress, and compliance (Atdjian & Vega, 2005). Helms (1995) suggests that among people of color, racial identity operates at a psychological level as a worldview to understand oneself as a racial being, to negotiate race-related discrimination, and to resolve internalized racist messages (Carter & Pieterse, 2006; Helms, 1995). Therefore, racial identity is not contingent on racial makeup itself, and individuals from the same racial group may vary in their level of racial identity. That is, all individuals, regardless of their race, ascribe different meanings to race. It is this meaning, which is often out of conscious awareness, that determines with whom one interacts, how one makes sense of the world, and how one makes sense of him- or herself.

Regardless of the client's and practitioner's racial makeup, their racial identities can have significant consequences on both engaging in treatment and building the therapeutic alliance (Atdjian & Vega, 2005). For example, if a woman color, who has a more mature racial identity and understands the meaning of race and its salience in her life, enters treatment with a practitioner who has a less mature racial identity and denies the existence or centrality of race, then she may feel uncomfortable discussing experiences of discrimination or racism if she becomes aware of the practitioner's cues (whether conscious or unconscious) revealing blindness to these issues. Thus, engagement in treatment is compromised and the potential for early termination is likely. However, if the practitioner also has a mature racial identity, then she/he will be able to acknowledge and incorporate racial/cultural issues in the client's healing.

Incorporating issues of discrimination and racism in treatment and understanding the impact of one's racial identity in our client's progress requires the practitioner to examine his/her own biases, assumptions, and worldview. It is also necessary both to acknowledge these biases and assumptions and to actively understand them. Engaging in self-reflection regarding these issues will assist practitioners to begin to understand themselves as racial-cultural beings and also to see how their biases influence the therapeutic relationship. Exploring biases and assumptions consists first of self-reflection and understanding of (1) the biases one holds about one's own groups (e.g., gender, race, social class, ethnic background, religion); (2) how those messages were communicated and by whom; (3) how these messages and beliefs influenced one's decisions and behaviors throughout life; (4) the emotional reactions to these biases; and (5) how these assumptions and worldviews influence one's understanding of illness, expectations of progress, and interactions with clients.

Once a practitioner has a better understanding of his/her own group, then he/she can gain a better understanding of the biases held against/for other groups by reflecting on the same aforementioned steps. It is also important for practitioners to know that there are many intragroup differences among each racial/ethnic group and that it would be helpful to tease apart their own biases as specifically as possible. The process of discovering our own biases and assumptions transcends a set of learned skills into a personal and lifelong journey. It is also not an easy journey and may stir up a range of feelings, some of which may be uncomfortable and difficult to understand. Therefore, having an outlet (e.g., supervision, psychotherapy, colleagues) to discuss and process these feelings in a trusted environment is recommended. Once practitioners engage in this self-discovery, then they will be able to see their clients' presenting problems and issues within a cultural context and further the clients' recovery.

Stigma

Stigma about physical and mental illnesses is another barrier to treatment, particularly among women of color. For example, Nadeem, Lange, Edge, Fongwa, Belin, and Miranda (2007) found that U.S.-born African American women were more likely to report stigma related to their depression compared to non-Hispanic White women. Similarly, they found that both U.S.-born African American and Hispanic American women were less likely to want mental health treatment and also more likely to express concerns about discussing mental health issues to practitioners compared to non-Hispanic White women (Van Hook, 1999). Black immigrant women, especially from the Caribbean, reported the most concerns regarding stigma compared to U.S.-born White women (Nadeem et al., 2007). Fears of misdiagnosis or "brainwashing" have also been expressed by African Americans in studies examining perceptions of mental health treatment (Sanders et al., 2004). As a result, African Americans tend to have cultural mistrust of health and mental health services (Bell & Tracey, 2006). Asian Americans also tend to underutilize health services as a result of shame associated with disclosing problems to outsiders and stigma regarding mental health treatment (Davey & Watson, 2008; Sue & Sue, 2008; Uba, 1994). For women of color with mental health problems, the negative effects of stigma related to their mental illness can be multiplied by stigma related to racial/ethnic heritage (Shim et al., 2009) and issues of sexism, racism, and discrimination, which may prevent some women of color from either seeking services or engaging in treatment due to perceived discrimination (Gary, 2005). For example, mistrust has resulted in African Americans being more likely to terminate treatment prematurely (DHHS, 2001). Therefore, practitioners must be able to discuss these issues with women of color, particularly immigrant women, and determine their impact on both engaging in treatment and their clinical presentation.

However, emerging research suggests the opposite; some minorities do report wanting treatment and are less embarrassed about it compared to non-Hispanic Whites (Diala et al., 2001). For example, Shim et al. (2009) found that African Americans were actually more likely than both Hispanics and non-Hispanic Whites to seek mental health services for their mental illness and less likely to report feeling embarrassed about seeking such services. Nadeem et al. (2007) also found that immigrant Hispanic women were more likely to want mental health services compared to U.S.-born White women. Both Nadeem et al. and Shim et al.'s findings contradict the notion that minorities are less likely to want professional help for their mental health problems. Therefore, it is possible that perceived discrimination or other factors may better explain the racial disparities in service utilization or premature termination from treatment. For example, as collectivist cultures, women of color may be more likely to seek services from primary care physicians, personal networks, or religious or spiritual healers (Cooper-Patrick et al., 1999). Therefore, practitioners must be willing to discuss these issues when women of color enter treatment and not interpret their struggle as resistance or pathology.

CULTURAL VALUES AND ENGAGEMENT

Cultural values also play a significant role in women of color entering treatment, establishing a therapeutic alliance, and continuing engagement. In a recent article on ethnocultural considerations in post-traumatic stress disorder (PTSD), Marcella (2010) provides an eloquent definition of culture we find useful in discussing cultural values—that is, values based on our cultural group:

> Shared learned behavior and meanings acquired in life activity contexts are passed on from one generation to another for purposes of promoting survival, adaptation, and adjustment. These behaviors and meanings are dynamic, and are responsive to change and modification in response to individual, societal, and environmental demands and pressures. Culture is represented *externally* in artifacts, roles, settings, and institutions. Culture is represented *internally* in values, beliefs, expectations, consciousness, epistemology (i.e., ways of knowing), ontology, and praxiology, personhood, and world views. (p. 19)

Cultural values, especially those that Marcella identified as internally represented, determine our reality, worldview, and beliefs about appropriate and deviant behavior. The United States is mainly characterized as an individualistic[6] culture that emphasizes values of independence, autonomy, and self-reliance (Stewart & Bennett, 1991). Individualist cultural values are woven throughout all conventional Western psychological therapies (e.g., importance of self-expression, individual therapy, self-actualization, differentiation from family as a milestone) and are oftentimes considered "normal" and appropriate for all clients. Clients who do not endorse these values run the risk of being pathologized or marginalized. It should be noted, however, that many Americans also identify with collectivist values (Constantine, Robinson, Wilton, & Caldwell, 2002), placing significant importance on interdependence, cooperation, family loyalty, and extended social support networks (Santiago-Rivera, Arredondo, & Gallardo-Cooper, 2002). For example, Hispanics, African Americans, and Asian Americans are typically considered collectivist cultures, while Western or Euro-Americans are typically considered individualist cultures.

With the growing number of racial/ethnic minorities in the United States, many researchers and scholars have been working toward expanding our current mental health practices to include cultural values. For example, researchers have found that as a result of endorsing collectivist values, some racial/ethnic minorities are more likely to resolve problems within their immediate social support network as opposed to seeking professional services for their mental illness (see Berdahl & Stone, 2009; Cabassa, 2007; Sanders Thompson et al., 2004). A client's perception of how connected her/his therapist is to the client's community has also been noted. For example, in a study of African Americans' perceptions of therapists, Sanders et al. found that it was important for clients to perceive that the therapist was in touch with or involved in the clients' community to be able to relate and understand the clients' experiences. This interconnectedness between the self and others is a salient characteristic of collectivist cultures, which may evaluate sense of worth, well-being, and satisfaction with life based on external sources (e.g., family expectations, quality of interpersonal relationships, and connection to social group).

Women of color who endorse collectivist values may also be more affected by stigma related to mental illnesses compared to those who endorse individualist values. For example, Schraufnagel and his colleagues (2006) found that racial/ethnic minorities may be less likely to obtain mental health treatment due to the negative messages about mental illnesses from their families or communities. While individualistic values emphasize taking care of one's "self" first and foremost, some racial/ethnic minority groups find that seeking mental health services is a sign of weakness (Sanders Thompson et al., 2004) and thus represents their inability to resolve their problems within the family and social support network. Considering that most practitioners continue to be non-Hispanic Whites, even when women of color do enter treatment, perceived cultural differences may result in feelings of discomfort in disclosing information regarding her mental health problems to a therapist who may be perceived as a member of her own group or social network.

Therefore, practitioners must make an effort to expand the boundaries of treatment and step outside the therapy or examination room and into their clients' community and context. While this may appear impractical for some practitioners, they must be willing, at a minimum, to "bring the family and the community" to the session. This contradicts many conventional psychological practices that focus on the individual in a vacuum—on their own thoughts, their own feelings, their own practices. However, to become a culturally competent practitioner means having the willingness to understand psychological distress in the context of clients' value systems and the ability to deliver interventions that include women of color's connection and interconnectedness to their family, extended social support network, and community.

Although ethical standards require practitioners to be knowledgeable about the cultural groups of their clients, at times this may also appear overwhelming and endless. Cultural values are dynamic, and not all people from one racial/ethnic group endorse all values or in the same way. Therefore, it is important for practitioners to be knowledgeable about the salient cultural values typically endorsed in the client's racial/ethnic group and be willing to examine their centrality in the individual client's worldview. Oftentimes, genuine questions that explore the client's beliefs and assumptions are enough to bring forth the client's worldview and also to engender trust and connection between the practitioner and her/his client. Caution, however, should be given regarding overreliance on the clients to help practitioners understand their culture since women of color (and men of color) are often burdened with the task of "teaching" and being the spokesperson for their entire racial/ethnic group. Similarly, questions that imply, whether intentionally or unintentionally, that clients are different, foreign, or alien (questions that include "those people" or "people of your race") can be forms of microaggressions that only foster feelings of alienation and marginality in clients and thus perpetuate the perception that practitioners are out of touch and disconnected. This, again, calls practitioners to be aware of their biases and assumptions and to process their reactions of racial and cultural issues in the same way that we would be asked to process countertransference.

Gender Roles

While every cultural group has specific gender roles, cultural values and social norms associated with these roles have been found particularly salient among racial/ethnic minority groups (Santiago-Rivera et al., 2002; Vandello & Cohen, 2003), which may impact how women of color engage in treatment. For example, Hispanic social norms characterize some Hispanic women as self-sacrificing for their families and the Hispanic males as protectors and courageous individuals (Valencia-Garcia, Starks, Strick, & Simoni, 2008). Therefore, it is possible that therapy with Hispanic women may focus heavily on their familial issues, which may be erroneously

interpreted as resistance to work on personal issues, enmeshment, or inability to assert and take care of the "self."

Asian American women often face social stigma, shame, and issues related to "saving face" (preserving public appearance of themselves and
their families for the sake of community propriety), which may prevent
them from seeking mental health services (Kramer, Kwong, Lee, & Chung,
2002) or exploring issues in treatment that would bring shame to their
families. In addition, Asian American women who have been socialized to
see emotional control as a sign of strength and emotional problems as
shameful (Sue & Sue, 2008) may also be at risk for being misinterpreted by
practitioners as suppressing their emotions and/or avoiding confrontation.
It is often the case that Western notions of healing emphasize verbal expression of feelings and emotional ailments (Marcella, 2010). However, for
some women of color, such as Asian American women, verbal expression
of feelings may be culturally inappropriate (Lin, 2000) and further her distress and discomfort in remaining in treatment.

Whereas Hispanic and Asian American women may be more typically
characterized as submissive or interdependent, African American women
have been characterized as self-reliant, strong, and responsible for forging
ahead in the face of adversity, with or without support from others and
without complaining. These characteristics, historically grounded in slavery, served as coping mechanisms to endure unthinkable abuse and
trauma, and are often described using the term "Strong Black Woman"
(Romero, 2000). While these characteristics demonstrate her resilience,
they may also prevent her from seeking services. Furthermore, while
African American women seek mental health services more than their
male counterparts do (Gonzalez, Alegria, & Prihoda, 2005), the pressure to
be strong and keep her "self" together may interfere with an African
American woman's ability to be vulnerable or engage in treatment.

While gender roles impact all women, the aforementioned values and
beliefs have been found more salient among women of color. However,
practitioners are warned not to overgeneralize these gender roles to all
women from a particular racial/cultural group simply because they be-
long to that group. For example, not all Asian American women may be
impacted by shame in the same way and some may not be impacted at
all. Therefore, practitioners should assess endorsement of these gender
roles, acknowledge that these can serve both as potential barriers and
resilient factors in their clients' lives, and be willing to discuss these in
treatment. Furthermore, practitioners who endorse individualistic values
may (whether intentionally or unintentionally) pathologize the client or
minimize how important her gender role may be to her psychological
well-being, which in essence should not be an issue that requires clinical
intervention. However, understanding how practitioners may or may
not endorse individualistic values requires that practitioners engage in

self-reflection and be aware of their biases and assumptions around these issues. In general, practitioners must be able to discuss and incorporate these critical issues in treatment. This would not only show women of color that they are respected and understood, but ultimately foster a stronger therapeutic alliance and better understanding of their cultural contexts.

Religion and Spirituality

Cultural values associated with religion and spirituality are also important to consider in treating women of color as they may dictate how she expresses herself, understands, and heals her mental illness. For example, racial/ethnic minorities have traditionally used song, dance, rituals, theater, poetry, and art to express themselves (Ciornai, 1983). As noted in previous sections of this chapter, some racial/ethnic minorities are less likely to seek conventional mental health treatment and instead resolve their problems within their social support network. The social network of many women of color includes religious or community healers such as clergy, pastors, curanderos, espiritistas, santerios, and shamans, who are often utilized for both spiritual and mental health services. Indigenous methods of healing include, for example, *Curanderismo*, often used by some Hispanics groups to heal folk illnesses. Among Asian Americans, women may first seek acupuncture or use traditional herbs for their illnesses, while others may concurrently seek folk healers to rid themselves of evil spirits. Seeking services from indigenous forms of treatment often entails the use of herbs, oils, incense, massages, and "homework" assignments, as well as practices of divination common in the African American, Asian, and Hispanic communities, which are in stark conflict to conventional interventions.

Furthermore, some racial/ethnic minority groups have also been shown to be guided by values of subjugation to nature and to endorse *fatalism* values (i.e., the belief that people have no control over their destiny, often associated with religiosity), which have been related to health status and help-seeking preferences (see Gallo, Penedo, Espinosa de los Monteros, & Arguelles, 2009). For example, Filipina women often avoid breast cancer screenings in fear that if they were meant to die of the disease, then a diagnosis would be part of God's plan (Nadal, 2011). Therefore, practitioners should be alert to implicit or explicit cues regarding fatalism values and how these may inhibit progress in treatment.

In general, practitioners working with women of color should be alert to the healing practices of their cultural groups, explore clients' own preferences for service type and how this may influence therapy, and be willing to build professional relationships with religious or spiritual leaders involved in the clients' lives. It should be noted, however, that while religious communities serve an integral part in the social support network of many women of color (Dana, 2000), some religious institutions may contribute to the stigma associated with mental illness (e.g., mental illness results from sinful behaviors, mistakes of previous life). For example, while Buddhist and Confucianist beliefs that emphasize interdependences and cooperation may explain lower suicide rates among Asian Americans, suicide may also be perceived as an appropriate course of action if it is deemed a method of protecting the family from shame (Suicide Prevention Resource Center, 2010).

Therefore, practitioners should assess the impact of religious/spiritual/ indigenous healing beliefs in serving both as risk and protective factors in their client's life and treatment. Discussing these critical issues would ensure that her values and preferences are respected and would also help the practitioner to understand the client's cultural context.

Symptom Manifestations and Culture-Bound Symptomotology

Understanding the different possible ways that women of color may understand their distress and manifest symptoms is another vital aspect of the culture that clinicians should be aware of. Emerging research in symptom manifestations of physical and mental illness suggests that some women of color (and men of color) may not be captured by psychiatric frameworks grounded in Western notions and classifications of distress (Atdjian & Vega, 2005). For example, some Asian American cultures emphasize interconnectedness among mind, body, and soul, and therefore Asian American women may express emotional distress through physical problems (Sue & Sue, 2008). Hispanic women are also more likely to present psychological distress in somatic representations (e.g, *ataque de nervios*; attack of the nerves) that include symptoms such as "headaches," stomach disturbances, and sleep difficulties. The physical manifestation of psychological distress may therefore explain why women of color are more likely to see a primary care physician than a mental health service provider. The extent to which cultural differences in expression of psychological distress are prevalent in today's society is made obvious in the appendix section of the *Diagnostic and Statistical Manual of Mental Disorders* (DSM-IV; American Psychiatric Association, 1994) with the inclusion of culture-bound syndromes. The *DSM-IV* describes several culture-bound syndromes that may not be captured by conventional psychological disorders; symptomontology that would otherwise be potentially dismissed or considered dysfunctional (Atdjian & Vega, 2005). For example, racial/ ethnic minorities, such as Asian Americans, whose prevalence of mental illness is reported to be lower when using traditional diagnostic criteria, have been found to endorse culture-bound syndromes, such as neurasthenia, which includes somatization, with higher rates (Sue & Chu, 2003). Thus, if culture-bound syndromes were included in research on prevalence of mental illness, then it is possible that some racial/ethnic minority groups may have higher unmet needs than are currently reported (Sue & Chu, 2003). The symptoms associated with the culture-bound syndromes can resemble a multitude of mental disorders that must be differentiated by contextual factors and incorporated in clinical formulations. However, the extent to which practitioners refer to these syndromes in clinical formulations remains unknown.

Although the index for culture-bound syndromes is marginalized to an appendix, which may minimize its credibility, the fact that the DSM-IV incorporated this index demonstrates awareness of the real need to understand and learn how to conceptualize women of color in a culturally sensitive way. Culture-bound syndromes reflect how some racial/ethnic minority individuals manifest stress and aversive experiences and are more commonly observed in women and older individuals, those with lower socioeconomic statuses, and those with lower educational levels (Falicov, 1998). Therefore, practitioners are encouraged to assess the way in which symptoms may manifest in women of color's cultural groups. Asking clients to speculate or guess about the emotional reasons for their physical ailments may be a useful way in determining the psychological meaning behind somatic symptoms. Incorporating these discussions in treatment would show women of color that their beliefs on health and healing practices are acknowledged and respected. Lastly, it provides practitioners rich information regarding how the client understands her experiences (her worldview) and the opportunity to generate culturally sensitive and relevant treatment interventions.

CONCLUSION

In conclusion, the theoretical and emerging body of research on ethnocultural factors relevant to racial/ethnic minorities in the United States highlights the importance of understanding these factors' impact in the treatment of women of color who have physical or mental health illnesses. Structural barriers, issues of stigma, gender roles, and religiosity have all been identified as salient ethnocultural considerations that can serve both as risk and protective factors and can impact clients' comfort level in seeking and remaining in treatment. The review of these considerations supports the importance of not only attending to racial and cultural preferences but also expanding traditional notions of healing. Practitioners who are aware of their own values, biases, and assumptions, who conceptualize clinical presentations in the context of the client's racial/cultural group, and who examine the role of the client's and their own worldviews throughout treatment will begin to reduce, and hopefully eliminate, underutilization of services and ensure that women of color receive culturally competent and relevant treatment.

NOTES

1. Portions of this chapter appeared in: Lundberg-Love, Nadal, and Paludi. (2012). *Women and mental disorders.* New York.

2. The term "racial/ethnic minority" is used broadly throughout this chapter to refer to groups of individuals who, due to their race or ethnicity, are marginalized, receiving differential and unequal treatment. We use the term Hispanic to identify people from Mexico, Cuba, Puerto Rico, Central America, and South America who are racially diverse. The term Asian American is used to identify people from diverse ethnic heritages and Asian countries (e.g., the Philippines, China, Korea, Japan, and India). African Americans are identified as Blacks born in the United States, unless otherwise noted in the chapter.

3. The terms non-Hispanic Whites and Whites are used interchangeably to identify individuals who are racially White but are not from Hispanic ancestry.

4. The terms "mental health services," "treatment," and "service" are used interchangeably throughout the chapter to refer to outpatient and inpatient services provided to individuals with mental disorders identified by the diagnostic categories in the DSM-IV.

5. The use of the term "practitioners" throughout this chapter describes individuals who are qualified through education and experience to practice in the field of psychology. These individuals include but are not limited to psychologists, psychiatrists, psychoanalysts, mental health professionals, clinical social workers, and master's level clinicians.

6. Throughout this chapter, we make reference to some racial ethnic minority groups endorsing collectivist values. Collectivism is characterized by several distinct values, and not all people of color endorse all these values equally. Therefore, while we compare collectivist and individualistic cultural values throughout the chapter, readers are warned not to overgeneralize these discussions. Similarly, collectivism and individualism are at the extreme poles of a spectrum, and significant within-group differences are found between both of these worldviews.

REFERENCES

American Psychiatric Association. (1994). *Diagnostic and statistical manual of mental disorders.* (4th ed.). Washington, DC: Author.

Atdjian, S., & Vega, W. A. (2005). Disparities in mental health treatment in the U.S. racial and ethnic minority groups: Implications for psychiatrists. *Psychiatric Services, 56,* 1600–1602.

Bell, T. J., & Tracey, T. J. G. (2006). The relation of cultural mistrust and psychological health. *Journal of Multicultural Counseling and Development, 34,* 2–14.

Berdahl, T., & Stone, T. (2009). Examining Latino differences in mental healthcare use: The roles of acculturation and attitudes towards healthcare. *Community Mental Health Journal, 45,* 393–403.

Biever, J. L., Castaño, M. T., de las Fuentes, C., González, C., Servín-López, S., & Sprowls, C. (2002). The role of language in training psychologists to work with Hispanic clients. *Professional Psychology: Research and Practice, 33,* 330–336.

Bradford, D. T., & Muñoz, A. (1993). Translation in bilingual psychotherapy. *Professional Psychology: Research and Practice, 24,* 52–61.

Breslau, J., Kendler, J. S., Sue, M., Gaxiolaaguilar, S., & Kessler, R. C. (2004). Lifetime risk and persistence of psychiatric disorders across ethnic groups in the United States. *Psychological Medicine, 35,* 317–327.

Cabassa, L. J. (2007). Latino immigrant men's perceptions of depression and attitudes toward help seeking. *Hispanic Journal of Behavioral Sciences, 29,* 492–509.

Carter, R. T., Forsyth, J., Mazzula, S. L., & Williams, B. (2005). Racial discrimination and race-based traumatic stress. In R. T. Carter (Vol. Ed.), *Handbook of racial-cultural psychology and counseling: Practice and training Vol. 2* (pp. 447–476). New York: Wiley & Sons, Inc.

Carter, R. T., & Pieterse, A. (2006). Race: A social and psychological analysis of the term and its meaning. In R. T. Carter (Vol. Ed.), *Handbook of racial-cultural psychology and counseling: Theory and research Vol. 1* (pp. 41–63). New York: Wiley & Sons, Inc.

Chow, J., Jaffee, K., & Snowden, L. (2003). Racial and ethnic disparities in the use of mental health services in poverty areas. *American Journal of Public Health, 93,* 792–797.

Ciornai, S. (1983). Art therapy with working class Latino women. *The Arts in Psychotherapy, 10, 2,* 63–77.

Constantine, M., Robinson, J., Wilton, L., & Caldwell, L. (2002). Collective self-esteem and perceived social support as predictors of cultural congruity among Black and Latino college students. *Journal of College Student Development, 43,* 307–316.

Cooper-Patrick, L., Gallo, J. J., Powe, N. R., Steinwachs, D. M., Eaton, W. W., & Ford, D. E. (1999). Mental health service utilization by African-Americans and Whites: The Baltimore Epidemilogic Catchment Area Follow-Up. *Medical Care, 37,* 1034–1045.

Dana, R. (2000). An assessment-intervention model for research and practice with multicultural populations. In R. Dana (Ed.), *Handbook of cross-cultural and multicultural personality assessment* (pp. 5–16). Mahwah, NJ: Lawrence Erlbaum.

Davey, M.P., & Watson, M. F. (2008). Engaging African-Americans in therapy: Integrating a public policy and family therapy perspective. *Contemporary Family Therapy, 30,* 31–47.

David, E. J. R. (2010). Cultural mistrust and mental health help-seeking attitudes among Filipino Americans. *Asian American Journal of Psychology, 1,* 57–66.

Diala, C. C., Muntaner, C., Walrath, C., Nickerson, K., LaVeist, T., & Leaf, P. (2001). Racial and ethnic differences in attitudes toward seeking professional mental health services. *American Journal of Public Health, 91,* 805–807.

Ecklund, K., & Johnson, B. (2007). The impact of a culture-sensitive intake assessment on the treatment of a depressed biracial child. *Clinical Case Studies, 6,* 468–482.

Falicov, C. J. (1998). *Latino families in therapy: A guide to multicultural practice.* New York: Guilford Press.

Gallo, L. C., Penedo, F. J., Espinosa de los Monteros, K., & Arguelles, W. (2009). Resiliency in the face of disadvantage: Do Hispanic cultural characteristics protect health outcomes? *Journal of Personality, 77,* 1707–1746.

Gary, F. A. (2005). Stigma: Barrier to mental health care among ethnic minorities. *Issues in Mental Health Nursing, 26,* 979–999.

González, H., Vega, W., Williams, P., Tarraf, W., West, P., & Neighbors, H. (2010). Depression care in the United States: Too little for too few. *Archives of General Psychiatry, 67,* 37–46.

Gonzalez, J. M., Alegria, M., & Prihoda, T. J. (2005). How do attitudes toward mental health treatment vary by age, gender, and ethnicity/race in young adults? *Journal of Community Psychology, 33,* 611–629.

Hays, P. A. (2001). *Addressing cultural complexities in practice. A framework for clinicians and counselors.* Washington, DC: American Psychological Association.

Helms, J. E. (1995). An update of Helms's white and people of color racial identity models. In Ponterotto, J. G., Casas, J. M., Suziki, L. A., & Alexander, C. M. (Eds.), *Handbook of multicultural counseling* (pp. 181–198). Thousand Oaks, CA: Sage Publications.

Kramer, E., Kwong, K., Lee, E., & Chung, H. (2002). Cultural factors influencing the mental health of Asian Americans. *Culture and Medicine, 176,* 227–231.

Lasser, K. E., Himmelstein, D. U., Woolhandler, S. J., McCormick, D., & Bor, D. H. (2002). Do minorities in the United States receive fewer mental health services than whites? *International Journal of Health Services, 32,* 567–578.

Lin, A. (2000). Why counseling and not Shou-Jing? *Cross-Cultural Psychology Bulletin, 34,* 10–15.

Marcella, A. J. (2010). Ethnocultural aspects of PTSD: An overview of concepts, issues, and treatment. *Traumatology, 16,* 17–26.

McRae, M. B., & Short, E. L. (2010). *Racial and cultural dynamics in group and organizational life: Crossing boundaries.* Thousand Oaks, CA: Sage Publications.

Nadal, K. L. (2011). *Filipino American psychology: A handbook of theory, research, and clinical practice.* New York: John Wiley and Sons.

Nadeem, E., Lange, J. M., Edge, D., Fongwa, M., Belin, T., & Miranda, J. (2007). Does stigma keep poor young immigrant and U.S.-born Black and Latina women from seeking mental health care? *Psychiatric Services, 58,* 1547–1554.

Nunez, A., & Robertson, C. (2006). Cultural competency. In Satcher, D., Pamies, R. J., & Woelfl, N. W. (Eds.), *Multicultural medicine and health disparities* (pp. 371–388). New York: McGraw-Hill Medical Publishing Division.

Ramos-Sánchez, L., Atkinson, D. R., & Fraga, E. (1999). Mexican Americans' bilingual ability, counselor bilingualism cues, counselor ethnicity, and perceived counselor credibility. *Journal of Counseling Psychology, 46,* 125–131.

Romero, R. E. (2000). The icon of the strong black woman: The paradox of strength. In Jackson, L. C., & Greene, B. (Eds.), *Psychotherapy with African-American women: Innovations in psychodynamic perspectives and practice* (pp. 225–238). New York: Guilford Press.

Sanders Thompson, V. L., Bazile, A., & Akbar, M. (2004). African-Americans' perceptions of psychotherapy and psychotherapists. *Professional Psychology: Research and Practice, 35*, 19–26.

Santiago-Rivera, A., Arredondo, P., & Gallardo-Cooper, M. (2002). *Counseling Latinos and La Familia: A practical guide.* Thousand Oaks, CA: Sage Publications.

Schraufnagel, T. J., Wagner, A. W., Miranda, J., & Roy-Byrne, P. P. (2006). Treating minority patients with depression and anxiety: What does the evidence tell us? *General Hospital Psychiatry, 28*, 27–36.

Shim, R. S., Compton, M. T., Rust, G., Druss, B. G., & Kaslow, N. J. (2009). Race-ethnicity as a predictor of attitudes toward mental health treatment seeking. *Psychiatric Services, 60*, 1336–1341.

Stewart, E. C., & Bennett, M. J. (1991*). American cultural patterns: A cross-cultural perspective* (2nd ed.). Yarmouth, ME: Intercultural Press, Inc.

Sue, D. W., & Sue, S. (2008). *Counseling the culturally diverse: Theory and practice* (5th ed.). New York: Wiley.

Sue, S., & Chu, J. Y. (2003). The mental health of ethnic minority groups: Challenges posed by the supplement to the surgeon general's report on mental health. *Culture, Medicine, and Psychiatry, 27*, 447–465.

Suicide Prevention Resource Center. (2010). Suicide among Asian Americans/ Pacific Islanders. Retrieved from http://www.sprc.org/library/asian.pi.facts .pdf.

Uba, L. (1994). *Asian Americans: Personality patterns, identity, and mental health.* New York: Guilford Press.

U.S. Department of Health and Human Services. (2001). *Mental health: Culture, race, and ethnicity: A supplement to mental health: A report of the Surgeon General. Executive Summary.* Retrieved from http://www.surgeongeneral.gov/ library/mentalhealth/cre.

Valenica-Garcia, D., Starks, H., Strick, L., & Simoni, J. M. (2008). After the fall from grace: Negotiation of new identities among HIV-positive women in Peru. *Culture, Health & Sexuality, 10, 7*, 739–752.

Vandello, J. A., & Cohen, D. (2003). Male honor and female fidelity: Implicit cultural scripts that perpetuate domestic violence. *Journal of Personality and Social Psychology, 84*, 997–1010.

Van Hook, M. P. (1999). Women's help seeking patterns for depression. *Social Work in Health Care, 29*, 15–34.

Williams, D. R., González, H. M., Neighbors, H., Nesse, R., Abelson, J. M., Sweetman, J., & Jackson, J. S. (2007). Prevalence and distribution of major depressive disorder in African-Americans, Caribbean Blacks, and non-Hispanic Whites. *Archives of General Psychiatry, 64*, 305–315.

Part III

Psychosocial Issues in Understanding and Treating Women's Cancers

Chapter 6

Psychosocial Aspects of Women's Reproductive Cancers

Joan C. Chrisler, Alexandra M. Nobel, and Jessica R. Newton

A cancer diagnosis is always a shock. It is a threat to physical and economic well-being; to bodily integrity and body image; to independence, privacy, autonomy, and control; to personal identity and self-concept; to life goals and future plans; to the course of one's relationships; indeed, in many cases, to life itself (Falvo, 1991). The intensity of the threat varies from person to person (Goodheart & Lansing, 1997) and from one type and stage of cancer to another. Reproductive cancers may be especially threatening to women in several ways: self-concept (e.g., Am I still a woman without my uterus or breast?), body image (e.g., Am I still attractive with surgical scars?), life goals (e.g., Will I be able to have children?), intimate relationships (e.g., Will my partner stay with me, or can I attract a partner, if I may not be able to have children?), privacy (e.g., What do I say when people ask me what type of cancer I have?). Although some women may find it embarrassing, or even taboo, to speak openly about reproductive cancer, they need the affection and support of their friends and family at least as much as other cancer patients do. We hope that the information in this chapter will help cancer patients and members of their social support network to understand reproductive cancer and how women have experienced it.

Women's reproductive cancers are uterine cancer, ovarian cancer, cervical cancer, vulvar cancer, vaginal cancer, fallopian tube cancer, and hydatidiform mole. Breast cancer is not classified as a reproductive cancer. Although breasts are important in nurturing infants, they are not necessary to conception, pregnancy, or giving birth—the physical functions known as reproduction. We will mention breast cancer from time to time when its effects are similar to those of reproductive cancers, but readers will find it described more thoroughly in chapter 3. We begin with a description of each type of cancer and its risk factors, its symptoms, and its treatments. Then we discuss psychosocial issues of concern to reproductive cancer patients. We end with some advice for coping and self-care and some suggestions for learning more about other women's experiences of reproductive and breast cancers.

THE REPRODUCTIVE CANCERS

Uterine Cancer

Uterine cancer is the most commonly diagnosed gynecological cancer in the United States, and it is the fourth most common cancer among women (U.S. Cancer Statistics Working Group, n.d.). The American Cancer Society (ACS, 2012a) estimated that in 2012 there would be more than 47,000 newly diagnosed cases and 8,000 deaths from uterine cancer. Cancerous cells most often begin to grow in the uterine lining, known as the endometrium. The most common endometrial cancers are endometrial carcinomas; the most common of these is known as endometrioid adenocarcinoma (ACS, 2012b). Carcinomas are malignant tumors that begin in epithelial cells; these cells line organs in the body, such as the uterus. When cancerous cells develop in the connective or muscular tissue of the uterus, these tumors are known as uterine sarcomas; these are much rarer than endometrial carcinomas and account for approximately 3–5 percent of uterine cancers (Thanopoulou & Judson, 2012).

The risk of uterine cancer increases with age, and it is most often diagnosed in postmenopausal women (ACS, 2012a). One of the most common signs of uterine cancer is irregular or abnormal bleeding. Because there is no routine test for uterine cancer, it is imperative that a woman make an appointment to see her gynecologist if she is experiencing abnormal bleeding or vaginal discharge, feelings of pain or pressure in her pelvis, pain during urination, or pain during intercourse (ACS, 2012a; CDC, 2012a). Despite its frequent occurrence, many women are unaware of the symptoms of and screening methods for uterine and other gynecological cancers (Cooper, Polonec, & Gelb, 2011).

Although rates of uterine cancer have declined steadily over the last several decades by more than 25 percent for European American women, the rates have increased by more than 15 percent for African American women (ACS, 2012a; NWHN, 1999). The survival rate for White women is about 7 percent higher than it is for Black women in the United States (ACS, 2012a). It is unclear exactly what risk factors contribute to this variability, but infrequent screening and delays in seeking medical care probably contribute to lower survival rates.

Another risk factor for uterine cancers is a higher than usual amount of estrogen in the body. This may be due to excess fat in the abdominal area (fat cells produce a form of estrogen) or exposure to estrogen therapy for perimenopausal symptoms (ACS, 2012a). Although use of estrogen-only therapy during perimenopause appears to increase a woman's risk of endometrial cancer, that does not seem to be the case for women who use the more typical estrogen plus progesterone therapy, although that carries other risks and side effects, including increased risk for breast cancer and coronary heart disease (Voda & Ashton, 2006).

Uterine cancers may be treated with surgery, chemotherapy, radiation therapy, or some combination of these, depending on the location and stage of the cancer (ACS, 2012a). Specific risks are associated with all of the above treatments. Chemotherapy alone has a number of potential side effects, including damage to gonadal cells that can affect a woman's fertility post-treatment (e.g., causing premature menopause). Radiation exposure can cause tissues to lose elasticity. When uterine tissue is exposed to radiation, infertility or infecundity (inability to carry a pregnancy to full term) may result. Results of the Childhood Cancer Survivor Study (Green et al., 2009), a multinational, retrospective study of tens of thousands of childhood cancer survivors, showed that those female patients who had radiation therapy for uterine or ovarian cancer at a dosage greater than 5 Gy (units of Gray) had a significantly lower chance than other patients of ever having been pregnant.

Surgery for uterine cancers may range from localized tumor resection to radical hysterectomy (i.e., removal of the uterus, cervix, upper vagina, and parametrium; this is done in cases where cancer cells have already, or are likely to, spread). Removal of the uterus (hysterectomy) and/or ovaries (oophorectomy) can have significant effects on women's sexual functioning (Williamson, 1992), as well as bring an end to their ability to conceive and bear children. It is possible that surgery alone may protect some women from the negative side effects on sexual functioning that may stem from chemotherapy or radiation therapy, although there are psychological effects of both surgeries and other treatments, which we will discuss later.

Ovarian Cancer

Ovarian cancers are most often identified within the tissue of the ovary (i.e., epithelial ovarian cancer) or within the gamete cells (i.e., germ cell tumors; ACS, 2012c; NCI, 2012a). Cancer cells of the ovary are heterogeneous; however, they have been grouped into two types (Kurman & Shih, 2010). Type I cancer cells are rather distinct, easy to identify, and typically diagnosed in early stages of development; these can be treated with a range of options. Type II cancer cells do not appear in ovarian tissue in an obvious fashion. By the time they are detected, they usually are at a higher stage of development and represent a poorer prognosis. Unfortunately, Type II ovarian cancer is diagnosed in about 75 percent of cases (Kurman & Shih, 2010). Known risk factors for ovarian cancer are age (40 years or older), family history of ovarian cancer, and never having given birth (CDC, 2012b). The highest incidence of ovarian cancer is in older European American women (median age at diagnosis is 63 years; NCI, 2012a). That rate is approximately 1.19 times that of Latinas and American Indian/Alaska Native women and 1.37 times more than African American and Asian American women. Although incidence rates reveal a higher prevalence of ovarian cancer in White women, racial minority women have higher mortality rates, as they are less likely to be screened and to receive the best available treatment (Harlan, Clegg, & Trimble, 2003). Current ovarian cancer screening methods are pelvic examination, ultrasonography, and identification of genetic tumor markers (Clarke-Pearson, 2009).

Ovarian cancer is often referred to as a "silent killer" because most cases are diagnosed in the late stages. Researchers are slowly beginning to understand the emergence of ovarian cancer and to refute the notion that all ovarian cancer patients are asymptomatic. A few of the most notable symptoms of ovarian cancer are abdominal bloating, lower abdominal or back pain, vaginal bleeding, sensation of being full quickly after eating, and increased urges to urinate or increased frequency of urination (ACS, 2012c). These symptoms overlap with those of a variety of other medical conditions (ACS, 2011c; Goff et al., 2011); thus they have low predictive value for ovarian cancer onset. Unfortunately, the cancer has usually progressed to a later staging by the time the symptoms become clearer and more salient (Rossing, Wicklund, Cushing-Haugen, & Weiss, 2010).

Surgery and chemotherapy are the main forms of treatment of ovarian cancer. Radiation therapy is sometimes employed, especially in low doses to treat recurring malignancies (Kunos et al., 2011). Surgery typically involves the removal of the ovaries, uterus, and fallopian tubes. Hysterectomy and oopherectomy are used as primary treatment for early-stage treatment or as a means of debulking cancer tumors in preparation for subsequent treatment in advanced stages of cancer development (Lanceley et al., 2011). Chemotherapy is typically used in advanced stages or in combination with surgery to ensure the complete removal of the cancer. Some recent research suggests that chemotherapy prior to surgery can also be effective (Vergote et al., 2010).

As with uterine cancer, chemotherapy for ovarian cancer can affect sexual functioning and cause patients to enter menopause prematurely (Buković et al., 2008; Stavraka et al., 2012). Oopherectomy means the end of ovulation, and hysterectomy precludes carrying a fetus. Thus, women who are still of reproductive age at the time of their diagnosis are unlikely to be able to have children in the future.

Cervical Cancer

Cervical cancer is diagnosed when cancer cells begin to grow on the tissue surface of the cervix. These abnormal cells are detected through routine screening via a Papanicolaou (Pap) test (ACS, 2012d). Women rely on screening by their health care providers because of the lack of symptoms during the early development of cervical cancer, which is known for its very slow growth. It can take as short as a few years to as long as a few decades to develop (Rogers & Cantu, 2009). This gradual progression allows physicians time to monitor abnormal cell growth and to take immediate action at the sighting of precancerous cells (ACS, 2012d). Because cervical cancer is usually detected in earlier stages, most patients have a good prognosis (Zeng, Li, & Loke, 2011). Although cervical cancer is seen throughout the female population, most cases are diagnosed in younger (i.e., teens to 20s) and older (i.e., more than 40 years) women (ACS, 2012d). Women in their 30s are most likely to get regular Pap tests and therefore are less likely to be diagnosed with cervical cancer (ACS, 2012d); African American women and Latinas (Smith et al., 2011; Owusu et al., 2005) have particularly high rates because they are less likely to get regular Pap tests.

Cervical cancer is seen as highly preventable by both physicians (e.g., by removal of precancerous cells) and by women themselves (e.g., through safe sex behavior, vaccination). There are a number of risk factors for cervical cancer including socioeconomic status (Paskett et al., 2010) and lifestyle behaviors (ACS, 2012d); however, researchers have found that a majority of cervical cancer patients are infected with the human papillomavirus (HPV; Bosch, Lorincz, Munoz, Meijer, & Shah, 2002). HPV, which is usually transmitted through sexual intercourse, is the key element in facilitating the development of cervical cancer (Bosch & de Sanjosé, 2007). Approximately one-third of the 30–40 identifiable HPV strains found in the mucosal epithelium are considered to be risk factors for cervical cancer (ACS, 2012d; Eaton et al., 2008); two strains (Types 16 and 18) have been consistently identified as causes of cervical cancer development (de Sanjose et al., 2010; Munoz et al., 2003), and vaccines to protect women from initial or recurrent exposure to them have recently been developed (Harper et al., 2004). Cervarix is a bivalent vaccine that attacks HPV Types 16 and 18; Gardasil is a quadrivalent vaccine that prevents the manifestation of Types 16 and 18 as well as Types 6 and 11, which cause the development of genital warts (SIGN, 2008). The prescription for both vaccines requires a series of three doses: The second dose must follow the first dose within 1–2 months, and the third dose must be received within 6 months of the first dose (CDC, 2012c). Cervarix is only prescribed to adolescent girls and to women, but Gardasil also can be administered to boys and men in order to prevent the transmission of those strains of HPV (CDC, 2012c).

During early stages of cancer cell development, surgery in the form of radical trachelectomy (i.e., removal of the cervix, also known as cervicectomy), simple hysterectomy, radical hysterectomy, and/or lymph node removal is typical (SIGN, 2008). Most side effects of surgery are minor and temporary, similar to those of other surgical procedures; patients generally will experience pain at the surgical site and possible complications in controlling their bladder (NCI, 2012b). The most serious side effect, like that of other gynecological cancers, is its impact on women's potential to bear children.

Nonsurgical medical treatment procedures are reserved for later cancer staging (SIGN, 2008). Radiation therapy is usually implemented in conjunction with chemotherapy (i.e., chemoradiotherapy), which is more effective in treating cervical cancer than is the singular use of chemotherapy or radiation therapy alone; combined treatment increases the survival rate by 12 percent (Green et al., 2009, as cited by SIGN, 2008). Radiation side effects can include pain during sexual intercourse (Lammerink, de Bock, Pras, Reyners, & Mourits, 2012), narrowing and tightening of the vaginal cavity, urinary incontinence, frequent urination (Greimel, Winter, Kapp, & Haas, 2009), and loss of fertility due to ovary damage (NCI, 2012b).

There are a number of effective and successful ways to treat precancerous cell development after an abnormal Pap test, such as laser surgery, cryosurgery, and the loop electrosurgical procedure (LEEP). Furthermore, once the risk of cervical cancer is perceived as more immediate and personally relevant, many patients choose to adhere to recommendations that diminish their risk of cervical cancer by practicing safer sex, seeking regular cervical screenings, and eliminating smoking (Kahn et al., 2005). Perhaps due to publicity for Gardasil and Cervarix, a recent study of women's understanding of abnormal Pap results and their emotional response to an HPV diagnosis showed that HPV was more likely to be associated with cancer than to be recognized as a curable sexually transmitted infection (STI; Kahn et al., 2005). Public health officials have noted the importance of addressing negative emotions associated with an HPV diagnosis as it can affect women's willingness to disclose infections to subsequent sexual partners and their continued engagement in high risk health behaviors. STIs remain a taboo topic, and Americans do not like to talk about them for fear of being stigmatized. Thus many women report that they have not received adequate education about either STI prevention or about cervical cancer screening and prevention (Dyer, 2010).

Vulvar Cancer

The vulva refers to the outer parts of the female genitalia, including the outer opening of the vagina, the vaginal lips, and the clitoris. The most commonly diagnosed vulvar cancers are squamous (i.e., skin) cell carcinomas (ACS, 2012e). These cancers are diagnosed by the appearance of a lump under the skin that may be biopsied. Other types of vulvar cancers include adenocarcinomas that begin in the gland cells of the vulva and, more rarely, melanomas. Vulvar cancers are relatively rare and account for approximately 4 percent of all gynecological cancers and approximately .6 percent of all cancers in women (ACS, 2012e). Vulvar cancer is typically found in elderly women, and it is generally diagnosed in early stages when the cancer is localized (Carter & Downs, 2012). Vulvar cancer usually can be treated conservatively by surgery only or surgery with radiation (Carter & Downs, 2012). Although these cancers are relatively rare, their presence indicates the importance of being familiar enough with one's outer genitalia to notice changes and the importance of continuing regular gynecology appointments beyond one's reproductive years.

Vaginal Cancer

Vaginal cancers also are rare compared to other forms of gynecological cancer. In the United States in 2008, 1,199 women were diagnosed with vaginal cancer, and 417 women died from it (ACS, 2012a). The majority of women (85%) diagnosed with vaginal cancer are older than age 40; abnormal bleeding and/or vaginal discharge are the primary signs of its presence (ACS, 2012f). The most common types of vaginal cancers are squamous cell carcinomas (70%), which are tumors of the epithelial cells of the vaginal wall, and adenocarcinomas (15%), which are glandular tumors; rarer types are sarcomas (9%) and melanomas (4%; ACS, 2012f).

Vaginal cancer is linked to the presence of HPV; research indicates that up to 90 percent of cases show traces of HPV cells (ACS, 2012f). Thus, although these cancers are rare, they are yet another reason for women and girls to discuss HPV vaccination with their health care providers. Other risk factors for vaginal cancer are HIV+ status and prenatal exposure to diethylstilbestrol (DES), given to women between 1940 and 1970 to prevent miscarriage (ACS, 2012f).

Although chemotherapy may be used with more advanced stages, the usual treatment for vaginal cancer is surgery with radiation (ACS, 2012f), which can cause scar tissue to build along the vaginal walls. This can lead to a condition called stenosis, which includes thinning of the vaginal walls and shortening of the vagina (cancer.org, 2012). Vaginal stenosis can make intercourse painful or nearly impossible. Some physicians recommend that women use a vaginal dilator either prophylactically to minimize the accumulation of scar tissue during treatment or to break up scar tissue post-treatment, but researchers (Cullen et al., 2012) have reported that some women found the use of this device to be as invasive as treatment itself. They described it as an embarrassing, painful, and aversive experience, which led them to limit or cease use of the dilator. In addition, some women choose not to follow advice to use a dilator because they are uncomfortable or embarrassed at the thought of touching the inside of their vaginas, as they may have been socialized to believe that such behavior is inappropriate or even sinful.

Fallopian Tube Cancer

Fallopian tube cancer, too, is rare. There were only 1,033 documented cases in the United States between 1988 and 2001 (Kosary, 2007). However, some research has shown that many ovarian cancers actually start in the fallopian tubes and then move to the ovaries (NCI, n.d.), which might mean that fallopian tube cancer is more common than experts think but tends to be diagnosed after it has spread. Black women have been found to have a slightly higher survival rate from fallopian tube cancer than White women. Survival rates overall are higher for women less than 50 years old; however, the majority (84%) of fallopian tube cancer patients are diagnosed after age 50 (Kosary, 2007).

One risk factor for fallopian tube cancer is a BRCA (i.e., breast cancer) gene mutation. However, women who carry a BRCA gene mutation are typically younger at age of diagnosis and may have a better survival rate than those without the mutation (Levine et al., 2003), perhaps because they undergo more frequent screening for cancers of various types, which could lead to earlier intervention. Some women who carry a BRCA mutation have chosen to undergo elective surgeries to remove at-risk organs; removal of the ovaries and fallopian tubes is known as salpingo-oophorectomy (NCI, 2009). It appears that women who have used oral contraceptives and those who have breastfed their children are at lower risk than other women of developing fallopian tube cancer (M. D. Anderson Cancer Center, 2012).

Surgery is the primary treatment for fallopian tube cancer, but it may be followed by chemotherapy and/or radiation depending on the success of the surgical procedure and the likelihood of the spread of cancerous cells. Surgery can range from a laparoscopic procedure, which is minimally invasive, to a radical hysterectomy, which entails removal of the fallopian tubes, ovaries, uterus, cervix, and nearby lymph nodes (M. D. Anderson Cancer Center, 2012).

Hydatidiform Mole

A hydatidiform mole (HM) is a type of gestational trophoblastic (i.e., excess growth of chorionic epithelium, which forms the placenta) disease, which appears as a growth developed on the uterine wall during the early stages of pregnancy. As the placenta begins to form, an overproduction of cells can grow into an abnormal mass on the uterus. HM, also known as molar pregnancy, can be partial or complete; that is, it can develop in the presence or absence of a fetus. The most predominant symptoms of HM are excessive vaginal bleeding during the first trimester of pregnancy, preeclampsia (i.e., high blood pressure developed during pregnancy), hyperthyroidism, and an enlarged uterus.

HM is a rare occurrence in Western countries (only .6 to 1.1 cases in 1,000 pregnancies in North America; Sermer & Macfee, 1995, as cited in Gerulath, Ehlen, Bessette, Jolicoeur, & Savoie, 2002), but it is more prevalent in East Asia (Sebire & Seckl, 2008). Most cases of HM are observed in adolescent girls and in women more than 39 years of age (Salehi, Eloranta, Johanssen, Bergström, & Lambe, 2011). The causes of HM development are not entirely known; however, a history of HM, smoking, alcohol consumption, STIs, and certain dietary factors (e.g., insufficient consumption of animal protein, low beta-carotene intake) may increase a woman's risk (Altieri, Franceschi, Ferlay, Smith, & Vecchia, 2003).

Because this condition is so rare and rather difficult to identify in the general population, many molar pregnancies are misdiagnosed as ectopic pregnancies and vice versa (Burton et al., 2001). Inability to recognize the presence of HM can have serious implications. Though many HMs are benign, women who have a history of HM, especially older women, are at a high risk for choriocarcinoma, a type of uterine cancer that develops from a complete HM (ACS, 2012g; Berkowitz & Goldstein, 1996; Salehi et al., 2011). Additional effects of untreated HM include uterine hemorrhage, uterine perforation, trophoblastic embolism (i.e., blood clots), and infection (WHO, 1983). If the condition is properly treated, then a history of HM should not affect the outcome of subsequent pregnancies (Kim, Park, Bae, Namkoong, & Kim, 1998). The usual treatment of HM is to remove the abnormal mass from the uterus via suction curettage (Gerulath et al., 2002). A hysterectomy is generally implemented only upon a request from the patient (International Society for the Study of Trophoblastic Diseases, 2012); chemotherapy is sometimes prescribed for patients whose human chorionic gonadotropin (hCG) levels do not stabilize in a timely manner (Agarwal et al., 2011).

PSYCHOSOCIAL ASPECTS OF CANCER DIAGNOSIS AND TREATMENT

Demographic and Developmental Issues

In our descriptions of the types of reproductive cancers, we mentioned demographic issues that might put women at greater risk of a cancer diagnosis or a poor prognosis. The reasons for the greater risk of some ethnic/racial groups are unclear. In some cases there may be genetic factors that ethnic groups share that put them at higher (or lower) risk. However, cultural (e.g., diet, belief in fate or God's will, comfort with seeking gynecological services) and economic (e.g., insurance coverage, availability of services near home, ability to take time from work to seek medical services) factors probably play a greater role. If lower-income women lack health insurance or have inadequate coverage (e.g., for preventive services, with high deductibles) or if they are unable to leave work for doctors' appointments and cannot find a doctor or clinic to see them after work hours, then they are unlikely to receive routine screenings that might find cancer in early stages, and thus they may have higher mortality rates. Women from cultural groups that promote excessive modesty often find it uncomfortable to do breast self-examination (e.g., Islam, Kwon, Senie, & Kathuria, 2006) or are unfamiliar with their genitalia (and so would not notice a vulvar lump), placing them at higher risk of a cancer diagnosis in a later stage. Furthermore, women who hold strong beliefs about the role of fate or God's will have been shown to be less likely to seek cancer (and other) screenings because they believe that there is not much that can be done about it (Abdullahi, Copping, Kessel, Luck, & Bonell, 2009; Farooqui et al., 2011); if they are ill, that was meant to be.

Women's age at the time of diagnosis is an important factor in her reaction to a diagnosis of reproductive cancer. Older women, who are at greater risk for uterine, ovarian, vulvar, and fallopian tube cancer, are more likely than younger women to have completed their reproductive plans (or to be postmenopausal) at the time of their diagnosis. Although they share many of the same worries and concerns as younger women do, they are not likely to be troubled by treatment side effects that result in infertility. Young and midlife women, who may not yet have had a chance to have children or who might have been considering another pregnancy, should consult their physicians about the possibility of fertility preservation, such as ovarian tissue cryopreservation and transposition (i.e., harvesting and freezing ova for later fertilization and implantation in one's own or a donor's uterus; Georgescu, Goldberg, du Plessis, & Agarwal, 2008; Kim, 2006).

Coping with Treatment Side Effects

Most cancer surgeries are invasive, but women may experience reproductive cancer surgeries as particularly invasive, as indicated by the lines from Goedicke's (1988) poem, which we quoted at the beginning of this chapter. Surgeries may result in pain and soreness, which can be treated with medication, rest, distraction, and relaxation techniques (e.g., meditation, deep breathing). Social support, such as emotional support/reassurance and task-related support (e.g., assistance with housework, child care, heavy lifting), are espe-cially useful to women recovering from major surgery (e.g., hysterectomy).

Chemotherapy and radiation therapy for reproductive cancer produce a range of side effects similar to those seen in other forms of cancer, such as fatigue, weakness, appetite and weight loss, nausea and vomiting, in-creased vulnerability to illness and infections, hair loss, and possible burns from radiation (Knight, 2004; NCI, 2012b). Nausea and fatigue appear to have the greatest effect on women's well-being, as they can cause women to feel sad, anxious, and passive (Badr, Basen-Engquist, Taylor, & de Moor, 2006). Fatigue and weakness are particularly problematic for employed women and women with caregiving responsibilities. A psychotherapist or counselor can help women to realize the importance of giving priority to their own needs during cancer treatment and recovery; teach them to ask for what they need from friends, family members, and coworkers; and reassure them that other people want to support and assist them. Even "superwomen" need to rest when they are ill. Furthermore, if women do not take care of themselves, then they cannot take care of others who depend on them.

Body Image Issues

Body image refers to people's appraisals of, and feelings about, their bodies and bodily functions (Cornwall & Schmitt, 1990). Psychologists think of it as a mental image or cognition (i.e., an internal representation or map) of physical appearance, sensation, motion, and other bodily expe-riences (Pruzinsky & Cash, 1990). Body image includes aspects such as weight consciousness; satisfaction or dissatisfaction with various parts of the body; energy and stamina; balance; understanding of one's skills and physical abilities; and adjustment to changes that result from illness, in-jury, or aging (Chrisler, 2007). Thus, body image is part of people's self-concept and one basis for their identity (Chrisler & Ghiz, 1993).

Treatments for reproductive cancers can result in changes to women's body image in a number of ways. First, surgical scars, hair loss, weight loss, and/or radiation burns alter the appearance of a woman's body—either temporarily or permanently. Women can cope by using fashion and acces-sories to hide the changes (e.g., hats, wigs, colorful scarves) or to draw attention away from them (e.g., fanciful jewelry, tattoos). Some women cope actively (e.g., choosing to shave their heads when their hair loss be-gins) in order to regain control. Use of humor (e.g., joking about their changed appearance); spirituality (e.g., meditation, realizing that life is more important than looks); positive reframing (e.g., our bodies change throughout life; no one looks the same way at 60 as she did at 20); and seeking social support from friends, family, and other cancer survivors are also good ways to cope.

Second, the very fact that she has been diagnosed with cancer can change the way a woman thinks about her body, especially if she is young and/or it is her first serious illness. Any patient who has been diagnosed with a serious illness or chronic condition "will never again return to the pre-illness sense of self, of options, of invulnerability, of obliviousness to the body's functioning" (Goodheart & Lansing, 1997, p. 3). Indeed, women may also become particularly sensitive to bodily functions and sensations after cancer treatment, which can cause them to monitor their bodies (sometimes excessively) due to concern about their health status (Hipkins, Whitworth, Tarrier, & Jayson, 2004). An open relationship with a health care provider who is willing to listen and provide reassurance can help women to learn what to watch for and what is not likely to be of concern. The loss of a sense of invulnerability, while a shock at first, can come to be seen as a benefit of having survived cancer (i.e., positive reframing). People who find meaning in cancer (e.g., it showed me how much my friends and family care; it made me appreciate my life; it led me to reorder my priorities to spend time on what matters most to me) have higher well-being scores and cope better with their treatment and its effects (Taylor, 1983).

Third, treatments for reproductive cancer in young and midlife women often result in menopause. The menopausal transition in this case (known as surgical, artificial, or premature menopause) is sudden, rather than gradual (as in natural menopause). Menopausal symptoms affect body image in a number of ways. For example, vasomotor instability (i.e., hot flashes, night sweats) may make a woman feel that her once reliable body is now out of control (Chrisler & Ghiz, 1993), and there is evidence that these symptoms are more severe in artificial, as opposed to natural, menopause (Voda, 1997). Dressing in layers, carrying a fan, standing in front of an air conditioner or open refrigerator door, using visual imagery (e.g., imagine swimming in a cool mountain lake or walking in a snow storm), using distraction, and avoiding known triggers of hot flashes (e.g., stress, alcohol, caffeine, spicy foods) are ways that women have successfully coped with vasomotor symptoms (Golub, 1992; Voda, 1997). Menopause is a major sign of aging in our culture, as it signals the close of reproductive life. Women who experience natural menopause around age 51 often think that they are "too young to be old," even though they have had time to adjust to the idea during perimenopause (Chrisler, 2007). Negative attitudes toward aging, particularly the double standard of aging, which considers older women more negatively than older men, complicate the menopausal transition for everyone, but perhaps especially for women who experience a sudden transition years before they had expected it. Seeking social support from older (i.e., postmenopausal) women friends and relatives, and perhaps psychotherapy or counseling, can help women adjust to their new physical status.

Fourth, surgery for reproductive cancer often involves not just the removal of the tumor, but the removal of the organ (and sometimes neighboring organs) in which the cancerous growth appeared. Loss of any part of the body (e.g., arm, leg, breast) affects body image and sometimes identity and self-worth. For example, women who have had hysterectomies have reported that the surgery led them to question their gender identity (Elson, 2002). Those who saw menstruation as particularly definitive of womanhood felt a loss of feminine identity, even in cases where the hysterectomy was to remove fibroid (noncancerous) tumors that caused painful menstruation. The women valued their ovaries greatly as symbols of womanhood and definitive of normality; thus, those who retained their ovaries coped better with their hysterectomies than those who did not (Elson, 2003). Women who hold strong cultural values about the importance of motherhood and fertility to self-worth (e.g., Latinas; Marván, Trujillo, & Karam, 2009) often find hysterectomy a difficult adjustment. Studies of Mexican women (Marván et al., 2009), Latinas (Ashing-Giwa et al., 2004), and African American women (Augustus, 2002) show that many are worried that male partners (or potential partners) may no longer find them desirable, as they will be seen as incomplete/no longer whole women. Thus, some may need particular reassurance that they are still valuable, worthy, and lovable women.

Sexuality and Fertility

Sexuality and fertility can be considered body image issues, but we discuss them in a separate section because of their high relevance to reproductive cancers. The sense of oneself as sexy, one's feelings of sexual desire and experience of sexual pleasure, and one's confidence in what one's body can do (e.g., sexual activity, conception) are all part of one's body image. Reproductive cancers and their treatments can affect all of these.

Side effects of chemotherapy (including sudden onset of menopause) can impact women's sexual functioning (Buković et al., 2008). For example, the more fatigue, nausea, and vaginal dryness women reported, the less sexual desire and sexual activity they reported (Taylor, Basen-Engquist, Shinn, & Bodurka, 2004). Radiation treatment for cervical cancer can result in changes to the vaginal walls that make sexual intercourse uncomfortable, which women reported decreased their sexual satisfaction and desire (Jensen et al., 2003). Vaginal stenosis, which can result from treatment of vaginal cancer, makes intercourse painful (Cullen et al., 2012), and, as we noted earlier, treatment of stenosis is also painful, which causes some women to discontinue it. Depression, anxiety, fear of painful intercourse, and worry about a second molar pregnancy have all been shown to interfere with women's sexual functioning post-treatment (Buković et al., 2008; Peterson, Ung, Holland, & Quinlivan, 2005). Informational support from health care providers, sex therapy, and/or couples counseling should assist women who experience dissatisfaction with their sexual functioning.

Most people assume that they will be able to have children whenever they are ready to do so. Thus, infertility—the realization that one cannot do what others seem to do so easily—is a shock and a threat, even to those who are otherwise healthy (Spector, 2004). In cancer patients infertility may cause women to feel that they are still ill, fragile, and flawed, even after their physicians have pronounced them well and cancer free; infertility is a daily reminder of cancer and its uncomfortable treatments for those who were of reproductive age at diagnosis and had not completed (or started) their childbearing plans. Infertility, like premature menopause and hysterectomy, can cause anxiety (especially about relationships), depression, and body image disturbances in women. It also can cause them to question their identity as women and force them to reevaluate their life goals. A sensitive psychotherapist or counselor can help women to work through these concerns and to consider other ways to achieve the happiness that is associated with childrearing (e.g., adoption, close interactions with young relatives or friends' and neighbors' children, employment or volunteer work with children or adolescents; Spector, 2004).

Stigma

Social scientists define stigma as a physical mark that sets some people apart from others because they have a physical defect or stain on their character that spoils their identity or makes them unfit company (Goffman, 1963). Controllability is an important part of people's attitudes toward stigmatized others; the more responsibility individuals are thought to have for their condition, the more they are disliked and rejected (Dovidio, Major, & Crocker, 2000). People prefer to avoid socializing with stigmatized individuals and discussing stigmatized topics.

A generation or two ago, cancer itself was a stigmatized condition. It was usually detected in later stages and thus had a high mortality rate. Patients were sometimes not told what was wrong with them because nothing could be done, and relatives whispered about "the c-word." Today, given all the medical advances in screening and treatment, many people survive cancer, and most people know others who have been diagnosed and treated successfully. Cancer has become a topic for polite conversation—in most cases. Reproductive cancers, especially in some communities, may still carry stigma that can prevent women from receiving the social support they need.

Many Americans are uncomfortable discussing sexuality and reproductive processes. For example, researchers have demonstrated that there is stigma associated with menstruation (Johnston-Robledo & Chrisler, 2013), pregnancy (Taylor & Langer, 1977), infertility (Maill, 1994; Spector,

2004), menopause (Chrisler, 2011), and hysterectomy (Marván et al., 2009). Stigma attached to sexuality in general and particularly to certain sexual behaviors that are considered immoral by some people is one reason why sex education is so poor in the United States (Taylor, 2009). Research has shown that many people blame women with cervical cancer for their condition because they believe that their sexual decision making led to their illness (Dyer, 2010). The association of gynecological cancers and their treatment with reproduction, premature menopause, infertility, hysterectomy, and, in the cases of cervical and vaginal cancer, with STIs (i.e., HPV, HIV) may make it difficult for a woman to tell others what type of cancer she has and for others to be willing to discuss the symptoms and treatment effects with her. Support groups may be especially helpful to women whose friends and family are uncomfortable and prefer to avoid discussing reproductive cancer. The American Cancer Society can help women to locate support groups in their communities and/or online.

Self-Care for Women with Reproductive Cancer

A cancer diagnosis is a shock and a threat, as we noted at the beginning of this chapter, but it can also be a challenge and an opportunity. Treatment for reproductive cancers has advanced in recent years, and many women survive, and even thrive, after their treatment. Yes, coping with symptoms, treatment, and treatment side-effects is a challenge, but with the support of a good medical team, the care and concern of family and friends, and a well of spiritual strength from which to draw, most women rise to the challenge. Stress management is important to all cancer patients, and women with reproductive cancer are no exception. It is important for them to take time to rest and recover, to spend time with the people who are most important to them, to listen to calming music, to meditate or pray, to breathe deeply, and to enjoy nature, including the company of dear pets.

It may seem odd to think of cancer as an opportunity, but many people report that they have come to see cancer and other forms of serious illness (e.g., heart disease, HIV, autoimmune disorders) as just that (Taylor, 2009). The diagnosis of cancer serves to remind us that life is precious, that every day is important, that we should take nothing (and no one) for granted, that we need to take good care of ourselves as well as others, and that we should treat our fragile bodies with kindness and respect (e.g., massage, warm baths). We encourage cancer patients to remember that life is more than work and that we all ought to, as best we can, "make time for time." Women may wish to keep a journal to help them focus on what is most important and precious in their lives and to consider their hopes and plans for the future. Mindfulness (i.e., a form of active meditation in which we focus on what we are doing/seeing/hearing and nothing else) is calming and invigorating, enhances the pleasures of the day, and helps to keep worries at bay.

Control and optimism have been shown repeatedly to be helpful in recovery from serious illnesses of all kinds (Taylor, 2009). Thus, it is important for women to learn as much as they can about the type of cancer they have and to take an active role in making decisions about their treatment and how they will manage their side-effects, rather than drifting along with suggestions and requests made by others. Women can learn more about cancer from their medical team, books like this one, and the websites of the American Cancer Society (www.cancer.org), National Cancer Institute (www.cancer.gov), Centers for Disease Control and Prevention (www.cdc.gov), and the National Women's Health Network (www.nwhn.org). It may be interesting to read illness narratives written by women who have had cancer (e.g., Clifford, 2002; Levine, 2001; Lifshitz, 1988; Stocker, 1991).

Cancer patients can stay optimistic by placing emphasis on the survival statistics for their type of cancer, taking care of themselves as best they can to build up their immune systems, and focusing on the positive aspects of life. Good moods promote optimism, so women should remember to laugh a lot and be sure to have some fun every day; they can watch comedies on television, post their favorite funny cartoons where they can see them regularly, read entertaining novels, play games and engage in hobbies, enjoy the antics of children and pets, and spend time with people who make them happy. Finally, we hope that women with reproductive cancer will remember that self-care and a positive approach to life are important not just during treatment, but beyond. To be a cancer survivor is a gift to be cherished.

REFERENCES

Abdullahi, A., Copping, J., Kessel, A., Luck, M., & Bonell, C. (2009). Cervical screening: Perceptions and barriers to uptake among Somali women in Camden. *Public Health, 123*, 680–685.

Agarwal, R., Teoh, S., Short, D., Harvey, R., Savage, P. M., & Seckl, M. J. (2011). Chemotherapy and human chorionic gonadotropin concentrations 6 months after uterine evacuation of molar pregnancy: A retrospective cohort study. *Lancet, 379*, 130–135.

Altieri, A., Franceschi, S., Ferlay, J., Smith, J., & Vecchia, C. L. (2003). Epidemiology and aetiology of gestational trophoblastic diseases. *Lancet Oncology, 4*, 670–678.

American Cancer Society [ACS]. (2012a). *Cancer facts & figures*. Atlanta, GA: American Cancer Society. Retrieved from http://www.cancer.org/acs/groups/content/@epidemiology surveilance/documents/document/acspc-031941.pdf.

American Cancer Society [ACS]. (2012b). *Endometrial (uterine) cancer*. Retrieved from http://www.cancer.org/cancer/endometrialcancer/detailedguide/endometrial-uterine-cancer-what-is-endometrial-cancer.

American Cancer Society [ACS]. (2012c). *Can ovarian cancer be found early?* Retrieved from http://www.cancer.org/cancer/ovariancancer/detailedguide/ovarian-cancer-detection.

American Cancer Society [ACS]. (2012d). *What is cervical cancer?* Retrieved from http://www.cancer.org/cancer/cervicalcancer/detailedguide/cervical-cancer-what-is-cancer.

American Cancer Society [ACS]. (2012e). *Vulvar cancer.* Retrieved from http://www.cancer.org/cancer/vulvarcancer/detailedguide/vulvar-cancer-what-is-vulvar-cancer.

American Cancer Society [ACS]. (2012f). *Vaginal cancer.* Retrieved from http://www.cancer.org/cancer/vaginalcancer/detailedguide/vaginal-cancer-risk-factors.

American Cancer Society [ACS]. (2012g). *What is gestational trophoblastic disease?* Retrieved from http://www.cancer.org/gestationaltrophoblasticdisease/detailedguide/gestational-trophoblastic-disease-what-is-g-t-d.

Ashing-Giwa, K. T., Kagawa-Singer, M., Padilla, G. V., Tejero, J. S., Hsiao, E., Chhabra, R., & Tucker, M. B. (2004). The impact of cervical cancer and dysplasia: A qualitative, multiethnic study. *Psycho-Oncology, 13,* 709–728.

Augustus, C. E. (2002). Beliefs and perceptions of African American women who have had hysterectomy. *Journal of Transcultural Nursing, 13,* 296–302.

Badr, H., Basen-Engquist, K., Taylor, C. L. C., & de Moor, C. (2006). Mood states associated with transitory physical symptoms among breast and ovarian cancer survivors. *Journal of Behavioral Medicine, 29,* 461–475.

Berkowitz, R. S., & Goldstein, D. P. (1996). Chorionic tumors. *New England Journal of Medicine, 335,* 1740–1748.

Bosch, F. X., & de Sanjosé, S. (2007). The epidemiology of human papillomavirus infection and cervical cancer. *Disease Markers, 23,* 213–227.

Bosch, F. X., Lorincz, A., Munoz, N., Meijer, C. J. L. M., & Shah, K. V. (2002). The causal relation between human papillomavirus and cervical cancer. *Journal of Clinical Pathology, 55,* 244–265.

Buković, D., Silovski, H., Silovski, T., Hojsak, I., Šakić, K., & Hrgović, Z. (2008). Sexual functioning and body image of patients treated for ovarian cancer. *Sexuality and Disability, 26,* 63–73.

Burton, J., Lidbury, E., Gillespie, A., et al. (2001). Overdiagnosis of hydatiform mole in early tubal ectopicpregnancy. *Histopathology, 38,* 409–414.

Cancer.org. (2012, June 28). *Radiation therapy for vaginal cancer.* Retrieved from http://www.cancer.org/cancer/vaginalcancer/detailedguide/vaginal-cancer-treating-radiation-therapy.

Carter, J. S., & Downs, L. S. (2012). Vulvar and vaginal cancer. *Obstetrics and Gynecology Clinics of North America, 39,* 213–231.

Centers for Disease Control and Prevention [CDC]. (2012a). *Uterine cancers.* Retrieved from http://www.cdc.gov/cancer/uterine/index.htm.

Centers for Disease Control and Prevention [CDC]. (2012b). *Ovarian cancer.* Retrieved from http://www.cdc.gov/cancer/ovarian/pdf/ovarian_facts.pdf.

Centers for Disease Control and Prevention [CDC]. (2012c). *Vaccine information statements.* Retrieved from http://www.cdc.gov/vaccines/pubs/vis.

Chrisler, J. C. (2007). Body image issues of women over 50. In V. Muhlbauer & J. C. Chrisler (Eds.), *Women over 50: Psychological perspectives* (pp. 6–25). New York: Springer.

Chrisler, J. C. (2011). Leaks, lumps, and lines: Stigma and women's bodies. *Psychology of Women Quarterly, 35,* 202–214.

Chrisler, J. C., & Ghiz, L. (1993). Body image issues of older women. *Women & Therapy, 14,* 67–75.

Clarke-Pearson, D. L. (2009). Screening for ovarian cancer. *New England Journal of Medicine, 361,* 170–177.

Clifford, C. (2002). *Cancer has its privileges: Stories of hope and laughter.* New York: Penguin.

Cooper, C. P., Polonec, L., & Gelb, C. A. (2011). Women's knowledge and awareness of gynecological cancer: A multi-site qualitative study in the United States. *Journal of Women's Health, 20,* 517–524.

Cornwall, C. J., & Schmitt, M. H. (1990). Perceived health status, self-esteem, and body image in women with rheumatoid arthritis or systemic lupus erythematosus. *Research in Nursing and Health, 13,* 99–107.

Cullen, K., Fergus, K., DasGupta, T., Fitch, M., Doyle, C., & Adams, L. (2012). From "sex toy" to intrusive imposition: A qualitative examination of women's experiences with vaginal dilator use following treatment for gynecological cancer. *Journal of Sexual Medicine, 9,* 1162–1173.

de Sanjose, S., Quint, W. G., Alemany, L., Geraets, D. T., Klaustermeier, J. E., Lloveras, B., . . . & Puras, A. (2010). Human papillomavirus genotype attribution in invasive cervical cancer: A retrospective cross-sectional worldwide study. *Lancet Oncology, 11,* 1048–1056.

Dovidio, J. F., Major, B., & Crocker, J. (2000). Stigma: Introduction and overview. In Heatherton, T. F., Kleck, R. E., Hebl, M. R., & Hull, J. G., (Eds.), *The social psychology of stigma* (pp. 1–28). New York: Guilford.

Dyer, K. E. (2010). From cancer to sexually transmitted infection: Explorations of social stigma among cervical cancer survivors. *Human Organization, 69,* 321–330.

Eaton, L., Kalichman, S., Cain, D., Cherry, C., Pope, H., Fuhrel, A., & Kaufman, M. (2008). Perceived prevalence and risks for human papillomavirus (HPV) infection among women who have sex with women. *Journal of Women's Health, 17,* 75–84.

Elson, J. (2002). Menarche, menstruation, and gender identity: Retrospective accounts from women who have undergone premenopausal hysterectomy. *Sex Roles, 46,* 37–48.

Elson, J. (2003). Hormonal hierarchy: Hysterectomy and stratified stigma. *Gender & Society, 17,* 750–770.

Falvo, D. R. (1991). *Medical and psychosocial aspects of chronic illness and disability.* Gaithersburg, MD: Aspen.

Farooqui, M., Hassali, M., Shatar, A. K., Shafie, A. A., Seang, T. B., & Farooqui, M. A. (2011). A qualitative exploration of Malaysian cancer patients' perspectives on cancer and its treatment. *BMC Public Health, 11,* 98–103.

Georgescu, E. S., Goldberg, J. M., du Plessis, S. S., & Agarwal, A. (2008). Present and future fertility preservation strategies for female cancer patients. *Obstetrical & Gynecological Survey, 63,* 725–732.

Gerulath, A. H., Ehlen, T. G., Bessette, P., Jolicoeur, L., & Savoie, R. (2002). Gestational trophoblastic disease. *Journal of Obstetrics and Gynaecology Canada, 24,* 434–439.

Goedicke, P. (1988). That was the fruit of my orchard. In L. H. Lifshitz (Ed.), *Her soul beneath the bone: Women's poetry on breast cancer* (pp. 20–21). Urbana, IL: University of Illinois Press.

Goff, B. A., Lowe, K. A., Kane, J. C., Robertson, M. D., Gaul, M. A., & Andersen, M. R. (2011). Symptom triggered screening for ovarian cancer: A pilot study of feasibility and acceptability. *Gynecologic Oncology, 124,* 230–235.

Goffman, E. (1963). *Stigma: Notes on the management of spoiled identity.* New York: Simon & Schuster.

Golub, S. (1992). *Periods: From menarche to menopause.* Newbury Park, CA: Sage.

Goodheart, C. D., & Lansing, M. H. (1997). *Treating people with chronic disease: A psychological guide.* Washington, DC: American Psychological Association.

Green, D. M., Kawashima, T., Stovall, M., Leisenring, W., Sklar, C. A., Mertens, A. C., . . . Robinson, L. L. (2009). Fertility of female survivors of childhood cancer: A report from the Childhood Cancer Survivor Study. *Journal of Clinical Oncology, 27,* 2677–2685.

Greimel, E. R., Winter, R., Kapp, K. S., & Haas, J. (2009). Quality of life and sexual functioning after cervical cancer treatment: A long-term follow-up study. *Psycho-Oncology, 18,* 476–482.

Harlan, L. C., Clegg, L. X., & Trimble, E. L. (2003). Trends in surgery and chemotherapy for women diagnosed with ovarian cancer in the United States. *Journal of Clinical Oncology, 21,* 3488–3494.

Harper, D. M., Franco, E. L., Wheeler, C., Ferris, D. G., Jenkins, D., Shuind, A., . . . Dubin, G. (2004). Efficacy of a bivalent L1 virus-like particle vaccine in prevention of infection with human papillomavirus Types 16 and 18 in young women: A randomized, controlled trial. *Obstetrical & Gynecological Survey, 60,* 303–305.

Hipkins, J., Whitworth, M., Tarrier, N., & Jayson, G. (2004). Social support, anxiety and depression after chemotherapy for ovarian cancer: A prospective study. *British Journal of Health Psychology, 9,* 569–581.

International Society for the Study of Trophoblastic Diseases. (2012). *The hydatidiform mole & choriocarcinoma information pamphlet for patients.* Retrieved from http://isstd.org/isstd/patients.html.

Islam, N., Kwon, S. C., Senie, R., & Kathuria, N. (2006). Breast and cervical cancer screening among South Asian women in New York City. *Journal of Immigrant and Minority Health, 8,* 211–221.

Jensen, P. T., Groenvold, M., Klee, M. C., Thranov, I., Petersen, M. A., & Machin, D. (2003). Longitudinal study of sexual function and vaginal changes after radiotherapy for cervical cancer. *International Journal of Radiation Oncology, Biology, and Physics, 15,* 937–949.

Johnston-Robledo, I., & Chrisler, J. C. (2013). The menstrual mark: Menstruation as social stigma. *Sex Roles, 68,* 9–18.

Kahn, J., Zimet, G., Bernstein, D., Riedesel, J., Lan, D., Huang, B., & Rosenthal, S. (2005). Pediatricians' intention to administer human papillomavirus vaccine: The role of practice characteristics, knowledge, and attitudes. *Journal of Adolescent Health, 37,* 502–510.

Kim, J. H., Park, D. C., Bae, S. N., Namkoong, S. E., & Kim, S. J. (1998). Subsequent reproductive experience after treatment for gestational trophoblastic disease. *Gynecologic Oncology, 71,* 108–112.

Kim, S. S. (2006). Fertility preservation in female cancer patients: Current developments and future directions. *Fertility and Sterility, 85,* 1–11.

Knight, S. J. (2004). Oncology and hematology. In P. Camic & S. Knight (Eds.), *Clinical handbook of health psychology* (pp. 233–261). Cambridge, MA: Hogrefe & Huber.

Kosary, C. L. (2007). Cancer of the fallopian tube. In Ries, L. A., Young, J. L., Keel, G. E., & Eisner, M. P., (Eds.), *Cancer survival among adults: U.S. SEER Program, 1988–2001—patient and tumor characteristics* (pp. 161–164). Bethesda, MD: National Cancer Institute.

Kunos, C. A., Sill, M. W., Buekers, T. E., Walker, J. L., Schilder, J. M., Yamada, S. D., . . . Fracasso, P. M. (2011). Low-dose abdominal radiation as a docetaxel chemosensitizer for recurrent epithelial ovarian cancer: A Phase I Study of the Gynecologic Oncology Group. *Gynecologic Oncology, 120,* 224–228.

Kurman, R. J., & Shih, I. M. (2010). The origin and pathogenesis of epithelial ovarian cancer—a proposed unifying theory. *American Journal of Surgical Pathology, 34,* 433–443.

Lammerink, E. A., de Bock, G. H., Pras, E., Reyners, A. K., & Mourits, M. J. (2012). Sexual functioning of cervical cancer survivors: A review with a female perspective. *Maturitas, 72,* 296–304.

Lanceley, A., Fitzgerald, D., Jones, V., Miles, T., Elliott, E., Darragh, L., & Peck, L. (2011). Ovarian cancer: Symptoms, treatment and long-term patient management. *Cancer Nursing Practice, 10,* 29–36.

Levine, D. A., Argenta, P. A., Yee, C. J., Marshall, D. S., Olvera, N., Bogomolniy, F., . . . Boyd, J. (2003). Fallopian tube and primary peritoneal carcinomas associated with BRCA mutations. *Journal of Clinical Oncology, 15,* 4222–4227.

Levine, M. (2001). *Surviving cancer.* New York: Crown.

Lifshitz, L. H. (1988). *Her soul beneath the bone: Women's poetry on breast cancer.* Urbana, IL: University of Illinois Press.

Maill, C. E. (1994). Community constructs of involuntary childlessness: Sympathy, stigma, and social support. *Canadian Review of Sociology and Anthropology, 31,* 392–421.

Marván, M. L., Trujillo, P., & Karam, M. A. (2009). Hysterectomy as viewed by Mexican women and men. *Sex Roles, 61,* 688–698.

M. D. Anderson Cancer Center. (2012). *Fallopian tube cancer.* Retrieved from http://www.mdanderson.org/patient-and-cancer-information/cancer-information/cancer-types/fallopian-tube-cancer/index.html.

Munoz, N., Bosch, F. X., de Sanjose, S., Herrero, R., Castellsagué, X., Shah, K. V., & Meijer, C. J. (2003). Epidemiologic classification of human papillomavirus types associated with cervical cancer. *New England Journal of Medicine, 348,* 518–527.

National Cancer Institute [NCI]. (n.d.). *Ovarian tumors traced to fallopian tubes.* Retrieved from http://www.cancer.gov/cancertopics/causes/ovarian/disease-source0408.

National Cancer Institute [NCI]. (2009). Removal of ovaries and fallopian tubes cuts cancer risk for BRCA1/2 gene carriers. *NCI Cancer Bulletin, 6.* Retrieved from http://www.cancer.gov/aboutnci/ncicancerbulletin/archive/2009/012709/page3.

National Cancer Institute [NCI]. (2012a). *Cancer of the ovary.* Retrieved from http://seer.cancer.gov/statfacts/html/ovary.html.

National Cancer Institute [NCI]. (2012b). *What you need to know about cervical cancer.* Retrieved from http://www.cancer.gov/cancertopics/wyntk/cervix/page8.

National Cancer Institute [NCI]. (2013). *Ovarian cancer screening.* Retrieved from http://cancer.gov.cancertopics/pdq/screening/ovarian/Patient/page3#Keypoint5.

National Women's Health Network [NWHN]. (1999, November 1). *Women's health snapshots: Uterine cancer.* Retrieved from http://nwhn.org/womens-health-snapshotsuterine-cancer.

Owusu, G. A., Eve, S. B., Cready, C. M., Koelln, K., Trevino, F., Urrutia-Rojas, X., & Baumer, J. (2005). Race and ethnic disparities in cervical cancer screening in a safety-net system. *Maternal and Child Health Journal, 9,* 285–295.

Paskett, E. D., McLaughlin, J. M., Reiter, P. L., Lehman, A. M., Rhoda, D. A., Katz, M. L., & Ruffin, M. T. (2010). Psychosocial predictors of adherence to risk-appropriate cervical cancer screening guidelines: A cross sectional study of women in Ohio Appalachia participating in the Community Awareness Resources and Education (CARE) project. *Preventive Medicine, 50,* 74–80.

Petersen, R. W., Ung, K., Holland, C., & Quinlivan, J. A. (2005). The impact of molar pregnancy on psychological symptomatology, sexual function, and quality of life. *Gynecologic Oncology, 97,* 535–542.

Pruzinsky, T., & Cash, T. F. (1990). Integrative themes in body image development, deviance, and change. In Cash, T. F., & Pruzinsky, T., (Eds.), *Body images: Development, deviance, and change* (pp. 337–349). New York: Guilford.

Rogers, N. M., & Cantu, A. G. (2009). The nurse's role in the prevention of cervical cancer among underserved and minority populations. *Journal of Community Health, 34,* 135–143.

Rossing, M. A., Wicklund, K. G., Cushing-Haugen, K. L., & Weiss, N. S. (2010). Predictive value of symptoms for early detection of ovarian cancer. *Journal of the National Cancer Institute, 102,* 222–229.

Salehi, S., Eloranta, S., Johanssen, A. L., Bergström, M., & Lambe, M. (2011). Reporting and incidence trends of hydatidiform mole in Sweden 1973–2004. *Acta Oncologica, 50,* 367–372.

Scottish Intercollegiate Guidelines Network [SIGN]. (2008). *Network management of cervical cancer: A national clinical guideline.* Edinburgh: Scottish Intercollegiate Guidelines Network.

Sebire, N. J., & Seckl, M. J. (2008). Gestational trophoblastic disease: Current management of hydatidiform mole. *British Medical Journal, 337,* 453–458.

Smith, A. M., Heywood, W., Ryall, R., Shelley, J. M., Pitts, M. K., Richters, J., & Patrick, K. (2011). Association between sexual behavior and cervical cancer screening. *Journal of Women's Health, 20,* 1091–1096.

Spector, A. R. (2004). Psychological issues and interventions with infertile patients. *Women & Therapy, 27,* 91–105.

Stavraka, C., Ford, A., Ghaem-Maghami, S., Crook, T., Agarwal, R., Gabra, H., & Blagden, S. (2012). A study of symptoms described by ovarian cancer survivors. *Gynecologic Oncology, 125,* 59–64.

Stocker, M. (1991). *Cancer is a woman's issue: Scratching the surface.* Chicago: Third Side Press.

Taylor, C. L. C., Basen-Engquist, K., Shinn, E. H., & Bodurka, D. C. (2004). Predictors of sexual functioning in ovarian cancer patients. *Journal of Clinical Oncology, 22,* 881–889.

Taylor, S. E. (1983). Adjustment to threatening events: A theory of cognitive adaptation. *American Psychologist, 41,* 1161–1173.

Taylor, S. E. (2009). *Health psychology* (8th ed.). New York: McGraw-Hill.

Taylor, S. E., & Langer, E. J. (1977). Pregnancy: A social stigma? *Sex Roles, 3,* 27–35.

Thanopoulou, E., & Judson, I. (2012). Hormonal therapy in gynecological sarcomas. *Expert Review of Anticancer Therapy, 12,* 885–894.

U.S. Cancer Statistics Working Group. (n.d.). *United States cancer statistics: 1999–2008 incidence and mortality web-based report.* Atlanta, GA: U.S. Department of Health and Human Services, Centers for Disease Control and Prevention, & National Cancer Institute. Retrieved from www.cdc.gov/uscs.

Vergote, I., Tropé, C. G., Amant, F., Kristensen, G. B., Ehlen, T., Johnson, N., & Reed, N. S. (2010). Neoadjuvant chemotherapy or primary surgery in stage IIIC or IV ovarian cancer. *New England Journal of Medicine, 363,* 943–953.

Voda, A. M. (1997). *Menopause, me and you.* New York: Harrington Park Press.

Voda, A. M., & Ashton, C. A. (2006). Fallout from the Women's Health Study: A short-lived vindication for feminists and the resurrection of hormone therapies. *Sex Roles, 54,* 401–411.

Williamson, M. L. (1992). Sexual adjustment after hysterectomy. *Journal of Obstetric, Gynecologic, and Neonatal Nursing, 21,* 42–47.

World Health Organization. (1983). *Gestational trophoblastic diseases.* Geneva: WHO. Retrieved from http://whqlibdoc.who.int/trs/WHO_TRS_692.pdf.

Zeng, Y. C., Li, D., & Loke, A. Y. (2011). Life after cervical cancer: Quality of life among Chinese women. *Nursing & Health Sciences, 13,* 296–302.

Chapter 7

Psychological Sequelae of Cancer in Women during the Acute Phase of Survival

Meagan A. Medina, Bridget R. Kennedy, Cecily A. Luft, Paula K. Lundberg-Love, and Jeanine M. Galusha

INTRODUCTION

Cancer is a serious worldwide health problem. More than 7.5 million people died of cancer in 2008, making it the world's leading cause of death (Ferlay et al., 2010). In that same year, there were a recorded 692,000 cancer cases among U.S. women (Ferlay et al., 2010). Moreover, research indicates that one in three women in the United States will be diagnosed with cancer in her lifetime (Siegel et al., 2012). Once diagnosed, patients must begin what is often a long and arduous battle against the disease with the primary goal of defeating cancer and achieving long-term survival. Survival can be broken down into four phases: acute, transitional, extended, and permanent (Mullan, 1985; Miller, Merry, & Miller, 2008). The acute period includes the initial cancer diagnosis and treatment. The transitional stage occurs when the patient completes active treatment and transitions to medical observation. Extended survival indicates when a patient is either living with cancer as a chronic disease or has achieved possible remission. Patients in the permanent survival phase are usually in remission, are asymptomatic, and have a lower chance of cancer recurrence (Mullan, 1985; Miller et al., 2008, Morgan, 2009). This chapter focuses primarily on the psychological sequelae of cancer in women who are currently in the acute phase of survivorship.

PSYCHOLOGICAL EFFECTS OF CANCER DIAGNOSIS

A cancer patient may struggle to find ways in which to cope with her diagnosis and the disease's numerous life-altering effects, such as fatigue, insomnia, pain, appetite changes, disruption of family and social functioning, and the possibility of death (Mock et al., 2005; Peckmann et al., 2009; Beatty, Oxlad, Koczwara, & Wade, 2008; Morgan, 2009). While cancer's toll on the body is certainly debilitating in the physical sense, a battle with this disease also negatively impacts one's social and emotional well-being. These areas of psychosocial concern are often referred to as survivorship issues. Immediately following diagnosis, women will likely struggle with distress, adjustment, acquiring coping skills, and grappling with their own mortality (Beatty et al., 2008). These problems are often compounded when women face complicated diagnostic issues like the development of cervical cancer due to a sexually transmitted disease or being diagnosed during pregnancy (Kahn et al., 2007; Henry, Huang, Sproule, & Cardonick, 2012). This section elaborates on some of the most widespread survivorship issues faced by women newly diagnosed with cancer.

Distress is a term widely used to refer to the continuum of psychological sequelae associated with cancer diagnosis. It is defined as "pain or suffering affecting the body, a bodily part, or the mind" (Merriam-Webster, 2012). The National Comprehensive Cancer Network uses the term *distress* to address the unpleasant emotional experiences (psychological, social, and/or spiritual) of individuals coping with cancer because network members view it as less stigmatizing than psychological terminology (2012). The continuum of distress that diagnosed individuals may experience ranges from common feelings of vulnerability, grief, and worry to clinically significant symptoms associated with psychological diagnoses, such as depression and anxiety (Evans et al., 2005; Stark et al., 2002). Beatty et al. (2008) noted that at diagnosis, it is common for women to react with anguish, shock, anger, fear, and even self-blame. Across different age and ethnicity groups, approximately one-third to one-half of individuals diagnosed with any type of cancer experience psychological distress (Derogatis, et al., 1983; Weiss, Weinberger, Holland, Nelson, & Moadel, 2012; Zabora, Brintzenhofeszoc, Curbow, Hooker, & Piantadosi, 2001). Research has indicated that distress varies by cancer site, with greater distress accompanying cancers that have a higher mortality rate. Other factors that may predict distress susceptibility are younger age, lack of adequate social support, and lower socioeconomic level.

In response to the distress of an initial diagnosis, it is common for women to react in different ways. For instance, some women openly deal with the emotions bombarding them, while others choose to repress them (Al-Azri, Al-Awisi, & Al-Moundhri, 2009; Drageset, Lindstrom, & Underlid, 2010). Coping strategies can be identified by naming their underlying themes. Some common approaches include "preparing for the worst," "step-by-step," "pushing away," "business as usual," and "enjoying life" (Drageset et al., 2010, p. 151). Women may "prepare for the worst" by allowing themselves to engage in pessimistic thoughts, such as imagining that the worst will happen. Conversely, women may utilize a "step-by-step" approach by ignoring problems that might arise in the future and instead focusing on the present situation. A "step-by-step" approach may help women reduce worry and minimize feelings of being overwhelmed by future concerns. "Pushing away" is characterized by distancing oneself emotionally from reality and pushing distressing thoughts out of one's mind. This strategy has been found to be ineffective for many women because often times distressing thoughts will return. Many women find comfort in using a "business as usual" approach in which they live life as usual and become absorbed in their ordinary routines. This strategy helps many women feel as though they have a sense of control in their lives. "Enjoying life" is characterized by focusing on what is truly important and participating in activities that help with the coping process. For women who utilize this coping approach, it may be important for them to take time off work to focus on more meaningful activities.

Since there are countless different ways in which patients can cope with a cancer diagnosis, researchers often group them according to their positions along an approach-avoidance continuum. According to Stanton, Revenson, and Tennen (2007), approach-oriented coping strategies "include information seeking, actively attempting to identify benefit in one's experience, and creating outlets for emotional expression," while those falling under the avoidance category include "cognitive strategies such as denial and suppression and behavioral strategies such as disengagement" (p. 576). Studies have revealed relationships between the use of avoidance coping strategies and higher levels of psychological distress, psychological maladjustment, and poorer quality of life (Hack & Degner, 2004; Stanton et al., 2007; Lehto, Ojanen, & Kellokumpu-Lehtinen, 2005). Avoidance coping also has been linked to fear of future cancer recurrence and may even place women at a higher risk of developing post-traumatic stress disorder (PTSD) (Mehnert, Berg, Henrich, & Herschbach, 2009). Research suggests that women may choose coping strategies that correspond to their attitude toward their cancer diagnoses. Franks and Roesch (2006) discovered that women who viewed their disease as a loss or harmful to their lives were more likely to employ avoidance-oriented coping strategies, but those who saw their cancer as more of a challenge used more approach-oriented strategies.

The coping strategy that a woman utilizes in response to the distress she experiences after a cancer diagnosis often affects her ongoing adjustment (Henselmans et al., 2010; Schou, Ekeberg, & Ruland, 2005). For example, Degner, Hack, O'Neil, & Kristjanson (2003) found that the meaning a woman ascribes to her cancer diagnosis could affect her mental health status at a three-year follow-up examination. Women who used negative words to describe the meaning of their diagnoses were more likely to report anxiety or depression and a poorer quality of life at their follow-up than were women who indicated a more positive meaning. Cancer patients who tend to cope by catastrophizing, or making a catastrophe out of the situation, are more likely to have increased levels of emotional distress, depression, anxiety, and pain intensity (Fischer, Villines, Kim, Epstein, & Wilkie, 2010; Sullivan et al., 2001). Despite the hardships that accompany a cancer diagnosis, a woman's ability to cope with her diagnosis in a positive or optimistic way may assuage the potential severity of her distress and improve her quality of life (Degner et al., 2003; Lehto et al., 2005).

The diagnosis of cervical cancer presents unique problems and stressors for women. According to the World Health Organization (2010), the human papillomavirus (HPV) affects many women throughout the world and is responsible for 99 percent of cervical cancer cases. Because HPV is a sexually transmitted infection, a cervical cancer diagnosis carries an extra stigma associated with perceived promiscuity and fear about transmitting the virus to future partners (Posner & Vessey, 1988; Clarke, Ebel, Catotti, & Stewart, 1996).

Research on the psychological effects of cervical cancer has focused primarily on women's reactions to obtaining abnormal results on a Pap smear. Wardle, Pernet, and Stephens (1995) found that women who received Pap smear results that indicated a need for further testing had higher levels of anxiety than women who had normal results according to the state anxiety scale of the Spielberger State-Trait Anxiety Inventory. In addition to higher anxiety, these women indicated that they felt worse about their general state of health and well-being as measured by the General Health Questionnaire. Waller, McCaffery, Kitchener, Nazroo, and Wardle (2007) followed up on women with one positive HPV test and found that their anxiety did resolve over time with education from the medical community and family support. However, a second positive result a year later led to much higher levels of anxiety and fear. Women in the study had a stated preference for definitive cancer screening over waiting on the results of a third HPV screening. Thus, the uncertainty of not knowing whether the HPV had caused cervical cancer was more distressing than the initial HPV diagnosis.

Kahn et al. (2007) examined the psychological reactions of adolescent and young adult women after receiving a diagnosis of HPV and/or abnormal Pap smear results. The study indicated that young women feared stigma from peers and sexual rejection by their partners in addition to the concerns that they had about their health and prognosis. The majority also placed blame on themselves alone for the diagnosis, experiencing self-directed guilt rather than shared guilt with a partner. Maissi et al. (2004) found that abnormal or borderline Pap smear results produced high levels of state anxiety in women even if subsequent testing showed that the woman was HPV negative. They emphasize the need for better education of women on the meaning of the tests and on risk factors for developing cervical cancer. A study of leaflets given out to patients after abnormal Pap smear results found that patient education materials that focused on giving accurate medical information as well as answering social questions such as how the results would impact future sexual partners did the most to alleviate their stress (Hall, Howard, & McCaffery, 2008).

Cancer diagnosis during pregnancy is another issue that can understandably amplify a patient's levels of distress. According to Henry et al. (2012), "When patients are diagnosed with cancer during pregnancy, feelings of hopelessness and fear of death can be intertwined with the joy and normal stresses of becoming a mother" (p. 448). Research has found that the presence of cancer during pregnancy often poses a risk to a patient's unborn child and even to her infant, which understandably increases distress in pregnant cancer patients (Henry et al., 2012). Some examples of situations that increase this risk include giving birth prematurely, being unable to produce sufficient breast milk, and undergoing surgery during or after pregnancy. Women who were advised to terminate their pregnancies due to cancer treatments, and therefore had to make decisions between their health and the life of the fetus, were more distressed than those who faced no such decision. In addition, women who conceived without fertility treatments before their cancer diagnosis were significantly more distressed than those who had utilized fertility assistance. It is speculated that the greater access to outside therapy and support provided to women undergoing fertility treatment may help to reduce their distress upon cancer diagnosis during pregnancy (Boivin, 2003; Henry et al., 2012). Due to the limited amount of research with this population, there is much room for further study on the psychological effects of cancer diagnosis during pregnancy.

PSYCHOLOGICAL SEQUELAE OF CANCER TREATMENT

Once a woman is diagnosed with cancer, she must carefully consider her treatment options. The most common treatments are one or a combination of the following: surgery, radiation, and chemotherapy (World

Health Organization, 2012). Much of the research on cancer's treatment effects has focused on women with breast cancer who have undergone either a full mastectomy or a lumpectomy and then followed with adjuvant chemotherapy and radiation in order to prevent the cancer from returning (Engel, Kerr, Schlesinger-Raab, Sauer, & Hölzel, 2004; King, Kenny, Shiell, Hall, & Boyages, 2001; Arora et al., 2001). Surgery, chemotherapy, and radiation often cause debilitating physical side effects that interrupt women's lives, such as fatigue, insomnia, nausea and vomiting, and pain (Montgomery, Schnur, Erblich, Diefenbach, & Bovbjerg, 2010; Engel et al., 2004). This section focuses on the psychological consequences, both negative and positive, that result from the treatment of cancer in women.

The widespread psychological sequelae of cancer treatments and their physical side effects include negatively impacting a woman's body image, sexual functioning, self-concept, and social and emotional well-being. Furthermore, due to the uncertainty surrounding her long-term prognosis and chance of survival even upon completion of treatment, it is typical for a woman to react with symptoms of distress, depression, anxiety, and the fear of future cancer recurrence (Beatty et al., 2008; Engel et al., 2004; Arora et al., 2001; Mock et al., 2005; Fischer et al., 2010; Norton et al., 2005).

Cancer treatments significantly impact survivors' body image and sexual functioning. Body image concerns are often a result of the physical side effects of treatment like scarring, hair loss, weight changes, and breast removal (Montgomery et al., 2010; Tierney, 2008; Beatty et al., 2008). These physical side effects can shake a woman's self-confidence and lead to feelings that she is unattractive. Cancer treatment's negative impact on a survivor's body image is just one way treatment can impact sexual functioning. Tierney (2008) focused on the physical, psychological, and social effects of how cancer and its treatment had negatively impacted cancer patients' sexuality. Chemotherapy, radiation, and surgeries that remove breasts and reproductive organs have been shown to affect women's ovaries and hormone levels, cause menopause and infertility, produce vaginal dryness and atrophy, diminish physical stamina, alter the cycle of sexual responses, reduce sexual desire, lower self-confidence, and strain sexual interpersonal relationships (Tierney, 2008; Cantinelli et al., 2006).

Surgery, chemotherapy, and radiation also have the power to alter a woman's self-concept. Beatty et al. (2008) found that many breast cancer survivors complained that they seemed to have lost sight of who they were. The women also observed that their roles at home and in the community had changed due to the physical side effects of cancer and its treatment, such as fatigue and weakness. They longed to regain normalcy in their daily lives and searched for new senses of self that could distinguish them from their public labels as cancer survivors.

Women's experiences of the physical and psychological consequences of cancer treatment are interrelated in various ways. Norton et al. (2005) found that an ovarian cancer survivor's level of psychological distress was related to the physical impairment she suffered from the cancer and its treatment. Similarly, cancer patients' levels of depression have been associated with their levels of physical discomfort stemming from the cancer and its treatment (Given et al.,1993). Moreover, So et al. (2009) analyzed the common symptom cluster of pain, fatigue, anxiety, and depression and found significant associations between all four symptom variables. According to Montgomery et al. (2010), a woman's psychological state can influence her subsequent experience of the physical side effects. The study discovered that a woman's expectancies about the outcomes of treatment along with the amount of distress she suffered before cancer surgery actually predicted her levels of post-surgery nausea, pain, and fatigue. This indicates that "patients with higher pre-surgery levels of expectancies and emotional distress appear to be at greater risk for experiencing higher levels of post-surgery side effects" (Montgomery et al., 2010, p. 1049). The authors of the study recommended implementing psychological interventions prior to surgery in an effort to decrease cancer patients' psychological distress and expectancies and therefore improve their recoveries. Since survivors' psychological concerns are often intertwined with their physical side effects, it is important to provide them with resources and interventions that aim to protect and nurture their psychological health in addition to their physical conditions.

Positive life changes, also referred to as benefit-finding or post-traumatic growth, often accompany the experiences of cancer treatment and diagnosis (Kucukkaya, 2010; Horgan, Holcombe, & Salmon, 2011; Lechner et al., 2003; Park, 2009; Taha, Matheson, & Anisman, 2012). Positive changes generally relate to a sense of personal growth resulting from the challenges of cancer. Personal growth can be shaped by one's self in relation to others, life philosophy, and/or one's perception of self. Specifically, positive changes may include increased resilience and self-reliance, improved relationships with friends and family, and enhanced appreciation for life.

Research has indicated that a large percentage of women treated for cancer experience positive life changes. Sears, Stanton, and Danoff-Burg (2003) found that 83 percent of women reported at least one benefit of their breast cancer experience. Cordova, Cunningham, Carlson, and Andrykowski (2001) revealed that breast cancer patients were more likely to experience post-traumatic growth than healthy controls after completion of treatment. In particular, breast cancer survivors demonstrated greater personal growth in relating to others, appreciation of life, and spiritual change. For example, a personal friend of one of the authors was recently diagnosed with coronary artery disease (CAD). Her response was that she had survived thyroid cancer and breast cancer and was not going to let

CAD kill her. Women also have been found to experience long-term positive changes following their cancer treatment. Carver and Antoni (2004) established a link between patients' initial benefit-finding and subsequent lower levels of distress and depression up to 8 years after a breast cancer diagnosis. Mols, Vingerhoets, Coebergh, and van de Poll-Franse (2009) found that 10 years after treatment, 79 percent of disease-free breast cancer survivors reported benefit-finding and significantly higher life satisfaction than controls. Similarly, Lelorain, Bonnaud-Antignac, and Florin (2010) reported that survivors of breast cancer, up to 15 years after treatment, continued to experience post-traumatic growth and a better appreciation of life. Recently, Schroevers, Kraaij, and Garnefski (2011) found that an individual's ability to acknowledge positive changes in her/his life as a result of cancer is related to his or her well-being, positive affect, and coping and goal-related strategies. They also reported that avoiding challenges rather than approaching them was associated with more negative life changes. The authors emphasized that patients can be assisted in learning to identify positive changes, approaching difficult situations, and creating meaningful life goals to support personal growth.

INTERVENTIONS AND SYMPTOM MANAGEMENT TECHNIQUES

Surgery, radiation, and chemotherapy are often supplemented with psychosocial interventions and hormone replacement therapy, which are designed to help a woman manage the psychological and physiological symptoms resulting from the disease and its treatment (Brem & Kumar, 2011). In addition to these intervention programs, research has revealed factors that may affect the psychological health and recovery of cancer patients. A few key mediating factors include social support, positive affect, spirituality, and the ability to return to work. This section will discuss the various intervention techniques and other factors that have been found to help alleviate disease and treatment-related symptoms and improve the quality of life of cancer patients.

There are many varieties of psychosocial intervention programs for cancer patients (Rehse & Pukrop, 2003). These programs include but are not limited to: group therapy, cognitive behavioral therapy, psychoeducational programs, mindfulness techniques, and telephone/internet counseling (McGregor & Antoni, 2009; Goodwin et al., 2001; Balabanovic, Ayers, & Hunter, 2012; Sheldon, Swanson, Dolce, Marsh, & Summers, 2008; Shennan, Payne, & Fenlon, 2011). Psychosocial interventions have been shown to improve the quality of life of adult cancer patients in a variety of ways. Moreover, research suggests that all programs, regardless of the specific type of intervention utilized, should be implemented for at least 12 weeks in order to maximize their effectiveness (Rehse & Pukrop, 2003).

Cognitive behavioral and stress management interventions are the most common programs used to help cancer patients who also suffer from depression and/or anxiety. Specific techniques include: guided imagery, progressive muscle relaxation, diaphragmatic breathing, and cognitive restructuring (McGregor & Antoni, 2009; Van den Beuken-van Everdingen et al., 2009). These types of interventions can help cancer patients adapt psychologically to their conditions, reduce their symptoms of anxiety and depression, and improve their health due to increased optimism, positive affect, and benefit-finding (McGregor & Antoni, 2009; Antoni et al., 2006; Antoni et al., 2001).

Consistently, studies have found that group treatment for women with cancer is associated with improvements in social functioning, mood, coping skills, and anxiety management (Balabanovic et al., 2012; Oz, Dil, Inci, & Kamisli, 2012). Group treatment even has been shown to reduce cancer patients' perception of pain after treatment (Goodwin et al., 2001). Additionally, research has indicated that telephone and Internet-based support groups could be an appropriate medium for some women battling cancer. A recent study by Sherman et al. (2012) found that participants of a telephone counseling group demonstrated decreased distress and side-effect severity. However, there was a decline in psychological well-being through the ongoing recovery phase, indicating that some adjustment issues were present during this period. Wiljer et al. (2011) found that women benefited from participation in an Internet-based support group. These benefits included the support of other members, increased emotional well-being, improved body image and sexuality, and comfort in discussing sexual issues online.

Psychoeducation, which refers to programs that provide patients with information regarding a cancer diagnosis and treatment, resources and providers, as well as self-care and symptom management, can have a positive impact on cancer patients (Sheldon et al., 2008). In a metastudy of psychoeducational approaches, Fors et al. (2011) found that the effect of psychoeducation varied with the type of program offered. Education programs that focused on prewritten or pretaped sessions reported little positive change, but face-to-face or telephone contact positively impacted quality of life measures and reduced anxiety and fatigue. Sherman et al. (2012) found that patients who received telephone counseling reported less distress during treatment. However, showing patients psychoeducational videotapes did not change their levels of distress significantly more than did standard care and the passage of time. The Breast Cancer Intervention Education program, which was tailored to the needs of the patients by trained psychoeducators, had both short- and long-term effects on the quality of life of the participants (Meneses et al., 2007). Women who completed the program reported better quality of life in physical, psychological, social, and spiritual areas as compared to baseline levels, while women in the control group had lower than baseline outcomes on those measures at both three months and six months after the program. Dolbeault et al. (2009) tested an eight-week psychoeducational program that included specific training on stress management and was based on such cognitive therapy techniques as cognitive restructuring. They found reductions in anxiety, anger, fatigue, and depression in women who participated in the program. Similarly, Sheldon et al. (2008) observed that psychoeducational interventions could aid in reducing and preventing anxiety. While psychoeducation is not a guarantee of better coping or psychological outcomes, well-developed programs that incorporate contact with the patient and follow-up can be quite beneficial for women in cancer treatment.

Mindfulness and its mediating effects on illness, including cancer, is a growing field of research. Mindfulness encompasses a wide range of ideas and practices. The most commonly studied mindfulness program utilized with cancer patients in treatment and recovery is the mindfulness-based stress reduction program (MBSR) (Shennan et al., 2011). MBSR, which has been adapted specifically for those suffering with breast cancer, is a group program that teaches mindfulness skills, such as sitting meditation, walking meditation, body scanning, and mindful movement, over an eight-week course. Breast cancer patients and survivors who participated in an MBSR program displayed several advantageous psychological and physiological effects, including augmented quality of life measures, improved coping skills, stress reduction, reduced blood pressure, lowered heart rate, and short-term cortisol reduction (Witek-Janusek et al., 2008; Matchim, Armer, & Stewart, 2011). MBSR also has been effective in reducing sleep disturbances and fatigue (Lengacher et al., 2012). Mindfulness-based cognitive therapy (MBCT) is another program emerging with promising research results. Originally created to treat depression and anxiety, MBCT has the same core components as the MBSR program but uses a smaller average group size and more structured meditation exercises (Shennan et al., 2011). Studies have shown that it is effective in decreasing depression, anxiety, distress, and treatment-related fatigue while at the same time increasing mindfulness and quality of life in cancer patients (Foley, Baillie, Huxter, Price, & Sinclair, 2010; van der Lee & Garssen, 2012).

One serious consequence of surgical, hormonal, and radiation therapy in women is the early onset of menopausal symptoms. According to a metastudy by King, Wynne, Assersohn, and Jones (2011), the menopausal symptoms brought on by cancer treatment are more severe and appear more rapidly than is usual with natural menopause. Women reported early onset of physical symptoms, such as hot flashes, weight gain, sleep disturbance, urinary problems, and sexual problems. Psychosocial symptoms are also common according to Befort and Klemp (2011), who cite growing evidence that menopausal status and/or age can predict severity of negative symptoms related to cancer treatment. These psychosocial symptoms include fear that cancer will recur, concerns about body image, depression, fear of death, changes in relationships with family members, and financial stress. Women who were premenopausal at the time of cancer treatment reported higher rates of these concerns than did older women who were postmenopausal at the time of initial treatment. Hormone replacement therapy may mediate some symptoms in women with early onset menopause, but further research into both its efficacy and long-term safety is needed (King et al., 2011).

Positive social support of family and friends appears to contribute to the well-being of women with cancer and has been associated with improved adaptation to the illness, emotional comfort, encouragement, material assistance, and generally increased quality of life (Bettencourt, Schlegel, Talley, & Molix, 2007; Nausheen, Gidron, Peveler, & Moss-Morris, 2009; Sandgren, Mullens, Erickson, Romanek, & McCaul, 2004; So et al., 2009). A study by Lutgendorf et al. (2005) has indicated that social support may even facilitate immune function and decrease the likelihood of cancer recurrence.

Conversely, studies have indicated that a lack of social support or unsupportive social interactions may have negative effects on women with cancer, including anxiety, depression, and intensified distress (Figueiredo, Fries, & Ingram, 2004; Iwamitsu et al., 2005; Manne, Winkel, Ostroff, Grana, & Fox, 2005). Recently, Jones, Hadjistavropoulos, and Sherry (2012) linked unsupportive social interactions to increased health anxiety. Similarly, Chan, Limoges, and Fung (2010) found that lower levels of functional social support were associated with major depression in a sample of adult cancer patients.

According to Arora, Rutten, Gustafson, Moser, and Hawkins (2007), women generally received high levels of support closely following their diagnoses, but this support significantly decreased over time. The authors speculated that this could be due to support-provider burnout, a misunderstanding as to how to provide support, or a patient's decreased desire for support. Results also indicated that helpful support at baseline was less likely to be reported by women of color, women with lower levels of education, and women who lacked private insurance.

Support from one's partner or spouse has particular importance and has been shown to greatly affect the lives of women battling cancer. Gremore et al. (2011) reported that daily spousal support contributed to the emotional and physical well-being of women with breast cancer. Wittenberg et al. (2010) found that while single marital status was associated with an increase in the reexperiencing of cancer-related symptoms, married women showed a greater increase in emotional well-being shortly after breast cancer diagnosis. These findings indicate that women who are not married or partnered may need more outside support than do those who have a partner.

While studies on cancer's psychological effects have shown the crucial role a patient's social support network plays in her ongoing recovery, it is important to acknowledge the impact that a woman's cancer has on the life of her partner. Baucom et al. (2012) reported that the well-being of male partners of women with early-stage breast cancer could be related to factors associated with their spouse's well-being. Factors identified by the authors included the female partner's well-being, physical symptoms, relationship functioning, and relationship duration. Similarly, it has been shown that spouses experienced equivalent levels of distress and had as much difficulty with social adjustment as did their wives who were battling cancer (Peleg-Oren & Sherer, 2001; Baider, Ever-Hadani, Godzweig, Wygoda, & Peretz, 2003). Conversely, male partners may also share the positive changes that result from their wives' cancer experiences, such as post-traumatic growth (Weiss, 2002). These studies indicate that cancer diagnosis and treatment are life-changing events for cancer patients and their partners. Therefore, it is necessary to care for the psychological health of both the patient and her social support network during this time of crisis (Peleg-Oren & Sherer, 2001).

Positive affect, defined as pleasant emotional states such as joy, excitement, peace, and contentment, may serve as an additional psychological buffer for cancer patients. Hou, Law, & Fu (2010) considered positive affect to be a psychosocial resource. They found that Chinese cancer patients with higher levels of positive affect, as measured by the Positive Affect subscale of the Chinese Affect Scale, reported lower incidences of depression during treatment, while those with lower positive affect reported significant increases in anxiety and depression. Hirsch, Floyd, and Duberstein (2012) indicated that positive affect was related to better perceived health in patients with lung cancer. Generally patients with positive affect showed better adaptive social functioning, fewer limitations based on emotions, and less severe bodily pain. Negative affect was associated with greater pain and reductions in overall quality of life. As such, psychosocial treatments that increase positive affect in patients may act as a protective factor against depressed mood, anxiety, severe bodily pain, and poor perceived health during and after treatment.

Researchers have sought to define the complex role that religion and spirituality play in how women cope with cancer, but these investigations have yielded very diverse results. Findings are predominantly split into two distinct groups: women who have more problems coping with cancer with increased religious participation, and women who find solace and acceptance through spiritual beliefs. Gall, Kristjansson, Charbonneau, and Florack (2009) studied the relationship between spirituality and long-term adjustment to breast cancer. They found that women who had a high level of religious or spiritual involvement prior to diagnosis reported lower levels of distress. Women who adopted a more religious belief system at or after diagnosis, however, reported increased difficulty with adjustment. Turning to religion during the stressful time of diagnosis and treatment, therefore, did not appear to be protective. Gall, Charbonneau, and Florack (2011) found that religious involvement prediagnosis was negatively correlated with measures of personal growth two years after diagnosis. They hypothesized that women who believed in the benevolence of God and the possibility of miraculous recovery from illness prior to cancer diagnosis may lose hope or belief when no miraculous cure is forthcoming. The authors also reported that negative views of God predicted poor growth, but that positive views of God did not predict increased growth. Some aspects of religious salience did increase growth, but on the whole there was little protective influence of religion and spirituality. However, other studies have found that some religions and belief systems may be more protective than others. Alferi, Culver, Carver, Arena, and Antoni (1999) found that Evangelical Christian Hispanic women had better coping and quality of life outcomes than Catholic Hispanic women when dealing with breast cancer. Increased church attendance predicted better coping in the Evangelical women, but led to greater distress in the Catholic women. Social support from their respective spiritual communities also was related to better coping in Evangelical women and poorer results for Catholic women. More research is needed to discover the cause of this dichotomy, but the authors speculated that it may be related to the Evangelical focus on trusting in a higher plan as opposed to the Catholic focus on good works and confession. Ching, Martinson, and Wong (2012) discovered that Chinese women who framed their experiences with breast cancer as outside their personal control and who adopted an attitude of "following the natural course" of the cancer had improved coping mechanisms over women who adopted a fighting attitude (p. 253). One of the most important of these mechanisms was a belief in a sustaining force that would make their suffering bearable. Ahmad, Muhammad, and Abdullah (2011) studied the role of religion in the coping of Malaysian Muslim women recovering from treatment for breast cancer. They found that Muslim spirituality, and specifically the concept of surrendering control to Allah, decreased distress and led to positive emotions about their experience with breast cancer. The women reported that they believed their cancer was a gift from Allah and allowed them to appreciate their lives more. These studies, though small and mostly qualitative, seem to indicate that relinquishing personal control over cancer treatment can reduce distress. Further testing, preferably with larger sample sizes, is required to confirm this effect.

A cancer survivor's ability to return to work often depends on the severity of her treatment. Generally as cancer treatments become more invasive, patients take longer to recover and experience more health and adjustment problems when they are able to go back to work. Although the physical and psychological effects of cancer and its treatment pose unique challenges for cancer survivors in the workplace, returning to work helps them regain a sense of normalcy and structure in their everyday lives (Rasmussen & Elverdam, 2008; Kennedy, Haslam, Munir, & Pryce, 2007). Going back to work after treatment is positively correlated with psychological health, satisfaction with work situation, current capacity in daily living, somatic health, global health satisfaction, and overall improvement in quality of life (Johnsson, Fornander, Rutqvist, & Olsson, 2011; Rasmussen & Elverdam, 2008). Despite the additional difficulties their treatments and recoveries pose, cancer survivors are productive and function well when they go back to their jobs (Bradley & Bednarek, 2002). In order to facilitate a reintegration that benefits both the cancer survivors and their workplaces, it is important for employers to be flexible, supportive, and accommodating to the needs of this population (Kennedy et al., 2007).

CONCLUSIONS

Since one in three American women will be diagnosed with cancer during her lifetime, it is likely that the readers of this chapter either know a woman who has been diagnosed with the disease or they have battled with cancer themselves (Siegel et al., 2012). A cancer diagnosis is a traumatic and life-altering event that affects a woman both physically and psychologically. Women in the acute phase of survival not only have to make critical choices regarding treatment, but they must also manage survivorship issues like distress, finding a way to cope, and considering their own mortality. In order to rid their bodies of this disease, cancer patients often undergo extensive treatments like surgery, chemotherapy, and radiation, which are necessary for survival but often negatively affect their body images, sexual functioning, concept of self, and social and emotional well-being.

Indeed, during the final revision of this chapter, one of the coauthors received information that she had a "suspicious" mammogram. Within three days she had another mammogram and an ultrasound procedure. It was determined that a biopsy should be performed. That occurred the following week. During those two weeks this coauthor engaged in many of the coping strategies outlined on page 4 of this chapter. The levels of anxiety and fear were overwhelming, even though this coauthor is a therapist and was utilizing various therapeutic interventions. While the results of the biopsy indicated that the tissue was benign and that there was probably a traumatic injury to the breast, this experience personally illustrated the information contained in this chapter. Our coauthor is scheduled for another mammogram in six months to clarify further whether these abnormalities are part of an inflammatory process or perhaps a malignancy.

Our chapter has sought to educate the reader on the complex psychological effects of the diagnosis and treatment of cancer as well as the interventions and mediating factors that can help alleviate these symptoms and improve survivors' physical, social, and emotional health. While progress is currently being made, research should continue to focus on further advances in cancer education and prevention programs, early detection and diagnosis, improvements in treatment, psychological interventions, and symptom management techniques in order to improve the quality of life of current cancer patients and protect future generations from this pervasive disease (World Health Organization, 2012; Siegel et al., 2012; Ganz, 2004).

REFERENCES

Ahmad, F., Muhammad, M., & Abdullah, A. A. (2011). Religion and spirituality in coping with advanced breast cancer: Perspectives from Malaysian Muslim women. *Journal of Religion and Health, 50,* 36–45.

Al-Azri, M., Al-Awisi, H., & Al-Moundhri, M. (2009). Coping with a diagnosis of breast cancer-literature review and implication for developing countries. *The Breast Journal, 15,* 615–622.

Alferi, S. M., Culver, J. L., Carver, C. S., Arena, P. L., & Antoni, M. H. (1999). Religiosity, religious coping, and distress: A prospective study of Catholic and Evangelical Hispanic women in treatment for early-stage breast cancer. *Journal of Health Psychology, 4,* 343–356.

Antoni, M. H., Lechner, S. C., Kazi, A., Wimberly, S. R., Sifre, T., Urcuyo, K. R., . . . Carver, C. S. (2006). How stress management improves quality of life after treatment for breast cancer. *Journal of Consulting and Clinical Psychology, 74,* 1143–1152.

Antoni, M. H., Lehman, J. M., Kilbourn, K. M., Boyers, A. E., Culver, J. L., Alferi, S. M., & Carver, C. S. (2001). Cognitive-behavioral stress management intervention decreases the prevalence of depression and enhances benefit finding among women under treatment for early-stage breast cancer. *Health Psychology, 20,* 20–32.

Arora, N. K., Gustafson, D. H., Hawkins, R. P., McTavish, F., Cella, D. F., Pingree, S., . . . Mahvi, D. M. (2001). Impact of surgery and chemotherapy on the quality of life of younger women with breast carcinoma: A prospective study. *Cancer, 92,* 1288–1298.

Arora, N. K., Rutten L. J. F., Gustafson, D. H., Moser, R., & Hawkins, R. P. (2007). Perceived helpfulness and impact of social support provided by family, friends, and health care providers to women newly diagnosed with breast cancer. *Psycho-Oncology, 16,* 474–486.

Baider, L., Ever-Hadani, P., Godzweig, G., Wygoda, M. R., & Peretz, T. (2003). Is perceived family support a relevant variable in psychological distress? A sample of prostate and breast cancer couples. *Journal of Psychosomatic Research, 55,* 453–460.

Balabanovic, J., Ayers, B., & Hunter, M. S. (2012). Women's experiences of group cognitive behaviour therapy for hot flushes and night sweats following breast cancer treatment: An interpretative phenomenological analysis. *Maturitas, 72,* 236–242.

Baucom, D. H., Kirby, J. S., Pukay-Martin, N. D., Porter, L. S., Fredman, S. J., Gremore, T. M., . . . Atkins, D. (2012). Men's psychological functioning in the context of women's breast cancer. *Journal of Marital and Family Therapy, 38,* 317–329.

Beatty, L., Oxlad, M., Koczwara, B., & Wade, T. D. (2008). The psychosocial concerns and needs of women recently diagnosed with breast cancer: A qualitative study of patient, nurse, and volunteer perspectives. *Health Expectations, 11,* 331–342.

Befort, C.A., & Klemp, J. (2011). Sequelae of breast cancer and the influence of menopausal status at diagnosis among rural breast cancer survivors. *Journal of Women's Health, 20,* 1307–1313.

Bettencourt, B. A., Schlegel, R. J., Talley, A. E., & Molix, L. A. (2007). The breast cancer experience of rural women: A literature review. *Psycho-Oncology, 16,* 875–887.

Boivin, J. A. (2003). A review of psychosocial interventions in infertility. *Social Science & Medicine, 57,* 2325–2341.

Bradley, C. J., & Bednarek, H. L. (2002). Employment patterns of long-term cancer survivors. *Psycho-Oncology, 11,* 188–198.

Brem, S., and Kumar, N. B. (2011). Management of treatment-related symptoms in patients with breast cancer: Current strategies and future directions. *Clinical Journal of Oncology Nursing, 15,* 63–71.

Cantinelli, F. S., Scaramboni, F., Camacho, R. S., Smaletz, O., Gonsales, B. K., Braguittoni, E., & Rennó Jr., J. (2006). The oncopsychiatric of breast cancer: Considerations about female questions. *Revista de Psiquiatria Clínica, 33,* 124–133.

Carver, C. S., & Antoni, M. H. (2004). Finding benefit in breast cancer during the year after diagnosis predicts better adjustment 5 to 8 years after diagnosis. *Health Psychology, 23,* 595–598.

Chan, E. K. H., Limoges, K. M., & Fung, T. S. (2010). Functional social support and major depression in cancer patients. *Psychology Journal, 7,* 46–50.

Ching, S. S. Y., Martinson, I. M., & Wong, T. K. S. (2012). Meaning making: Psychological adjustment to breast cancer by Chinese women. *Qualitative Health Research, 22,* 250–262.

Clarke, P., Ebel, C., Catotti, D. N., & Stewart, S. (1996). The psychosocial impact of human papillomavirus infection: Implications for health care providers. *International Journal of STD and AIDS, 7,* 197–200.

Cordova, M. J., Cunningham, L. L. C., Carlson, C. R., & Andrykowski, M. A. (2001). Posttraumatic growth following breast cancer: A controlled comparison study. *Health Psychology, 20,* 176–185.

Degner, L., Hack, T., O'Neil, J., & Kristjanson, L. J. (2003). A new approach to eliciting meaning in the context of breast cancer. *Cancer Nursing 26,* 169–178.

Derogatis, L. R., Morrow, G. R., Fetting, J. H., Penman, D., Piasetsky, S., Schmale, A. M., . . . Carniche, C. L. (1983). The prevalence of psychiatric disorders among cancer patients. *The Journal of the American Medical Association, 249,* 751–757.

Dolbeault, S., Cayrou, S., Bredart, A., Viala, A. L., Desclaux, B., Saltel, P., . . . Dickes, P. (2009). The effectiveness of a psycho-educational group after early-stage breast cancer treatment: Results of a randomized French study. *Psycho-Oncology, 18,* 647–656.

Drageset, S., Lindstrom, T. C., & Underlid, K. (2010). Coping with breast cancer: Between diagnosis and surgery. *Journal of Advanced Nursing, 66,* 149–158.

Engel, J., Kerr, J., Schlesinger-Raab, A., Sauer, H., & Hölzel, D. (2004). Quality of life following breast-conserving therapy or mastectomy: Results of a 5-year prospective study. *The Breast Journal, 10,* 223–231.

Evans, D. L., Charney, D. S., Lewis, L., Golden, R. N., Gorman, J. M., Krishnan, K. R. R., . . . Valvo, W. J. (2005). Mood disorders in the medically ill: Scientific review and recommendations. *Biological Psychiatry, 58,* 175–189.

Ferlay, J., Shin, H. R., Bray, F., Forman, D., Mathers, C., & Parkin, D. M. (2010). GLOBOCAN 2008 v1.2: Cancer incidence and mortality worldwide. IARC CancerBase No. 10. Lyon, France: International Agency for Research on Cancer. Retrieved from http://globocan.iarc.fr/.

Figueiredo, M. I., Fries, E., & Ingram, K. M. (2004). The role of disclosure patterns and unsupportive social interactions in the well-being of breast cancer patients. *Psycho-Oncology, 13,* 96–105.

Fischer, D. J., Villines, D., Kim, Y. K., Epstein, J. B., & Wilkie, D. J. (2010). Anxiety, depression, and pain: Differences by primary cancer. *Support Cancer Care, 18,* 801–810.

Foley, E., Baillie, A., Huxter, M., Price, M., & Sinclair, E. (2010). Mindfulness-based cognitive therapy for individuals whose lives have been affected by cancer: A randomized controlled trial. *Journal of Consulting and Clinical Psychology, 78,* 72–79.

Fors, E. A., Bertheussen, G. F., Thune, I., Juvet, L. K., Elvsaas, I. K., Oldervalle, L., . . . Leivseth, G. (2011). Psychosocial interventions as part of breast cancer rehabilitation programs? Results from a systematic review. *Psycho-Oncology, 20,* 909–918.

Franks, H. M., & Roesch, S. C. (2006). Appraisals and coping in people living with cancer: A meta-analysis. *Psycho-Oncology, 15,* 1027–1037.

Gall, T. L., Charbonneau, C., & Florack, P. (2011). The relationship between religious/ spiritual factors and perceived growth following a diagnosis of breast cancer. *Psychology and Health, 26,* 287–305.

Gall, T. L., Kristjansson, E., Charbonneau, C., & Florack, P. (2009). A longitudinal study on the role of spirituality in response to the diagnosis and treatment of breast cancer. *Journal of Behavioral Medicine, 32,* 174–186.

Ganz, P. A. (2004). Quality of life at the end of primary treatment of breast cancer: First results from the moving beyond cancer randomized trial. *Journal of the National Cancer Institute, 96,* 376–387.

Given, C. W., Stommel, M., Given, B., Osuch, J., Kurtz, M. E., & Kurtz, J. C. (1993). The influence of cancer patients' symptoms and functional states on patients' depression and family caregivers' reaction and depression. *Health Psychology, 12,* 277–285.

Goodwin, P. J., Leszcz, M., Ennis, M., Koopmans, J., Vincent, L., Guther, H., . . . Hunter, J. (2001). The effect of group psychosocial support on survival in metastatic breast cancer. *New England Journal of Medicine, 345,* 1719–1726.

Gremore, T. M., Baucom, D. H., Porter, L. S., Kirby, J. S., Atkins, D. C., & Keefe, F. J. (2011). Stress buffering effects of daily spousal support on women's daily emotional and physical experiences in the context of breast cancer concerns. *Health Psychology, 30,* 20–30.

Hack, T. F., & Degner, L. F. (2004). Coping responses following breast cancer diagnosis predict psychological adjustment three years later. *Psycho-Oncology, 13,* 235–247.

Hall, B., Howard, K., & McCaffery, K. (2008). Do cervical cancer screening patient information leaflets meet the HPV information needs of women? *Patient Education and Counseling, 72,* 78–87.

Henry, M., Huang, L. N., Sproule, B. J., & Cardonick, E. H. (2012). The psychological impact of a cancer diagnosed during pregnancy: Determinants of long-term distress. *Psycho-Oncology, 21,* 444–450.

Henselmans, I., Helgeson, V. S., Seltman, H., de Vries, J., Sanderman, R., & Ranchor, A. V. (2010). Identification and prediction of distress trajectories in the first year after breast cancer diagnosis. *Health Psychology, 29,* 160–168.

Hirsch, J. K., Floyd, A. R., & Duberstein, P. R. (2012). Perceived health in lung cancer patients: The role of positive and negative affect. *Quality of Life Research: An International Journal of Quality of Life Aspects of Treatment, Care & Rehabilitation, 21,* 187–194.

Horgan, O., Holcombe, C., & Salmon, P. (2011). Experiencing positive change after a diagnosis of breast cancer: A grounded theory analysis. *Psycho-Oncology, 20,* 1116–1125.

Hou, W. K., Law, C. C., & Fu, Y. T. (2010). Does change in positive affect mediate and/or moderate the impact of symptom distress on psychological adjustment after cancer diagnosis? A prospective analysis. *Psychology and Health, 25,* 417–431.

Iwamitsu, Y., Shimoda, K., Abe, H., Tani, T., Okawa, M., & Buck, R. (2005). The relation between negative emotional suppression and emotional distress in breast cancer diagnosis and treatment. *Journal of Health Communication, 18,* 201–215.

Johnsson, A., Fornander, T., Rutqvist, L. E., & Olsson, M. (2011). Work status and life changes in the first year after breast cancer diagnosis. *Work, 38,* 337–346.

Jones, S. L., Hadjistavropoulos, H. D., & Sherry, S. B. (2012). Health anxiety in women with early-stage breast cancer: What is the relationship to social support? *Canadian Journal of Behavioural Science, 44,* 108–116.

Kahn, J. A., Slap, G. B., Bernstein, D. I., Tissot, A. M., Kollar, L. M., Hillard, P. A., & Rosenthal, S. L. (2007). Personal meaning of human papillomavirus and Pap test results in adolescent and young adult women. *Health Psychology, 26,* 192–200.

Kennedy, F., Haslam, C., Munir, F., & Pryce, J. (2007). Returning to work following cancer: A qualitative exploratory study into the experience of returning to work following cancer. *European Journal of Cancer Care, 16,* 17–25.

King, J., Wynne, C. H., Assersohn, L., & Jones, A. (2011). Hormone replacement therapy and women with premature menopause—A cancer survivorship issue. *European Journal of Cancer, 47,* 1623–1632.

King, M. T., Kenny, P., Shiell, A., Hall, J., & Boyages, J. (2001). Quality of life three months and one year after first treatment for early stage breast cancer: Influence of treatment and patient characteristics. *Quality of Life Research, 9,* 789–800.

Kucukkaya, P. G. (2010). An exploratory study of positive life changes in Turkish women diagnosed with breast cancer. *European Journal of Oncology Nursing, 14,* 166–173.

Lechner, S. C., Zakowski, S. G., Antoni, M. H., Greenhawt, M., Block, K., & Block, P. (2003). Do sociodemographic and disease-related variables influence benefit-finding in cancer patients? *Psycho-Oncology, 12,* 491–499.

Lehto, U-S., Ojanen, M., & Kellokumpu-Lehtinen, P. (2005). Predictors of quality of life in newly diagnosed melanoma and breast cancer patients. *Annals of Oncology, 16,* 805–816.

Lelorain, S., Bonnaud-Antignac, A., & Florin, A. (2010). Long-term posttraumatic growth after breast cancer: Prevalence, predictors, and relationships with psychological health. *Journal of Clinical Psychology in Medical Settings, 17,* 14–22.

Lengacher, C. A., Reich, R. R., Post-White, J., Moscoso, M., Shelton, M. M., Barta, M., . . . Budhrani, P. (2012). Mindfulness-based stress reduction in posttreatment breast cancer patients: An examination of symptoms and symptom clusters. *Journal of Behavioral Medicine, 35,* 86–94.

Lutgendorf, S. K., Sood, A. K., Anderson, B., McGinn, S., Maiseri, H., Dao, M., . . . Lubaroff, D. M. (2005). Social support, psychological distress, and natural killer cell activity in ovarian cancer. *Journal of Clinical Oncology, 23,* 7105–7113.

Maissi, E., Marteau, T., Hankins, M., Moss, S., Legood, R., & Gray, A. (2004). Psychological impact of human papillomavirus testing in women with borderline or mildly dyskaryotic cervical smear test results: Cross sectional questionnaire study. *British Medical Journal, 328,* 1293.

Manne, S. L., Winkel, G., Ostroff, J., Grana, G., & Fox, K. (2005). Partner unsupportive responses, avoidant coping, and distress among women with early stage breast cancer: Patient and partner perspectives. *Health Psychology, 24,* 635–641.

Matchim, Y., Armer, J. M., & Stewart, B. R. (2011). Effects of mindfulness-based stress reduction (MBSR) on health in breast cancer survivors. *Western Journal of Nursing Research, 33,* 996–1016.

McGregor, B. A., & Antoni, M. H. (2009). Psychological intervention and health outcomes among women treated for breast cancer: A review of stress pathways and biological mediators. *Brain, Behavior, and Immunity, 23,* 159–166.

Mehnert, A., Berg, P., Henrich, G., & Herschbach, P. (2009). Fear of cancer progression and cancer-related intrusive cognitions in breast cancer survivors. *Psycho-Oncology, 18,* 1273–1280.

Meneses, K. D., McNees, P., Loerzel, V. W., Su, X., Zhang, Y., & Hassey, L. A. (2007). Transition from treatment to survivorship: Effects of psychoeducational intervention on quality of life in breast cancer survivors. *Oncology Nursing Forum, 34,* 1007–1016.

Merriam-Webster. (2012) *Merriam-Webster Dictionary.* Retrieved from http://www .merriam-webster.com/dictionary/distress.

Miller, K., Merry, B., & Miller, J. (2008). Seasons of survivorship revisited. *Cancer, 14,* 369–374.

Mock, V., Frangakis, C., Davidson, N. E., Ropka, M. E., Pickett, M., Poniatowski, B., . . . McCorkle, R. (2005). Exercise manages fatigue during breast cancer treatment: A randomized controlled trial. *Psycho-Oncology, 14,* 464–477.

Mols, F., Vingerhoets, Ad, J. J. M., Coebergh, J. W., & van de Poll-Franse, L. V. (2009). Well-being, posttraumatic growth, and benefit finding in long-term breast cancer survivors. *Psychology and Health, 24,* 583–595.

Montgomery, G. H., Schnur, J. B., Erblich, J., Diefenbach, M. A., & Bovbjerg, D. H. (2010). Presurgery psychological factors predict pain, nausea, and fatigue one week after breast cancer surgery. *Journal of Pain and Symptom Management, 39,* 1043–1052.

Morgan, M. A. (2009). Cancer survivorship: History, quality-of-life issues, and the evolving multidisciplinary approach to implementation of cancer survivorship care plans. *Oncology Nursing Forum, 36,* 429–436.

Mullan, F. (1985). Seasons of survival: Reflections of a physician with cancer. *New England Journal of Medicine, 313,* 270–273.

National Comprehensive Cancer Network. (2012). *NCCN clinical practice guidelines in oncology (NCCN Guidelines®): Distress management, version 3.2012.* Retrieved from http://www.nccn.org/professionals/physician_gls/PDF/ distress.pdf.

Nausheen, B., Gidron, Y., Peveler, R., & Moss-Morris, R. (2009). Social support and cancer progression: A systemic review. *Journal of Psychosomatic Research, 67,* 403–415.

Norton, T. R., Manne, S. L., Rubin, S., Hernandez, E., Carlson, J., Bergman, C., & Rosenblum, N. (2005). Ovarian cancer patients' psychological distress: The role of physical impairment, perceived unsupportive family and friend behaviors, perceived control, and self-esteem. *Health Psychology, 24,* 143–152.

Oz, F., Dil, S., Inci, F., & Kamisli, S. (2012). Evaluation of group counseling for women with breast cancer in Turkey. *Cancer Nursing, 35,* E27–E34.

Park, C. L. (2009). Overview of theoretical perspectives. In Park, C. L., Lechner, S., Antoni, M. H., & Stanton, A., (Eds.), *Positive life change in the context of medical illness: Can the experience of serious illness lead to transformation?* (pp. 11–30). Washington, DC: American Psychological Association.

Peckmann, V., Ekholm, O., Rasmussen, N. K., Groenvold, M., Christiansen, P., Moller, S., . . . Sjogren, P. (2009). Chronic pain and other sequelae in long-term breast cancer survivors: Nationwide survey in Denmark. *European Journal of Pain, 13,* 478–485.

Peleg-Oren, N., & Sherer, M. (2001). Cancer patients and their spouses: Gender and its effect on psychological and social adjustment. *Journal of Health Psychology, 6,* 329–338.

Posner, T., & Vessey, M. (1988). Psychosexual trauma of an abnormal cervical smear. *British Journal of Obstetrics and Gynaecology, 95,* 729.

Rasmussen, D. M., & Elverdam, B. (2008). The meaning of work and working life after cancer: An interview study. *Psycho-Oncology, 17,* 1232–1238.

Rehse, B., & Pukrop, R. (2003). Effects of psychosocial interventions on quality of life in adult cancer patients: Meta analysis of 37 published controlled outcome studies. *Patient Education and Counseling, 50,* 179–186.

Sandgren, A. K., Mullens, A. B., Erickson, S. C., Romanek, K. M., & McCaul, K. D. (2004). Confidant and breast cancer patient reports of quality of life. *Quality of Life Research: An International Journal of Quality of Life Aspects of Treatment, Care & Rehabilitation, 13,* 155–160.

Schou, I., Ekeberg, O., & Ruland, C. M. (2005). The mediating role of appraisal and coping in the relationship between optimism-pessimism and quality of life. *Psycho-Oncology, 14,* 718–727.

Schroevers, M. J., Kraaij, V., & Garnefski, N. (2011). Cancer patients' experience of positive and negative changes due to the illness: Relationships with psychological well-being, coping, and goal reengagement. *Psycho-Oncology, 20,* 165–172.

Sears, S. R., Stanton, A. L., & Danoff-Burg, S. (2003). The yellow brick road and the Emerald City: Benefit finding, positive reappraisal coping, and posttraumatic growth in women with early-stage breast cancer. *Health Psychology, 22,* 487–497.

Sheldon, L. K., Swanson, S., Dolce, A., Marsh, K., & Summers, J. (2008). Putting evidence into practice: Evidence-based interventions for anxiety. *Clinical Journal of Oncology Nursing, 12,* 789–797.

Shennan, C., Payne, S., & Fenlon, D. (2011). What is the evidence for the use of mindfulness-based interventions in cancer care? A review. *Psycho-Oncology, 20,* 681–697.

Sherman, D. W., Haber, J., Hoskins, C. N., Budin, W. C., Maislin, G., Shukla, S., . . . Roth, A. (2012). The effects of psychoeducation and telephone counseling on the adjustment of women with early-stage breast cancer. *Applied Nursing Research, 25,* 3–16.

Siegel, R., DeSantis, C., Virgo, K., Stein, K., Mariotto, A., Smith, T., . . . Ward, E. (2012). Cancer treatment and survivorship statistics, 2012. *CA: A Cancer Journal for Clinicians, 62,* 220–241.

So, W. K. W., Marsh, G., Ling, W. M., Leung, F. Y., Lo, J. C. K., Yeung, M., & Li, G. K. H. (2009). The symptom cluster of fatigue, pain, anxiety, and depression and the effect on the quality of life of women receiving treatment for breast cancer: A multicenter study. *Oncology Nursing Forum, 36,* E205–E214.

Stanton, A. L., Revenson, T. A., & Tennen, H. (2007). Health psychology: Psychological adjustment to chronic disease. *Annual Review of Psychology, 58,* 565–592.

Stark, D., Kiely, M., Smith, A., Velikova, G., House, A., & Selby, P. (2002). Anxiety disorders in cancer patients: Their nature, associations, and relation to quality of life. *Journal of Clinical Oncology, 20,* 3137–3148.

Sullivan, M. J., Thorn, B., Haythornthwaite, J. A., Keefe, F., Martin, M., Bradley, L. A., & Lefebvre, J. C. (2001). Theoretical perspectives on the relation between catastrophizing and pain. *Clinical Journal of Pain, 17,* 52–64.

Taha, S. A., Matheson, K., & Anisman, H. (2012). Everyday experiences of women posttreatment after breast cancer: The role of uncertainty, hassles, uplifts, and coping on depressive symptoms. *Journal of Psychosocial Oncology, 30,* 359–379.

Tierney, D. K. (2008). Sexuality: A quality-of-life issue for cancer survivors. *Seminars in Oncology Nursing, 24,* 71–79.

Van den Beuken-van Everdingen, M. H., de Rijke, J. M., Kessels, A. G., Schouten, H. C., van Kleef, M., & Patijn J. (2009). Quality of life and non-pain symptoms in patients with cancer. *Journal of Pain and Symptom Management, 38,* 216–233.

van der Lee, M. L., & Garssen, B. (2012). Mindfulness-based cognitive therapy reduces chronic cancer-related fatigue: A treatment study. *Psycho-Oncology, 21,* 264–272.

Waller, J., McCaffery, K., Kitchener, H., Nazroo, J., & Wardle, J. (2007). Women's experiences of repeated HPV testing in the context of cervical cancer screening: A qualitative study. *Psycho-Oncology, 16,* 196–204.

Wardle, J., Pernet, A., & Stephens, D. (1995). Psychological consequences of positive results in cervical cancer screening. *Psychology and Health, 10,* 185–194.

Weiss, T. (2002). Posttraumatic growth in women with breast cancer and their husbands: An intersubjective validation study. *Journal of Psychosocial Oncology, 20,* 65–80.

Weiss, T., Weinberger, M. I., Holland, J., Nelson, C., & Moadel, A. (2012). Falling through the cracks: A review of psychological distress and psychosocial service needs in older Black and Hispanic patients with cancer. *Journal of Geriatric Oncology, 3,* 163–173.

Wiljer, D., Urowitz, S., Barbera, L., Chivers, M. L., Quartey, N. K., Ferguson, S. E., & Classen, C. (2011). A qualitative study of an internet-based support group for women with sexual distress due to gynecologic cancer. *Journal of Cancer Education, 26,* 451–458.

Witek-Janusek, L., Alburquerque, K., Chroniak, K. R., Chroniak, C., Durazo-Arvizu, R., & Mathews, H. L. (2008). Effects of mindfulness-based stress reduction on immune function, quality of life, and coping in women newly diagnosed with early stage breast cancer. *Brain, Behavior, and Immunity, 22,* 969–981.

Wittenberg, L., Yutsis, M., Taylor, S., Giese-Davis, J., Bliss-Isberg, C., Star, P., & Spiegel, D. (2010). Marital status predicts change in distress and well-being in women newly diagnosed with breast cancer and their peer counselors. *The Breast Journal, 16,* 481–489.

World Health Organization. (2010). Human papillomavirus (HPV). Retrieved from http://www.who.int/immunization/topics/hpv/en/.

World Health Organization. (2012). Cancer Fact Sheet 297. Retrieved from http://www.who.int/mediacentre/factsheets/fs297/en/.

Zabora, J., Brintzenhofeszoc, K., Curbow, B., Hooker, C., & Piantadosi, S. (2001). The prevalence of psychological distress by cancer site. *Psycho-Oncology, 10,* 19–28.

Chapter 8

Mind-Body Health Promotion and Women's Cancers

Ricardo Joao Texeira and Maria da Graca Pereira

INTRODUCTION

Cancer is known as a spectrum of diseases that occur in all societies and in all places of the world. In humans, it is known that this disease has existed from immemorial times until modern communities. However, the most prevalent types of cancer in a community vary with age and distribution by gender and race, as well as with geographic, economic, and environmental context, and customs of people, including their diets (Stephens & Aigner, 2009). In developed countries, cancer is responsible for about 25–30 percent of deaths, being the second leading cause of death after cardiovascular disease. Although cancer can occur at any stage of the life cycle, it is relatively uncommon before the age of 40, but as people get older, the risk of cancer increases progressively (Stephens & Aigner, 2009).

According to Marques and Pimentel (1995), one in four Europeans will suffer from an oncological disease during their lifetime, and one in each five will die from it, and this is true for North Americans as well. Because cancer is a chronic disease that requires ongoing and often prolonged care, it usually incapacitates wholly or partially the patient and the family. Cancer is a health problem of extreme importance to health services and remains a challenge for most health care professionals who have to deal with this disease (Virgo et al., 2013).

Recently, in the field of oncology, specific therapies and biological treatments have been introduced that offer the possibility of effective treatment with fewer side effects (Baselga & Hammond, 2002; Van der Poel, 2004). However, both cancer and its treatments often cause significant physical and psychological morbidity. Almost half of cancer patients suffer from moderate to severe psychological distress and face serious difficulties in dealing with the disease (Carlson et al., 2004; Spiegel, 1996; Zabora, Brintzenhofeszoc, Curbow, Hooker, & Piantadosi, 2001). There are many potential sources of distress, such as the anticipation of suffering, compliance with treatment regimens, difficulties in facing and dealing with life changes, and adjustment to the inherent uncertainty and uncontrollability of the disease (Carlson, Ursuliak, Goodey, Angen, & Speca, 2001).

Standard cancer treatments include surgery, radiotherapy, chemotherapy, and hormone therapy, and are intended to remove, delay, or kill tumor cells (Pitot, 2002). Oncologists and other health professionals may also recommend other types of treatment in order to improve overall health and well-being. These interventions are often referred to as "complementary," since they are coadjutant with the usual therapies (Dreher, 2003; Hilsden & Verhoef, 1999; Verhoef, Hilsden, & O'Beirne, 1999). For patients seeking complementary therapies, making decisions about their use provides significant opportunities to take some control over their disease during cancer treatment and recovery (Truant & Bottorff, 1999; Verhoef et al., 1999).

The symptoms of cancer, and its treatment side effects, vary in intensity, duration, and severity. They are associated with a number of factors, such as type, location, and extent of the disease, as well as the specific course of treatment(s) and the patients' previous health state (Stephens & Aigner, 2009). After the diagnosis, many patients face difficult choices concerning treatment options, weakness, and an uncertain future. Very often, cancer exceeds the coping resources of patients and their families, and as the burden increases, daily routines change, and issues concerning the confrontation with the inevitability of death emerge. Understandably, emotional stress following a diagnosis of cancer is common (Kangas, 2013). Fears about the future, changes in social roles, and physical symptoms or functional losses resulting from the illness or treatments contribute to an experience that is usually described as an "emotional rollercoaster" (Fox, 1995).

Among the population of cancer patients, there is a growing interest in mind-body medicine and complementary therapies, sustained by a desire to be proactive and assume initiatives for personal treatment (Weiger et al., 2002). The current interest of many cancer patients in interventions to reduce stress through relaxation techniques, meditation, and yoga stems from the belief that cancer can be caused or aggravated by stress, emotions, and other psychological factors, although causal relationships among these factors and the initiation and progression of cancer have not been clearly demonstrated in the literature (Fox, 1995; Spahn et al., 2013; Tomatis, 2001).

THE MIND-BODY APPROACH AND ITS APPLICABILITY IN ONCOLOGY

The very existence of the placebo effect, in which suggestions and expectancy can induce biological changes, demonstrates the connection between mind and body (Benedetti, 2013). The potential to influence health with one's mind is an appealing concept and an underutilized opportunity. Mind-body therapies have been practiced in different parts of the world for thousands of years, especially in the Eastern Hemisphere, where the importance of the mind in illness and healing has been integrated for more than 2,000 years (Carlson & Bultz, 2008). These therapies are defined as a variety of techniques to enhance the mind's capacity to affect bodily function and symptoms. Its practices include relaxation techniques, hypnosis, visualization, meditation, biofeedback, cognitive-behavioral therapies, support groups, autogenic training, spirituality, and expressive therapies such as art, music, or dance. These therapies are likely to have a strong effect through a mind-body connection and, as such, are included in a discipline called "mind-body medicine" (Carlson & Bultz, 2008). Some of these therapies are no longer considered "alternative," being perfectly integrated into conventional medicine. As research progresses in this field, treatments showing benefits tend to integrate with conventional medical care (Chandwani, Chaoul-Reich, Biegler, & Cohen, 2008; Rodrick et al., 2013).

Many of these therapies have been included in the care of cancer patients. In the United States, a national study found that 30 percent of adults indicated never having used a mind-body technique, and 19 percent had used one of these techniques in the past year (Wolsko, Eisenberg, Davis, & Phillips, 2004). For example, in California, one study with adults (including cancer patients and people without cancer), found that 26 percent of the participants resorted to mind-body techniques (Goldstein et al., 2005). Mind-body practices such as meditation and yoga have become extremely popular as a way to reduce stress and promote spiritual growth, and this is especially noticeable in medical populations. Many cancer patients believe that stress plays a role in the etiology and progression of the disease, and this belief is sustained by some research. For example, results of Chen et al.'s (1995) study suggested that stressful life events might contribute to the incidence and progression of cancer. However, Petticrew, Fraser, and Regan's (1999) study found no such association. Despite these results, depression, which is a common physiological response to stressful events or circumstances of life, has been associated with an increased risk of cancer and disease progression (Penninx et al., 1998; Watson, Haviland, Greer, Davidson, & Bliss, 1999).

Extensive research supports the association between stress and depression, clarifying that it actually causes cellular immunosuppression (Cohen et al., 2012; Irwin et al., 1990; Rabin, 1999) and increases angiogenesis in human and animal studies (Lutgendorf et al., 2002; Thaker et al., 2006), both important factors involved in metastatic processes. A particularly important discovery in this context emerged from prospective and cross-sectional studies with breast cancer patients, revealing that emotional distress is negatively correlated with the number and function of immune cells, after controlling for age and stage of the disease (Andersen et al., 1998; Tjemsland, Soreide, Matre, & Malt, 1997). Furthermore, an association was found between the survival rate of patients with breast cancer, the activity of the sympathetic nervous system, and the mental health of these patients (Sephton, Sapolsky, Kraemer, & Spiegel, 2000; Watson et al., 1999). However, the clinical and biological significance concerning the influence of psychosocial factors on the biological mechanisms of this disease is still very premature.

An effective management of the effects and consequences of a cancer diagnosis, and its treatment, is becoming an increasingly important priority to health policies, considering the auspicious survival rates of cancer patients. Certain symptoms are very common after a cancer treatment, making it necessary to undertake measures for maintaining and promoting health in this adverse situation. In this sense, this chapter aims to report some fundamental aspects of the mind-body approach and its influence on promoting the health and quality of life of cancer patients.

DISTRESS AND CANCER RECOVERY

In addition to the reported prevalence of clinical depression and other behavioral health problems, many cancer survivors report feelings of distress, daily or episodic. Distress is considered an unpleasant emotional experience, multidetermined, with a psychological (cognitive, behavioral, emotional), social, and/or spiritual nature, which can interfere with the ability to cope effectively with cancer, its physical symptoms, and treatment (Carlson & Speca, 2007). According to the National Comprehensive Cancer Network (NCCN, 2002), the distress in cancer patients is distributed on a continuum, ranging from common feelings of vulnerability and sadness, to depression, anxiety, panic, social isolation, and spiritual crisis. Although not as serious as a psychiatric diagnosis of anxiety or depression, the prevalence rates of distress are higher in cancer patients (Grassi et al., 2013).

Zabora's et al. (2001) study with 4,496 cancer patients found an overall prevalence of significant distress (35.1%), with the highest distress in patients with lung cancer (43.4%), followed by brain cancer, Hodgkin's disease, pancreatic cancer, lymphoma, liver cancer, head and neck cancer, breast cancer, leukemia, melanoma, colon cancer, prostate cancer, and finally, gynecological cancer. Another large-scale study, which aimed to assess all patients who visited a cancer center in Canada (with more than 3,000 patients), found that 37 percent meet the criteria of significant distress using the Brief Symptom Inventory—BSI (Carlson et al., 2004). In the same study, patients who just moved to the center for follow-up appointments showed high levels of distress, with 34.4 percent scoring above the cutoff for overall significant distress. But this is not a unique phenomenon among cancer patients in North America, since similar overall rates were found in several European countries (Dolbeault et al., 2003; Gil, Travado, Tomamichel, & Grassi, 2003; Grassi et al., 2013; Mehnert, 2004), in the Middle East (Isikhan et al., 2001; Montazeri, Sajadian, Fateh, Haji-Mahmoodi, & Ebrahimi, 2004; Sadeh-Tassa, Yagil, & Stadler, 2004), in South America (Santos, 2004), and in Asia (Fielding, Lam, & Ho, 2004; Shimizu, Akechi, Okamura, Akizuki, & Uchitomi, 2004).

These results highlight the need to pay attention to symptoms of distress among cancer survivors as they progress in their recovery. Based on these and other data, distress was considered the sixth vital sign in cancer treatment, after temperature, respiration, heart rate, blood pressure, and pain (Bultz & Carlson, 2006; NCCN, 2002; Van Halteren, Bongaerts, & Wagener, 2004).

PROBLEM SOLVING AND HEALTH: IMPLICATIONS FOR PSYCHO-ONCOLOGY

Problem solving in real life situations, often referred to as "social problem solving," is considered an important psychological variable that restricts the impact of cancer (Nezu, Nezu, Felgoise, & Zwick, 2003). In this context, Nezu, Nezu, Friedman, Faddis, and Houts (1998) define "problem solving" as a general coping strategy that can help people manage stressful situations, thereby enhancing their flexibility and perceived control, in order to reduce emotional suffering, even in adverse situations. Therefore, people with training in problem-solving techniques, in stressful situations show a decrease of emotional distress and present a higher quality of life. This hypothesis was considered valid in a wide variety of clinical populations, ages, and psychological difficulties (Nezu, 2004). The conceptual relevance of the problem-solving model for cancer patients, developed by Nezu et al. (1998), is incorporated into a general problem-solving model for stress, in which the experience of cancer is designed both as a major negative life event as well as an inducer of stressful daily problems (Nezu, Nezu, Felgoise, McClure, & Houts, 2003; Nezu, Nezu, Houts, Friedman, & Faddis, 1999). Both sources of stress increase the likelihood of a cancer patient to suffer from significant psychological distress, including depression and anxiety. However, the problem-solving ability is conceptualized as an important moderator of this relationship, whereby an effective problem-solving capacity reduces the difficulties associated with the relationship between cancer and distress.

The key assumptions of the problem-solving model have been supported by research findings with undergraduates but also with several clinical samples (Brack, LaClave, & Wyatt, 1992; Cheng, 2001; Frye & Goodman, 2004; Goodman, Gravitt, & Kaslow, 1995; Nezu, Nezu, Saraydarian, Kalmar, & Ronan, 1986; Nezu, Nezu, Faddis, DelliCarpini, & Houts, 1995; Nezu et al., 1999; Nezu & Ronan, 1985, 1988), including cancer patients (Nezu et al., 1995; Nezu, Nezu, Felgoise, McClure et al., 2003; Nezu et al., 1999). For example, in a study with 105 patients newly diagnosed with cancer, the authors found that participants who were characterized by a lower efficiency in problem solving also had higher levels of anxiety and depressive symptoms, as well as a larger number of cancer-related physical problems (Nezu et al., 1999). In a second study, the same authors sought to evaluate how problem-solving capacities predicted cancer-related distress, in a sample of 64 mastectomized women, in the 1–13 years before their participation in the research. The results indicate that problem solving was a significant negative predictor of psychological distress (Nezu et al., 1999). In a previous study, the authors found similar levels of cancer-related distress in patients characterized as having more difficulties in solving problems, and that they reported higher levels of depression when compared to a group without difficulties in problem solving (Nezu et al., 1995). More recently, the authors (Nezu, Nezu, Felgoise, McClure et al., 2003) proved the efficacy of problem-solving therapy in reducing psychological distress in a 132 adult cancer patients sample (and a significant other). Improvements in problem solving were found to correlate significantly with lower psychological distress and higher overall quality of life, and these effects were maintained one year post-treatment. These results are consistent with the biobehavioral model of cancer stress and disease course proposed by Andersen, Kiecolt-Glaser, and Glaser (1994) and Andersen (2001). Previous research that identified problem-solving techniques as an effective clinical intervention for a variety of psychological disorders (Nezu, D'Zurilla, Zwick, & Nezu, 2004), particularly for major depression (Arean et al., 1993; Nezu et al., 1986; Nezu & Perri, 1989), provide further support for the assumption that these techniques should include effective interventions aiming to reduce distress in adult cancer patients.

RECIPROCAL RELATIONSHIP BETWEEN MIND AND BODY: EFFECTS OF IMAGERY IN CANCER PATIENTS

Visualization corresponds to the mental representation of an event, an object, or a sensation, in their physical absence (Cabete, Cavaleiro, & Pinteus, 2003). It is a simple but powerful technique that directs the imagination and attention to produce symptomatic relief. "Positive visualization," as a form of treatment, can potentiate some physiological benefits, such as lowering blood pressure and heart rate (Cassileth & Gubili, 2009). For Bazzo and Moeller (1999), the use of visualization in psychological interventions corresponds to a process of "guided imagery," where the concentration focus is retained on the images formed in the mind. In the context of oncology, the Simontons (Simonton & Matthews-Simonton, 1981; Simonton, Simonton, & Creighton, 1978) are an unavoidable reference, wherein the authors associated relaxation to visualization in the medical treatment of cancer cells, adding a further training in assertive expression of feelings, the results of which showed an increased survival rate and improved quality of life. In one of their key studies, with 159 patients considered "terminal" (i.e., with a life expectancy of approximately 12 months), the authors compared a treatment of meditation with visualization, whereas in the control group they used exclusively supportive therapy. Two years later, in the experimental group, they found very high incidences of partial regressions (19%), clinical complete regressions (22%), and stabilizations (27%), and only 32% of the cases were registered as a cancer progression (Simonton et al., 1978). Despite these appealing results, however, the authors never published the results of any well-designed study testing their ideas. Although they taught cancer patients to imagine their cancer being destroyed by their white blood cells, there is no evidence that white cells actually attack cancer cells in this manner or that "immune suppression" is a factor in the development of common cancers (American Cancer Society, 1982).

A study carried out by Walker et al. (1999), with a group of 96 women with breast cancer who were treated with relaxation training and visualization during chemotherapy, showed an improvement in quality of life and in the ability to relax. Similarly, the study by Kolcaba and Fox (1999) with guided imagery showed an increased perception of comfort in a group of 54 patients with breast cancer in chemotherapy. A review of 67 published studies conducted by Mundy, DuHamel, and Montgomery (2003) indicated that relaxation, visualization, and suggestion had an impact on cancer pain.

Imagery can also be effective in nausea control. In a study with 110 patients with breast cancer undergoing bone marrow transplantation, participants were randomly chosen to receive usual treatments vs. cognitive restructuring and relaxation with visualization. The experimental group showed significantly less nausea and anxiety (Gaston-Johansson et al., 2000). Cabete et al. (2003) conclude that imagery has already demonstrated important results, with low costs and significant benefits, and should be given an increasingly important place in psychological intervention with cancer patients.

IMPORTANCE OF SOCIAL SUPPORT IN PSYCHO-ONCOLOGY

In a sample of 282 couples in which the wife had breast cancer, assessed one year after diagnosis, 42 percent of couples agreed that cancer had approached the couple, 16 percent reported an impact on the closeness of social relationships, 34 percent were discordant (i.e., only one member of the couple reported a feeling of closeness), and only 7 percent of the couples reported a perception of greater distance in one or both members (Dorval et al., 2005). Although reports of improved relationships are still inconsistent, some data suggest that the enhancement of intimate relationships may be more prevalent in married than in unmarried patients (Aizer et al., in press, 2013; Rieker, Edbril, & Garnick, 1985; Rieker et al., 1989).

In the study of Curbow, Somerfield, Baker, Wingard, and Legro (1993), with bone marrow transplantation survivors studied between 6 and 149 months after transplantation, the authors also found more positive relationship changes than negative ones with different family members, including siblings, parents, children, and spouses.

COPING AND CANCER: IS THERE MORE TO SAY?

The individual significance of a cancer diagnosis, and its treatments, promote a set of stressors on personal and family lives. Cancer is a disease extended in time, which leads to a deterioration of the individual's physical and social resources, affecting the effectiveness of coping strategies (Varela & Leal, 2007). Weisman and Worden (1985) point out that the most effective coping strategies are those that reflect the acceptance of cancer and are followed by strategies to respond to issues related to the disease and its consequences, realistically. Patients who respond more willingly to changes that are raised by their disease tend to develop coping strategies and deal better with their health conditions. Thus, individuals who use coping strategies more appropriate to the circumstances, who maintain high expectations regarding the results of their actions, and who feel control over the disease process report a better quality of life (Ogden, 2012).

Post-traumatic growth is an interesting research field (e.g., Cordova & Andrykowski, 2003; Teixeira & Pereira, 2013; Tomich & Helgeson, 2012). The reasons for why some patients, and their caregivers, are able to perceive the cancer experience as positive, with interpersonal benefits, is a field of great current interest and may eventually illuminate the concept of distress and coping in cancer patients, which could lead to better interventions in this area. Despite the promising data, the studies on the relationship between coping and adaptation are still limited. For example, the nonexpression of negative feelings (e.g., anger, anxiety, depression) has been associated with greater mood disturbance (Classen, Koopman, Angell, & Spiegel, 1996). On the other hand, an attitude focused on overcoming cancer has been associated with a lower mood disturbance (Classen et al., 1996; Steptoe, Sutcliffe, Allen, & Coombes, 1991).

The effectiveness of the attitude entitled "fighting spirit" suggests that active attempts to manage the disease may be beneficial. For example, in a study carried out by Burgess, Morris, and Pettingale (1988), the authors report that increased levels of anxiety corresponded to a poor adjustment in response to diagnosis, including helplessness, hopelessness, and a low internal locus of control. Thus, anxiety and emotional suppression may be determining factors in the psychological adjustment to cancer.

The study of the relationship between personality traits and the diagnosis and progression of cancer has raised in the coping literature concepts such as "fighting spirit" and "fatalism" (Ranchor & Sanderman, 2006). The famous study of Greer, Morris, and Pettingale (1979) promoted the idea that coping and personality traits may have an influence on the survival of cancer patients. The authors found that "fighting spirit" was associated with improved survival in women with breast cancer. Petticrew, Bell, and Hunter (2002) conducted a review to investigate the relationship between coping and personality traits and found 26 studies. However, a large percentage had small samples, and only 4 studies had samples of more than 200 patients. The authors created clusters with the following coping styles: (1) fighting spirit; (2) helplessness/hopelessness; (3) denial or avoidance; (4) stoic acceptance and fatalism; (5) anxious concern (anxious coping); (6) depressive coping; (7) active or problem-focused coping; and (8) suppression of emotions (emotion-focused coping). Considering the results of all the reviewed studies, the authors concluded that there is insufficient evidence to support an association between survival and the mentioned concepts. More recently, a 10-year longitudinal study conducted by Watson, Homewood, Haviland, and Bliss (2005), with an initial sample of 578 patients with breast cancer, found that the coping strategy of helplessness/hopelessness was associated with shorter survival periods. Also Watson et al. (1991) conducted an investigation concerning the relationship among emotional control, adjustment to cancer, and levels of anxiety and depression in 380 women diagnosed (between 1 and 3 months) with breast cancer. The authors found that a "fighting spirit" was associated with lower levels of anxiety and depression, while helplessness, worry, and fatalism were associated with an increase in disturbance.

Despite the inconclusiveness of these studies about the role of personality and adjustment in cancer progression, the influence of personality traits on psychological adjustment should be considered in interventions with patients (Hodges & Winstanley, 2012). However, in clinical practice, this influence should be approached with caution, since there is no clear evidence that cancer can actually be controlled through psychological factors (Ranchor & Sanderman, 2006).

MARITAL RELATIONSHIPS IN PSYCHO-ONCOLOGY

In Northouse, Templin, and Mood's (2001) study, adjustment was assessed at three different stages (at diagnosis, two months later, and one year later), showing moderate high correlations between patients and partners, in all disease stages. The level of adjustment of husbands after one year had a direct effect on their wives' adjustment level (at the same stage). Furthermore, as reported by Carter and Carter (1993), two to three years after diagnosis and treatment, wives and husbands still had similar levels of emotional adjustment.

The couple influences the coping responses in a reciprocal manner, thus influencing the quality of support the two provide each other. Some key examples of research in this field involve: (1) the use of problem-focused strategies by partners (Ptacek, Ptacek, & Dodge, 1994); (2) the use of external coping control/resignation by partners (Hannum, Giese-Davis, Harding, & Hatfield, 1991); and (3) the use of active relational coping strategies by partners (Kuijer et al., 2000). Women with cancer are more likely to experience distress when their partners use unrealistic cognitions to deal with the disease (Ptacek et al., 1994), when they use denial or optimism (Hannum et al., 1991), and when they are overprotective (Kuijer et al., 2000). Likewise, the women's coping strategies to deal with cancer influence the adjustment of their partners. Thus, partners adapt better when women use optimism as a coping style (Hannum et al., 1991), when they use more problem-focused coping and less avoidance, and when they use less unrealistic cognitions (Ptacek et al., 1994). These results illustrate the significant relationship between the coping of the couple's adaptation to cancer. Partners employ a shared approach toward the disease, and communication support is improved to the extent that they not only recognize and validate each other's feelings, but they also tend to view a stressful situation as "their problem," sharing the burdens and responsibilities in a way that balances the individual and relational needs (Kayser & Scott, 2008).

While it is the desire of most couples to talk openly about issues that bother them, several obstacles may stand in the way of couples dealing with oncological diseases. For example, the fear of overloading the partner, often referred to as a "conspiracy of silence" (Keller, Henrich, Sellschopp, & Beutel, 1996; Zhang & Siminoff, 2003), is very recurrent. Couples can avoid the topic of cancer in order to keep life as it was before the diagnosis or with the intention to prevent the patient from getting upset or sad (Koocher & Pollin, 2001). In addition, there is uncertainty in what to do, or say, that could be actually useful in dealing with the disease. Even if the couple has had a relationship with good communication before the diagnosis, it can still be very difficult to address the issue because of the fear associated with cancer (Dorval et al., 2005). In a qualitative study with 20 couples in which the wife had breast cancer, Skerrett (1998) found that the communication between "problematic" couples occurred in one of two identified patterns: one of the partners was restricted to silence or followed a pattern of communication characterized by "telling all." Resilient couples spoke openly about cancer but did not allow that communication about the disease to dominate everyday life. Thus, there seems to be an optimal amount of communication that lies between these two extremes: total silence and constant talk about cancer.

THE ADAPTIVE EFFECT OF EMOTIONAL EXPRESSION IN CANCER PATIENTS

Correlation studies vary in demonstrating a positive or negative relationship between emotional expression and adjustment to cancer, according to how the emotional expression is conceptualized and assessed. In a sample of 80 patients with breast cancer, in the six months after diagnosis, Compas et al. (1999) found that emotional ventilation, used as a coping strategy, was associated with a decrease in distress, leading to the conclusion that the expression of emotions in response to breast cancer leads to a greater understanding and regulation of emotions, being thus adaptive.

When assessed with measures directly related to distress, emotional expression predicted a more positive adjustment in patients with cancer. For example, in a longitudinal study carried out by Stanton et al. (2000) with 92 women who had undergone medical treatment for primary breast cancer, the authors (having investigated emotion-focused coping) found a better adjustment of women within three months involving a purposeful expressive processing of emotions under stress conditions. The authors conceptualized emotional processing as active, or as intentional attempts to recognize, explore meanings, and come to an understanding of emotions (and emotional expression) in regard to a stressor, either in an intrapersonal (e.g., writing for a newspaper) or an interpersonal way (Stanton, Kirk, Cameron, & Danoff-Burg, 2000).

Emotional-expression coping is related to an improved quality of life in women with cancer who perceive their social contexts as highly receptive. Stanton et al. (2000) found that women with cancer who express their emotions about cancer, at baseline, had fewer medical appointments to address cancer-related psychological morbidity (e.g., pain), better perception of physical health and energy, and decreased distress within three months, when compared with less expressive women. Furthermore, the authors showed that emotional expression, compared to emotional processing, seems to be more useful toward a persistent stressor. In Stanton et al.'s (2000) study, women had been diagnosed with cancer about six months before the study, and the good results in coping through emotional processing may reflect: (1) an incapacity to reach a satisfactory understanding of feelings around the cancer experience; or (2) rumination, which has been associated with an increase of distress (e.g., Morrow & Nolen-Hoeksema, 1990). It is also possible that distress is only reduced to the extent that emotional processing is associated with a persistent emotional expression. Additional analyses suggested that emotion-focused coping can facilitate alignment and clarification of goals, as revealed by the significant effects (mediator and moderator) of coping between emotional expression and dispositional hope (a construct that involves a sense toward goals and the ability to generate plans to achieve those goals) (Stanton, Danoff-Burg et al., 2000). For example, through the expression of feelings about the loss of control associated with a diagnosis of cancer, women may begin to distinguish what they can/cannot control based on their experience with the disease (and life in general), attempt to seek attainable goals, and work toward the acceptance of dimensions of the disease experience that are less controllable (Stanton & Danoff-Burg, 2002).

Indirect evidence of the utility of emotional expression resides in the study of the relationship between emotional suppression (or avoidance) and adjustment to the disease. In a study with metastatic breast cancer or recurrent cancer in women, Classen et al. (1996) found that a high control of emotional expression was associated with greater intensity of distress. Numerous studies about avoidance-oriented coping provide indirect evidence that more approaching-oriented strategies (and less avoidance) of cancer-related cognitions and emotions can cause greater benefits (Myers et al., 2008). Although studies with samples of noncancer patients suggest that avoidance of emotions can be useful in some circumstances (e.g., Bonanno, Znoj, Siddique, & Horowitz, 1999), longitudinal studies (e.g., Carver et al., 1993; Stanton & Snider, 1993) with breast cancer patients have revealed that avoidance-centered coping predicts increasing distress over time.

All together, correlational and longitudinal studies reveal that intentional attempts of cancer patients to address their emotions through emotional expression are associated with important benefits (Stanton & Danoff-Burg, 2002).

QUALITY OF LIFE AFTER A CANCER DIAGNOSIS: REALITY OR AN ILLUSION?

Quality of life is a subjective, dynamic, multidimensional, and very personal concept that reflects numerous factors, with subtle or clearer interactions between physical, psychological, social, and spiritual domains (Canavarro et al., 2006; Ferrell & Dow, 1997; Ferrell, Dow, & Grant, 1995; Fleck, 2006). According to the World Health Organization (WHO), quality of life corresponds to the individual perception of the position in life, contextualized in physical, cultural, and social domains where each person lives in relation to his or her goals, expectations, standards, and concerns (WHOQOL-Group, 1994, 1998).

Despite current scientific advances that allow patients to face oncological disease with greater hope, this issue still has huge implications on their lives and their families, labor or social contexts (Zebrack, Yi, Peterson, & Ganz, 2007). According to Pimentel (2006), the success of cancer therapy is usually described in terms of survival, complications, and recurrence rates. Using only these parameters, the complexity of oncological diseases is not fully addressed. The perception that patients have about all the events related to their cancer is more globalized and assumes a central role in their existence. But even with great advances in this field, cancer patients are still seen as true survivors, despite the incongruity of quality-of-life definition and its operationalization (Bloom, Kang, Petersen, & Stewart, 2007).

The five-year post-diagnosis is considered a reference mark regarding quality of life studies in the 1980s. In fact, Gotay and Muraoka's (1998) review of 34 publications describes the concept of "long-term survivors" as those adult patients who had completed treatment for at least five years after diagnosis. However, according to Pinto and Pais Ribeiro (2006), only in the mid-1990s was the term "psychological adaptation" replaced by "quality of life."

In oncology, the quality of life of cancer patients is defined as the assessment/satisfaction of patients with their level of functioning, when compared to what they perceive as possible or ideal (Fayers & Machin, 2007). Since quality of life derives from the personal subjective evaluation of each patient, multiple measures were created, mirroring the multidimensionality of the concept. But according to Pinto and Pais Ribeiro (2006), only one instrument of quality of life is specific to cancer survivors, the *Quality of Life in Cancer Survivors* (QOL-CS; [Ferrell et al., 1995]), which includes four domains: physical, psychological, spiritual, and social.

In a functional and social adaptation perspective, oncology should not ultimately aim to prolong the life of patients with cancer but to "give life to years," a fundamental challenge introduced by the WHO and directly related to an investment in a person's quality of life (Walker, 2002). Thus, a "good" quality of life means physical, psychological, and social health, and not an absence of disease. Thus, studies in quality of life can be a landmark in identifying specific needs of cancer survivors in a dynamic perspective, since these are changeable throughout the cycle of survival, being also a challenge for health promotion (Becker, Kang, & Stuifbergen, 2012).

The concerns of the survivors are considerably different in the early stage of the disease and after treatment(s). However, as Kornblith (1998) sustains, some initial problems may remain over time. For example, symptom-related concerns such as pain and fatigue may continue to rise (Dow, Ferrell, Leigh, Ly, & Gulasekaram, 1996), as well as sexual functioning concerns (Dorval, Maunsell, Deschenes, Brisson, & Masse, 1998; Perz, Ussher, & Gilbert, 2013) and body image preoccupations (Ferrell, Dow, Leigh, Ly, & Gulasekaram, 1995; Przezdziecki et al., 2013). Years after the diagnosis, there may be concerns about the future of the family, as well as the fear of recurrence (Dow et al., 1996; Ferrell, Dow, Leigh et al., 1995; Jones, Hadjistavropoulos, & Gullickson, in press, 2013; Thewes et al., in press, 2013), job discrimination, financial problems, and difficulty in dealing with late side effects of the treatment (Carver, Smith, Petronis, & Antoni, 2006; Veach, Nicholas, & Barton, 2002).

Cancer is still highly stigmatized in society, particularly toward the patient and family, since it is still associated with significant mortality, even though the disease stage is an important variable to take into consideration. This, coupled with the frequent uncertainty of the diagnosis, prognosis, and the physical and psychological suffering, raises important issues/challenges for quality of life. Therefore, psychological support and care should involve specific issues to maximize quality of life (Mehnert & Koch, 2008).

CONCLUSION

Clinical practice in all disciplines related to health is increasingly being shaped by the ethical imperative of the evidence of effectiveness of interventions offered to patients (Grol & Grimshaw, 2003). Mind-body approaches to health promotion include a variety of treatments designed to improve the emotional well-being and physical health of patients and have shown great potential for improving their quality of life. By reducing the effects of stress, mind-body techniques may help to prevent disease or reverse certain underlying disease processes, thereby fostering health promotion. There is no conclusive evidence that personality type or stressful events predispose a person toward cancer. Support groups and other psychological approaches may help, particularly with the psychological morbidity that is so common in cancer patients. Some patients may become so anxious and depressed that they are unable to pursue their cancer treatment. For those patients there is some evidence that relaxation, guided imagery, meditation, hypnosis, and other behavioral techniques can help with the side effects of cancer and are valuable coadjuvant techniques to conventional medicine

We are still in the beginning stages of understanding the intricate relationship between mind and body. The challenge ahead is to understand what are the psychological events that have the greatest impact on health on the one hand, and how they physiologically affect the body, on the other. Future research needs to integrate these mind-body techniques and use rigorous designs to show their efficacy, particularly in preventing disease recurrence and improving quality of life in chronic illness such as cancer.

REFERENCES

Aaronson, N. K. (1991). Methodological issues in assessing the quality of life of cancer patients. *Cancer, 67*(Suppl. 3), 844–850.

Aaronson, N. K., Meyerowitz, B. E., Bard, M., Bloom, J. R., Fawzy, F. I., Feldstein, M., . . . Lowman, J. T. (1991). Quality of life research in oncology. Past achievements and future priorities. *Cancer, 67*(Suppl. 3), 839–843.

Aizer, A. A., Chen, M. H., McCarthy, E. P., Mendu, M. L., Koo, S., Wilhite, T. J., . . . Nguyen, P. L. (in press, 2013). Marital status and survival in patients with cancer. *Journal of Clinical Oncology.*

American Cancer Society. (1982). Unproven methods of cancer management: O. Carl Simonton, M.D. *CA: A Cancer Journal for Clinicians, 32*(1), 58–61.

Andersen, B. L. (2001). A biobehavioral model for cancer interventions. In Baum, A., & Andersen, B. L. (Eds.), *Psychosocial Interventions for Cancer* (pp. 119–129). Washington DC: American Psychological Association.

Andersen, B. L., Farrar, W. B., Golden-Kreutz, D., Kutz, L. A., MacCallum, R., Courtney, M. E., & Glaser, R. (1998). Stress and immune responses after surgical treatment for regional breast cancer. *Journal of the National Cancer Institute, 90*(1), 30–36.

Andersen, B. L., Kiecolt-Glaser, J. K., & Glaser, R. (1994). A biobehavioral model of cancer stress and disease course. *The American Psychologist, 49*(5), 389–404.

Andrykowski, M. A., Brady, M. J., & Hunt, J. W. (1993). Positive psychosocial adjustment in potential bone marrow transplant recipients: Cancer as a psychological transition. *Psycho-Oncology, 2*(4), 261–276.

Arean, P. A., Perri, M. G., Nezu, A. M., Schein, R. L., Christopher, F., & Joseph, T. X. (1993). Comparative effectiveness of social problem-solving therapy and reminiscence therapy as treatments for depression in older adults. *Journal of Consulting and Clinical Psychology, 61*(6), 1003–1010.

Avis, N. E., Crawford, S., & Manuel, J. (2005). Quality of life among younger women with breast cancer. *Journal of Clinical Oncology, 23*(15), 3322–3330.

Baselga, J., & Hammond, L. A. (2002). HER-targeted tyrosine-kinase inhibitors. *Oncology, 63*(Suppl. 1), 6–16.

Bazzo, D., & Moeller, R. (1999). Imagine this! Infinite uses of guided imagery in women's health. *Journal of Holistic Nursing, 17*(4), 317–330.

Becker, H., Kang, S. J., & Stuifbergen, A. (2012). Predictors of quality of life for long-term cancer survivors with preexisting disabling conditions. *Oncology Nursing Forum, 39*(2), 122–131.

Benedetti, F. (2013). Placebo and the new physiology of the doctor-patient relationship. *Physiological Reviews, 93*(3), 1207–1246.

Blanchard, C. G., Albrecht, T. L., & Ruckdeschel, J. C. (1997). The crisis of cancer: Psychological impact on family caregivers. *Oncology, 11*(2), 189–194.

Bloom, J. R., Kang, S. H., Petersen, D. M., & Stewart, S. L. (2007). Quality of life in long-term cancer survivors. In Feuerstein, M. (Ed.), *Handbook of Cancer Survivorship* (pp. 43–65). New York: Springer.

Bonanno, G. A., Znoj, H., Siddique, H. I., & Horowitz, M. J. (1999). Verbal-autonomic dissociation and adaptation to midlife conjugal loss: A follow-up at 25 months. *Cognitive Therapy and Research, 23*(6), 605–624.

Brack, G., LaClave, L., & Wyatt, A. S. (1992). The relationship of problem solving and reframing to stress and depression in female college students. *Journal of College Student Development, 33*(2), 124–131.

Bultz, B. D., & Carlson, L. E. (2006). Emotional distress: The sixth vital sign—future directions in cancer care. *Psycho-Oncology, 15*(2), 93–95.

Burgess, C., Morris, T., & Pettingale, K. W. (1988). Psychological response to cancer diagnosis, II: Evidence for coping styles. *Journal of Psychosomatic Research, 32*(3), 263–272.

Burman, B., & Margolin, G. (1992). Analysis of the association between marital relationships and health problems: An interactional perspective. *Psychological Bulletin, 112*(1), 39–63.

Cabete, D. G., Cavaleiro, A. M., & Pinteus, M. T. (2003). Visualização: Uma intervenção possível em psicologia da saúde [Visualization: A possible intervention in health psychology]. *Análise Psicológica, 2*(21), 195–200.

Canavarro, M. C., Vaz Serra, A., Pereira, M., Simões, M. R., Quintais, L., Quartilho, M. J., . . . Paredes, T. (2006). Desenvolvimento do instrumento de avaliação da qualidade de vida da Organização Mundial de Saúde (WHOQOL100) para português de Portugal [Development of an instrument for assessing World Health Organization quality of life (WHOQOL100) to Portuguese of Portugal]. *Psiquiatria Clínica, 27*(1), 15–23.

Carlson, L. E., Angen, M., Cullum, J., Goodey, E., Koopmans, J., Lamont, L., . . . Bultz, B. D. (2004). High levels of untreated distress and fatigue in cancer patients. *British Journal of Cancer, 90*(12), 2297–2304.

Carlson, L. E., & Bultz, B. D. (2008). Mind-body interventions in oncology. *Current Treatment Options in Oncology, 9*(2-3), 127–134.

Carlson, L. E., & Speca, M. (2007). Managing daily and long-term stress. In Feuerstein, M. (Ed.), *Handbook of Cancer Survivorship* (pp. 339–360). New York: Springer.

Carlson, L. E., Ursuliak, Z., Goodey, E., Angen, M., & Speca, M. (2001). The effects of a mindfulness meditation-based stress reduction program on mood and symptoms of stress in cancer outpatients: 6-month follow-up. *Supportive Care in Cancer, 9*(2), 112–123.

Carter, R. E., & Carter, C. A. (1993). Individual and marital adjustment in spouse pairs subsequent to mastectomy. *American Journal of Family Therapy, 21*(4), 291–300.

Carver, C. S., Porn, C., Harris, S. D., Noriega, V., Scheier, M. F., Robinson, D. S., . . . Clark, K. C. (1993). How coping mediates the effect of optimism on distress: A study of women with early-stage breast cancer. *Journal of Personality and Social Psychology, 65*(2), 375–390.

Carver, C. S., Smith, R. G., Petronis, V. M., & Antoni, M. H. (2006). Quality of life among long-term survivors of breast cancer: Different types of antecedents predict different classes of outcomes. *Psycho-Oncology, 15*(9), 749–758.

Cassidy, J., Bissett, D., Spence, R., & Payne, M. (2011). *Oxford handbook of oncology* (3rd ed.). London: Oxford University Press.

Cassileth, B., & Gubili, J. (2009). Integrative oncology: Complementary therapies in cancer care. In Ettinger, D. S. (Ed.), *Supportive Care in Cancer Therapy* (pp. 269–277). New Jersey: Humana Press.

Cella, D. F., Tulsky, D. S., Gray, G., Sarafian, B., Linn, E., Bonomi, A., . . . Brannon, J. (1993). The Functional Assessment of Cancer Therapy scale: Development and validation of the general measure. *Journal of Clinical Oncology, 11*(3), 570–579.

Chandwani, K. D., Chaoul-Reich, A., Biegler, K. A., & Cohen, L. (2008). Mind-body research in cancer. In Cohen, L., & Markman, M. (Eds.), *Integrative Oncology: Incorporating Complementary Medicine into Conventional Cancer Care* (pp. 139–160). New Jersey: Humana Press.

Chen, C. C., David, A. S., Nunnerley, H., Michell, M., Dawson, J. L., Berry, H., . . . Fahy, T. (1995). Adverse life events and breast cancer: Case-control study. *British Medical Journal, 311*(7019), 1527–1530.

Cheng, S. K. (2001). Life stress, problem solving, perfectionism, and depressive symptoms in Chinese. *Cognitive Therapy and Research, 25*(3), 303–310.

Classen, C., Koopman, C., Angell, K., & Spiegel, D. (1996). Coping styles associated with psychological adjustment to advanced breast cancer. *Health Psychology, 15*(6), 434–437.

Cohen, L., Cole, S. W., Sood, A. K., Prinsloo, S., Kirschbaum, C., Arevalo, J. M., . . . Pisters, L. (2012). Depressive symptoms and cortisol rhythmicity predict survival in patients with renal cell carcinoma: Role of inflammatory signaling. *PLoS One, 7*(8), e42324.

Cohen, L., Warneke, C., Fouladi, R. T., Rodriguez, M. A., & Chaoul-Reich, A. (2004). Psychological adjustment and sleep quality in a randomized trial of the effects of a Tibetan yoga intervention in patients with lymphoma. *Cancer, 100*(10), 2253–2260.

Compas, B. E., Stoll, M. F., Thomsen, A. H., Oppedisano, G., Epping-Jordan, J. E., & Krag, D. N. (1999). Adjustment to breast cancer: Age-related differences in coping and emotional distress. *Breast Cancer Research and Therapy, 54*(3), 195–203.

Cordova, M. J., & Andrykowski, M. A. (2003). Responses to cancer diagnosis and treatment: Posttraumatic stress and posttraumatic growth. *Seminars in Clinical Neuropsychiatry, 8*(4), 286–296.

Curbow, B., Somerfield, M. R., Baker, F., Wingard, J. R., & Legro, M. W. (1993). Personal changes, dispositional optimism, and psychological adjustment to bone marrow transplantation. *Journal of Behavioral Medicine, 16*(5), 423–443.

Deimling, G. T., Kahana, B., Bowman, K. F., & Schaefer, M. L. (2002). Cancer survivorship and psychological distress in later life. *Psycho-Oncology, 11*(6), 479–494.

Dolbeault, S., Mignot, V., Gauvain-Piquard, A., Mandereau, L., Asselain, B., & Medioni, J. (2003). Evaluation of psychological distress and quality of life in French cancer patients: Validation of the French version of the memorial distress thermometer. *Psycho-Oncology, 12*(4), S225.

Dorval, M., Guay, S., Mondor, M., Masse, B., Falardeau, M., Robidoux, A., . . . Maunsell, E. (2005). Couples who get closer after breast cancer: Frequency and predictors in a prospective investigation. *Journal of Clinical Oncology, 23*(15), 3588–3596.

Dorval, M., Maunsell, E., Deschenes, L., Brisson, J., & Masse, B. (1998). Long-term quality of life after breast cancer: Comparison of 8-year survivors with population controls. *Journal of Clinical Oncology, 16*(2), 487–494.

Dow, K. H., Ferrell, B. R., Leigh, S., Ly, J., & Gulasekaram, P. (1996). An evaluation of the quality of life among long-term survivors of breast cancer. *Breast Cancer Research and Treatment, 39*(3), 261–273.

Dreher, H. (2003). *Mind-body unity: A new vision for mind-body science and medicine.* London: The John Hopkins University Press.

D'Zurilla, T. J., & Nezu, A. M. (2006). *Problem-solving therapy: A positive approach to clinical intervention* (3rd ed.). New York: Springer.

Elkins, G. R., Cheung, A., Marcus, J., Palamara, L., & Rajab, H. (2004). Hypnosis to reduce pain in cancer survivors with advanced disease: A prospective study. *Journal of Cancer Integrative Medicine, 2*(4), 167–172.

Fayers, P. M., & Machin, D. (2007). *Quality of life: The assessment, analysis, and interpretation of patient-reported outcomes* (2nd ed.). West Sussex: John Wiley & Sons.

Ferrell, B., & Dow, K. (1997). Quality of life among long-term cancer survivors. *Oncology, 11*(4), 565–576.

Ferrell, B. R., Dow, K. H., & Grant, M. (1995). Measurement of the quality of life in cancer survivors. *Quality of Life Research, 4*(6), 523–531.

Ferrell, B. R., Dow, K. H., Leigh, S., Ly, J., & Gulasekaram, P. (1995). Quality of life in long-term cancer survivors. *Oncology Nursing Forum, 22*(6), 915–922.

Fielding, R., Lam, W. W., & Ho, E. (2004). Factors predicting psychological morbidity in Chinese women following breast cancer surgery. *Psycho-Oncology, 13*(Suppl. 1), S53.

Fleck, M. (2006). O projecto WHOQOL: Desenvolvimentos e aplicações [The WHOQOL project: Developments and applications]. *Psiquiatria Clínica, 27*(1), 5–13.

Fox, B. H. (1995). The role of psychological factors in cancer incidence and prognosis. *Oncology, 9*(3), 245–253.

Frye, A. A., & Goodman, S. H. (2004). Which social problem-solving components buffer depression in adolescent girls? *Cognitive Therapy and Research, 24*(6), 637–650.

Gaston-Johansson, F., Fall-Dickson, J. M., Nanda, J., Ohly, K. V., Stillman, S., Krumm, S., & Kennedy, M. J. (2000). The effectiveness of the comprehensive coping strategy program on clinical outcomes in breast cancer autologous bone marrow transplantation. *Cancer Nursing, 23*(4), 277–285.

Gil, F., Travado, L., Tomamichel, M., & Grassi, L. (2003). Visual analogue scales (VAS) and hospital anxiety depression (HAD) scale as tools for evaluating distress in cancer patients: A multi-centre southern European study. *Psycho-Oncology, 12*, S257.

Golden-Kreutz, D. M., & Andersen, B. L. (2004). Depressive symptoms after breast cancer surgery: Relationships with global, cancer-related and life event stress. *Psycho-Oncology, 13*(3), 211–220.

Goldstein, M. S., Brown, E. R., Ballard-Barbash, R., Morgenstern, H., Bastani, R., Lee, J., . . . Ambs, A. (2005). The use of complementary and alternative medicine among California adults with and without cancer. *Evidence Based Complementary & Alternative Medicine, 2*(4), 557–565.

Goodman, S. H., Gravitt, G. W., & Kaslow, N. J. (1995). Social problem solving: A moderator of the relation between negative life stress and depression symptoms in children. *Journal of Abnormal Child Psychology, 23*(4), 473–485.

Gotay, C. C., & Muraoka, M. (1998). Quality of life in long-term survivors of adult-onset cancers. *Journal of the National Cancer Institute, 90*(9), 656–667.

Grassi, L., Johansen, C., Annunziata, M. A., Capovilla, E., Costantini, A., Gritti, P., . . . Italian Society of Psycho-Oncology Distress Thermometer Study Group. (2013). Screening for distress in cancer patients: A multicenter, nationwide study in Italy. *Cancer, 119*(9), 1714–1721.

Greer, S., Morris, T., & Pettingale, K. W. (1979). Psychological response to breast cancer: Effect on outcome. *Lancet, 2*(8146), 785–787.

Grol, R., & Grimshaw, J. (2003). From best evidence to best practice: Effective implementation of change in patients' care. *Lancet, 362*(9391), 1225–1230.

Hack, T. F., & Degner, L. F. (2004). Coping responses following breast cancer diagnosis predict psychological adjustment three years later. *Psycho-Oncology, 13*(4), 235–247.

Hannum, J. W., Giese-Davis, J., Harding, K., & Hatfield, A. K. (1991). Effects of individual and marital variables on coping with cancer. *Journal of Psychosocial Oncology, 9*(2), 1–20.

Hilsden, R. J., & Verhoef, M. J. (1999). Complementary therapies: Evaluating their effectiveness in cancer. *Patient Education and Counseling, 38*(2), 101–108.

Hodges, K., & Winstanley, S. (2012). Effects of optimism, social support, fighting spirit, cancer worry, and internal health locus of control on positive affect in cancer survivors: A path analysis. *Stress and Health, 28*(5), 408–415.

Hodges, L., Humphris, G., & Macfarlane, G. (2005). A meta-analytic investigation of the relationship between the psychological distress of cancer patients and their caregivers. *Social Science & Medicine, 60*(1), 1–12.

Irwin, M., Patterson, T., Smith, T. L., Caldwell, C., Brown, S. A., Gillin, J. C., & Grant, I. (1990). Reduction of immune function in life stress and depression. *Biological Psychiatry, 27*(1), 22–30.

Isikhan, V., Guner, P., Komurcu, S., Ozet, A., Arpaci, F., & Ozturk, B. (2001). The relationship between disease features and quality of life in patients with cancer–I. *Cancer Nursing, 24*(6), 490–495.

Jones, S. L., Hadjistavropoulos, H. D., & Gullickson, K. (in press, 2013). Understanding health anxiety following breast cancer diagnosis. *Psychology, Health & Medicine.*

Kangas, M. (2013). DSM-5 trauma and stress-related disorders: Implications for screening for cancer-related stress. *Frontiers in Psychiatry, 4*(122), 1–3.

Kayser, K., & Scott, J. L. (2008). *Helping couples cope with women's cancers: An evidence-based approach for practitioners.* New York: Springer.

Keller, M., Henrich, G., Sellschopp, A., & Beutel, M. (1996). Between distress and support: Spouses of cancer patients. In Baider, L., Cooper, C. L., & Kaplan De-Nour, A. (Eds.), *Cancer and the Family* (pp. 187–223). Chichester, England: John Wiley & Sons.

Kolcaba, K., & Fox, C. (1999). The effects of guided imagery on comfort of women with early stage breast cancer undergoing radiation therapy. *Oncology Nursing Forum, 26*(1), 67–72.

Koocher, G. P., & Pollin, I. S. (2001). Preventive psychosocial intervention in cancer treatment: Implications for managed care. In Baum, A., & Andersen, B. L. (Eds.), *Psychosocial Interventions for Cancer* (pp. 363–374). Washington, DC: American Psychological Association.

Kornblith, A. B. (1998). Psychosocial adaptation of cancer survivors. In Holland, J. (Ed.), *Psycho-Oncology* (1st ed., pp. 223–254). New York: Oxford University Press.

Kuijer, R. G., Buunk, B. P., De Jong, G. M., Ybema, J. F., & Sanderman, R. (2004). Effects of a brief intervention program for patients with cancer and their partners on feelings of inequity, relationship quality, and psychological distress. *Psycho-Oncology, 13*(5), 321–334.

Kuijer, R. G., Ybema, J. F., Buunk, B. P., DeJong, G. M., Thijs-Boer, F., & Sanderman, R. (2000). Active engagement, protective buffering, and overprotection: Three ways of giving support by intimate partners of patients with cancer. *Journal of Social and Clinical Psychology, 19*(2), 256–275.

Lepore, S. J., & Ituarte, P. H. (1999). Optimism about cancer enhances mood by reducing negative social relations. *Cancer Research Therapy and Control, 8,* 165–174.

Li, Q., & Loke, A. Y. (2013, in press). A literature review on the mutual impact of the spousal caregiver-cancer patients dyads: "Communication," "reciprocal influence," and "caregiver-patient congruence." *European Journal of Oncology Nursing.*

Lichtman, R. R., Taylor, S. E., Wood, J. V., Bluming, A. Z., Dosik, G. M., & Leibowitz, R. L. (1984). Relations with children after breast cancer: The mother-daughter relationship at risk. *Journal of Psychosocial Oncology, 2*(3-4), 1–19.

Lutgendorf, S. K., Johnsen, E. L., Cooper, B., Anderson, B., Sorosky, J. I., Buller, R. E., & Sood, A. K. (2002). Vascular endothelial growth factor and social support in patients with ovarian carcinoma. *Cancer, 95*(4), 808–815.

Manne, S. L. (1998). Cancer in the marital context: A review of the literature. *Cancer Investigation, 16*(3), 188–202.

Manne, S. L., Taylor, K. L., Dougherty, J., & Kemeny, N. (1997). Supportive and negative responses in the partner relationship: Their association with psychological adjustment among individuals with cancer. *Journal of Behavioral Medicine, 20*(2), 101–125.

Marques, H., & Pimentel, F. (1995). *Oncologia para clínicos gerais [Oncology for general practitioners].* Porto: Mevlor.

McCaul, K. D., Sandgren, A. K., King, B., O'Donnell, S., Branstetter, A., & Foreman, G. (1999). Coping and adjustment to breast cancer. *Psycho-Oncology, 8*(3), 230–236.

Mehnert, A. (2004). Prevalence of post-traumatic stress disorder, anxiety, and depression in a representative sample of breast cancer patients. *Psycho-Oncology, 13,* S62.

Mehnert, A., & Koch, U. (2008). Psychological comorbidity and health-related quality of life and its association with awareness, utilization, and need for psychosocial support in a cancer register-based sample of long-term breast cancer survivors. *Journal of Psychosomatic Research, 64*(4), 383–391.

Montazeri, A., Sajadian, A., Fateh, A., Haji-Mahmoodi, M., & Ebrahimi, M. (2004). Factors predicting psychological distress in cancer patients. *Psycho-Oncology, 13,* S62.

Moorey, S., Frampton, M., & Greer, S. (2003). The cancer coping questionnaire: A self-rating scale for measuring the impact of adjuvant psychological therapy on coping behaviour. *Psycho-Oncology, 12*(4), 331–344.

Moreira, H., & Canavarro, M. C. (2013). Psychosocial adjustment and marital intimacy among partners of patients with breast cancer: A comparison study with partners of healthy women. *Journal of Psychosocial Oncology, 31*(3), 282–304.

Morrow, J., & Nolen-Hoeksema, S. (1990). Effects of responses to depression on the remediation of depressive affect. *Journal of Personality and Social Psychology, 58*(3), 519–527.

Mundy, E. A., DuHamel, K. N., & Montgomery, G. H. (2003). The efficacy of behavioral interventions for cancer treatment related side effects. *Seminars in Clinical Neuropsychiatry, 8*(4), 253–275.

Myers, L. B., Burns, J. W., Derakshan, N., Elfant, E., Eysenck, M. W., & Phipps, S. (2008). Current issues in repressive coping and health. In Vingerhoets, J. J., Nyklícek, I., & Denollet, J. (Eds.), *Emotion Regulation: Conceptual and Clinical Issues* (pp. 69–86). New York: Springer.

National Comprehensive Cancer Network [NCCN]. (2002). *Practice Guidelines in Oncology—v.1.2002: Distress Management (Version 1)*. National Comprehensive Cancer Network, Inc.

Neuling, S. J., & Winefield, H. R. (1988). Social support and recovery after surgery for breast cancer: Frequency and correlates of supportive behaviours by family, friends, and surgeon. *Social Science & Medicine, 27*(4), 385–392.

Nezu, A. M. (2004). Problem solving and behavior therapy revisited. *Behavior Therapy, 35*(1), 1–33.

Nezu, A. M., D'Zurilla, T. J., Zwick, M. L., & Nezu, C. M. (2004). Problem-solving therapy for adults. In Chang, E. C., D'Zurilla, T. J., & Sanna, L. J. (Eds.), *Social Problem Solving: Theory, Research, and Training* (pp. 171–191). Washington, DC: American Psychological Association.

Nezu, A. M., Nezu, C. M., Faddis, S., DelliCarpini, L. A., & Houts, P. S. (1995). *Social problem solving as a moderator of cancer-related stress.* Paper presented at the Association for Advancement of Behavior Therapy, Washington, DC.

Nezu, A. M., Nezu, C. M., Felgoise, S. H., McClure, K. S., & Houts, P. S. (2003). Project Genesis: Assessing the efficacy of problem-solving therapy for distressed adult cancer patients. *Journal of Consulting and Clinical Psychology, 71*(6), 1036–1048.

Nezu, A. M., Nezu, C. M., Felgoise, S. H., & Zwick, M. L. (2003). Psychosocial oncology. In Nezu, A. M., Nezu, C. M., & Geller, P. A. (Eds.), *Health Psychology* (pp. 267–292). New York: Wiley.

Nezu, A. M., Nezu, C. M., Friedman, S. H., Faddis, S., & Houts, P. S. (1998). *Helping cancer patients cope: A problem-solving approach.* Washington, DC: American Psychological Association.

Nezu, A. M., Nezu, C. M., Houts, P. S., Friedman, S. H., & Faddis, S. (1999). Relevance of problem-solving therapy to psychosocial oncology. *Journal of Psychosocial Oncology, 16*(3-4), 5–26.

Nezu, A. M., Nezu, C. M., Saraydarian, L., Kalmar, K., & Ronan, G. F. (1986). Social problem solving as a moderating variable between negative life stress and depression. *Cognitive Therapy and Research, 10*(5), 489–498.

Nezu, A. M., & Perri, M.G. (1989). Social problem-solving therapy for unipolar depression: An initial dismantling investigation. *Journal of Consulting and Clinical Psychology, 57*(3), 408–413.

Nezu, A. M., & Ronan, G. F. (1985). Life stress, current problems, problem solving, and depressive symptoms: An integrative model. *Journal of Consulting and Clinical Psychology, 53*(5), 693–697.

Nezu, A. M., & Ronan, G. F. (1988). Problem solving as a moderator of stress-related depressive symptoms: A prospective analysis. *Journal of Counseling Psychology, 35*(2), 134–138.

Nezu, C. M., Nezu, A. M., Friedman, S. H., Houts, P. S., DelliCarpini, L. A., Bildner, C., & Faddis, S. (1999). Cancer and psychological distress: Two investigations regarding the role of problem solving. *Journal of Psychosocial Oncology, 16*(3-4), 27–40.

Nordin, K., & Glimelius, B. (1998). Reactions to gastrointestinal cancer variation in mental adjustment and emotional well-being over time in patients with different prognoses. *Psycho-Oncology, 7*(5), 413–423.

Northouse, L. L., Templin, T., & Mood, D. (2001). Couples' adjustment to breast disease during the first year following diagnosis. *Journal of Behavioral Medicine, 24*(2), 115–136.

Northouse, L. L., Templin, T., Mood, D., & Oberst, M. (1998). Couples' adjustment to breast cancer and benign breast disease: A longitudinal analysis. *Psycho-Oncology, 7*(1), 37–48.

Oberst, M. T., & Scott, D. W. (1988). Post-discharge distress in surgically treated cancer patients and their spouses. *Research in Nursing and Health, 11,* 223–233.

Ogden, J. (2012). *Health psychology: A textbook.* New York: Open University Press.

Penninx, B. W., Guralnik, J. M., Pahor, M., Ferrucci, L., Cerhan, J. R., Wallace, R. B., & Havlik, R. J. (1998). Chronically depressed mood and cancer risk in older persons. *Journal of the National Cancer Institute, 90*(24), 1888–1893.

Perz, J., Ussher, J. M., & Gilbert, E. (2013). Constructions of sex and intimacy after cancer: A methodology study of people with cancer, their partners, and health professionals. *BMC Cancer, 270,* 1–13.

Petticrew, M., Bell, R., & Hunter, H. (2002). Influence of psychological coping on survival and recurrence in people with cancer: Systematic review. *British Medical Journal, 325*(7372), 1066–1075.

Petticrew, M., Fraser, J. M., & Regan, M. F. (1999). Adverse life-events and risk of breast cancer: A meta analysis. *British Journal of Health Psychology, 4*(1), 1–17.

Pimentel, F. L. (2006). *Qualidade de vida e oncologia [Quality of life and oncology].* Coimbra: Almedina.

Pinto, C., & Pais Ribeiro, J. L. (2006). Qualidade de vida dos sobreviventes de cancro [Quality of life of cancer survivors]. *Revista Portuguesa de Saúde Pública, 24*(1), 37–56.

Pistrang, N., & Barker, C. (1995). The partner relationship in psychological response to breast cancer. *Social Science & Medicine, 40*(6), 789–797.

Pitot, H. C. (2002). *Fundamentals of oncology.* New York: Marcel Dekker, Inc.

Przezdziecki, A., Sherman, K. A., Baillie, A., Taylor, A., Foley, E., & Stalgis-Bilinski, K. (2013). My changed body: Breast cancer, body image, distress and self-compassion. *Psycho-Oncology, 22*(8), 1872–1879.

Ptacek, J. T., Ptacek, J. J., & Dodge, K. L. (1994). Coping with breast cancer from the perspectives of husbands and wives. *Journal of Psychosocial Oncology, 12*(3), 47–72.

Quartana, P. J., Schmaus, B. J., & Zakowski, S. G. (2005). Gender, neuroticism, and emotional expressivity: Effects on spousal constraints among individuals with cancer. *Journal of Consulting and Clinical Psychology, 73*(4), 769–776.

Rabin, B. S. (1999). *Stress, immune function, and health: The connection.* New York: Wiley-Liss & Sons.

Ranchor, A. V., & Sanderman, R. (2006). The role of personality in cancer onset and survival. In Vollrath, M. E. (Ed.), *Handbook of Personality and Health* (pp. 35–49). England: John Wiley & Sons.

Rieker, P. P., Edbril, S. D., & Garnick, M. B. (1985). Curative testis cancer therapy: Psychosocial sequelae. *Journal of Clinical Oncology, 3*(8), 1117–1126.

Rieker, P. P., Fitzgerald, E. M., Kalish, L. A., Richie, J. P., Lederman, G. S., Edbril, S. D., & Garnick, M. B. (1989). Psychosocial factors, curative therapies, and behavioral outcomes. A comparison of testis cancer survivors and a control group of healthy men. *Cancer, 64*(11), 2399–2407.

Rodrick, J. R., Poage, E., Wanchai, A., Stewart, B. R., Cormier, J. N., & Armer, J. M. (2013). Complementary, alternative, and other non-complete decongestive therapy (CDT) treatment methods in the management of lymphedema: A systematic search and review. *PM&R: The Journal of Injury, Function, and Rehabilitation, S1934-1482*(13), 1082–1084.

Sadeh-Tassa, D., Yagil, Y., & Stadler, J. (2004). A comparison between first occurrence and recurrent breast cancer: Anxiety, depression, PTSD. *Psycho-Oncology, 13*(Suppl. 4), S66.

Santos, F. R. (2004). Symptoms of post-traumatic stress disorder in patients with malignant hematologic disease. *Psycho-Oncology, 13*(Suppl. 1), S67.

Schou, I., Ekeberg, O., Ruland, C. M., Sandvik, L., & Karesen, R. (2004). Pessimism as a predictor of emotional morbidity one year following breast cancer surgery. *Psycho-Oncology, 13*(5), 309–320.

Sears, S. R., Stanton, A. L., & Danoff-Burg, S. (2003). The yellow brick road and the Emerald City: Benefit finding, positive reappraisal coping, and posttraumatic growth in women with early-stage breast cancer. *Health Psychology, 22*(5), 487–497.

Sellick, S. M., & Zaza, C. (1998). Critical review of 5 nonpharmacologic strategies for managing cancer pain. *Cancer Prevention & Control, 2*(1), 7–14.

Sephton, S. E., Sapolsky, R. M., Kraemer, H. C., & Spiegel, D. (2000). Diurnal cortisol rhythm as a predictor of breast cancer survival. *Journal of the National Cancer Institute, 92*(12), 994–1000.

Shimizu, K., Akechi, T., Okamura, M., Akizuki, N., & Uchitomi, Y. (2004). Feasibility and usefulness of the distress and impact thermometer as a brief screening tool to detect psychological distress in clinical oncology practice. *Psycho-Oncology, 13*(Suppl. 2), S68–S69.

Simonton, O. C., & Matthews-Simonton, S. (1981). Cancer and stress: Counseling the cancer patient. *Medical Journal of Australia, 1*(27), 679–683.

Simonton, S., Simonton, O. C., & Creighton, J. C. (1978). *Getting well again: A step-by-step, self-help guide to overcoming cancer for patients and their families.* New York: Bantam Books.

Skerrett, K. (1998). Couple adjustment to the experience of breast cancer. *Families, Systems & Health, 16*(3), 281–298.

Spahn, G., Choi, K. E., Kennemann, C., Lüdtke, R., Franken, U., Langhorst, J., . . . Dobos, G. J. (2013). Can a multimodal mind-body program enhance the treatment effects of physical activity in breast cancer survivors with chronic tumor-associated fatigue? A randomized controlled trial. *Integrative Cancer Therapies, 12*(4), 291–300.

Speca, M., Carlson, L. E., Goodey, E., & Angen, M. (2000). A randomized, wait-list controlled clinical trial: The effect of a mindfulness meditation-based stress reduction program on mood and symptoms of stress in cancer outpatients. *Psychosomatic Medicine, 62*(5), 613–622.

Spiegel, D. (1996). Cancer and depression. *British Journal of Psychiatry, 168*(Suppl. 30), 109–116.

Spiegel, D. (2013, in press). Minding the body: Psychotherapy and cancer survival. *British Journal of Health Psychology.*

Stanton, A., Bower, J. E., & Low, C. A. (2005). Posttraumatic growth after cancer. In Calhoun, L., & Tedeschi, R. (Eds.), *The Handbook of Posttraumatic Growth: Research and Practice* (pp. 138–175). Mahwah, NJ: Lawrence Erlbaum Associates.

Stanton, A. L., & Danoff-Burg, S. (2002). Emotional expression, expressive writing, and cancer. In Lepore, S. J., & Smyth, J. M. (Eds.), *The Writing Cure: How Expressive Writing Promotes Health and Emotional Well-being* (pp. 31–51). Washington, DC: American Psychological Association.

Stanton, A. L., Danoff-Burg, S., Cameron, C. L., Bishop, M., Collins, C. A., Kirk, S. B., . . . Twillman, R. (2000). Emotionally expressive coping predicts psychological and physical adjustment to breast cancer. *Journal of Consulting and Clinical Psychology, 68*(5), 875–882.

Stanton, A. L., Kirk, S. B., Cameron, C. L., & Danoff-Burg, S. (2000). Coping through emotional approach: Scale construction and validation. *Journal of Personality and Social Psychology, 78*(6), 1150–1169.

Stanton, A. L., & Snider, P. (1993). Coping with a breast cancer diagnosis: A prospective study. *Health Psychology, 12*(1), 16–23.

Stephens, F. O., & Aigner, K. R. (2009). *Basics of oncology.* New York: Springer.

Steptoe, A., Sutcliffe, I., Allen, B., & Coombes, C. (1991). Satisfaction with communication, medical knowledge, and coping style in patients with metastatic cancer. *Social Science & Medicine, 32*(6), 627–632.

Teixeira, R. J., & Pereira, M. G. (2013). Factors contributing to posttraumatic growth and its buffering effect in adult children of cancer patients undergoing treatment. *Journal of Psychosocial Oncology, 31*(3), 235–265.

Thaker, P. H., Han, L. Y., Kamat, A. A., Arevalo, J. M., Takahashi, R., Lu, C., . . . Sood, A. K. (2006). Chronic stress promotes tumor growth and angiogenesis in a mouse model of ovarian carcinoma. *Nature Medicine, 12*(8), 939–944.

Thewes, B., Bell, M. L., Butow, P., Beith, J., Boyle, F., Friedlander, M., & McLachlan, S. A. (2013, in press). Psychological morbidity and stress but not social factors influence level of fear of cancer recurrence in young women with early breast cancer: Results of a cross-sectional study. *Psycho-Oncology.*

Thornton, A. A. (2002). Perceiving benefits in the cancer experience. *Journal of Clinical Psychology in Medical Settings, 9*(2), 153–165.

Thornton, A. A., & Perez, M. A. (2007). Interpersonal relationships. In Feuerstein, M. (Ed.), *Handbook of Cancer Survivorship* (pp. 191–210). New York: Springer.

Thornton, A. A., Perez, M. A., & Meyerowitz, B. E. (2004). Patient and partner quality of life and psychosocial adjustment following radical prostatectomy. *Journal of Clinical Psychology in Medical Settings, 11*(1), 15–30.

Tjemsland, L., Soreide, J. A., Matre, R., & Malt, U. F. (1997). Preoperative psychological variables predict immunological status in patients with operable breast cancer. *Psycho-Oncology, 6*(4), 311–320.

Tomatis, L. (2001). Between the body and the mind: The involvement of psychological factors in the development of multifactorial diseases. *European Journal of Cancer, 37*(Suppl. 8), 148–152.

Tomich, P. L., & Helgeson, V. S. (2012). Posttraumatic growth following cancer: Links to quality of life. *Journal of Traumatic Stress, 25*(5), 567–573.

Trask, P. C., & Pearman, T. (2007). Depression. In Feuerstein, M. (Ed.), *Handbook of Cancer Survivorship* (pp. 173–189). New York: Springer.

Truant, T., & Bottorff, J. L. (1999). Decision making related to complementary therapies: A process of regaining control. *Patient Education and Counseling, 38*(2), 131–142.

Van der Poel, H. G. (2004). Smart drugs in prostate cancer. *European Urology, 45*(1), 1–17.

Van Halteren, H. K., Bongaerts, G. P., & Wagener, D. J. (2004). Cancer and psychosocial distress: Frequent companions. *Lancet, 364*(9437), 824–825.

Varela, M., & Leal, I. (2007). Estratégias de coping em mulheres com cancro da mama [Coping strategies in women with breast cancer]. *Análise Psicológica, 3*(25), 479–488.

Veach, T., Nicholas, D., & Barton, M. (2002). *Cancer and the family life cycle: A practitioner's guide.* New York: Brunner-Routledge.

Verhoef, M. J., Hilsden, R. J., & O'Beirne, M. (1999). Complementary therapies and cancer care: An overview. *Patient Education and Counseling, 38*(2), 93–100.

Virgo, K. S., Bromberek, J. L., Glaser, A., Horgan, D., Maher, J., & Brawley, O. W. (2013). Health care policy and cancer survivorship. *Cancer, 119*(Suppl 11), 2187–2199.

Walker, A. (2002). The evolving meaning of retirement: A strategy for active aging. *International Social Security Review, 55,* 121–139.

Walker, L. G., Walker, M. B., Ogston, K., Heys, S. D., Ah-See, A. K., Miller, I. D., . . . Eremin, O. (1999). Psychological, clinical, and pathological effects of relaxation training and guided imagery during primary chemotherapy. *British Journal of Cancer, 80*(1-2), 262–268.

Watson, M., Greer, S., Rowden, L., Gorman, C., Robertson, B., Bliss, J. M., & Tunmore, R. (1991). Relationships between emotional control adjustment to cancer and depression and anxiety in breast cancer patients. *Psychological Medicine, 21*(1), 51–57.

Watson, M., Haviland, J. S., Greer, S., Davidson, J., & Bliss, J. M. (1999). Influence of psychological response on survival in breast cancer: A population-based cohort study. *Lancet, 354*(9187), 1331–1336.

Watson, M., Homewood, J., Haviland, J., & Bliss, J. M. (2005). Influence of psychological response on breast cancer survival: 10-year follow-up of population-based cohort. *European Journal of Cancer, 41*(12), 1710–1714.

Weiger, W., Smith, M., Boon, H., Richardson, M., Kaptchuk, T., & Eisenberg, D. (2002). Advising patients who seek complementary and alternative medical therapies for cancer. *Annals of Internal Medicine, 137*(11), 889–903.

Weisman, A. D., & Worden, J. W. (1985). The emotional impact of recurrent cancer. *Journal of Psychosocial Oncology, 3*(4), 5–16.

WHOQOL-Group. (1994). Development of the WHOQOL: Rationale and current status. *International Journal of Mental Health, 23*(3), 24–56.

WHOQOL-Group. (1998). The World Health Organization Quality of Life Assessment (WHOQOL): Development and general psychometric properties. *Social Science & Medicine, 46*(12), 1569–1585.

Wolsko, P. M., Eisenberg, D. M., Davis, R. B., & Phillips, R. S. (2004). Use of mind-body medical therapies. *Journal of General Internal Medicine, 19*(1), 43–50.

Zabora, J., Brintzenhofeszoc, K., Curbow, B., Hooker, C., & Piantadosi, S. (2001). The prevalence of psychological distress by cancer site. *Psycho-Oncology, 10*(1), 19–28.

Zebrack, B., Yi, J., Peterson, L., & Ganz, P. (2007). The impact of cancer and quality of life for long-term survivors. *Psycho-Oncology, 17*(9), 891–900.

Zhang, A., & Siminoff, L. A. (2003). Silence and cancer: Why do families and patients fail to communicate? *Health Communication, 15*(4), 415–429.

Chapter 9

Coping with Long-Term and Late Effects: Challenges Facing Female Survivors of Childhood, Adolescent, and Young Adult Cancer

Anne Moyer, Elisbeth Santore, and
Allison Marziliano

Fortunately, success in the treatment of cancers in younger individuals over recent decades has resulted in a dramatic rise in the proportion of those affected living to be adult survivors, and they now number in the hundreds of thousands (Hewitt, Weiner, & Simone, 2003). Unfortunately, a significant percentage of these individuals cope with complications related to heart, lung, hormonal, and neurocognitive functioning, and muscular and bone health, as well as the threat of second cancers (IOM & NRC, 2003). These long-term effects (those that begin while being treated for cancer and last for five years or more) and late effects (those that begin after completion of treatment) vary due to many disease- and treatment-related factors, but are more likely to affect females (Stein, Syrjala, & Andrykowski, 2008). One prevalent example is the risk for breast cancer following chest radiotherapy in young female survivors of Hodgkin's disease (Bhatia et al., 1996; Travis et al., 2003). This chapter outlines the myriad ways in which childhood, adolescent, and young adult cancer's aftereffects influence several domains of functioning, from the physical, social, and psychological, to the practical (Patenaude & Kupst, 2005).

We emphasize the ways in which, for female survivors in particular, the new normal that they must adjust to, even following successful treatment of their illness, can be especially challenging.

THE REACH AND AFTEREFFECTS OF CHILDHOOD, ADOLESCENT, AND YOUNG ADULT CANCER

There are currently 12 million Americans with a history of cancer, which includes both survivors and those who still have cancer (ACS, 2012). Once diagnosed, a person is considered a survivor until the end of his or her life. The American Cancer Society (2012) asserts that anyone touched by cancer, including patients, caregivers, and supporters, can be referred to as a survivor. Cancer is commonly known to have physical effects; however, in more recent years a larger focus on the psychological and social effects has emerged. For young people, who are still developing in these areas, the disease and its aftermath are likely to impact them to a greater extent.

Although cancer is associated with aging, it does not only affect those who are older (Yang, 2008). There are an estimated 12,060 new cases of cancer affecting children between the ages of 0 and 14 each year (Yang, 2008). About 1,340 deaths from childhood cancer will occur in this age bracket, with 67.4 percent due to cancer relapse and 21.3 percent due to treatment-related adverse effects (Hewitt et al., 2003). The most common cancer among this age group is leukemia, with an overall percentage of 34 percent (Hewitt et al., 2003). Other types of cancers that affect young people include brain and other nervous system cancers, neuroblastoma, Wilms tumor, non-Hodgkin and Hodgkin lymphoma, rhabdomyosarcoma, retinoblastoma, osteosarcoma, and Ewing sarcoma.

With improved treatments available for those with cancer, survival rates have increased. The five-year survival rate for childhood cancers is now 83 percent, which has risen from 58 percent in the mid-1970s (ACS, 2012). Between 2001 and 2007, the five-year survival rate for those aged 0–14 for Hodgkin lymphoma was 95 percent; Wilms tumor, 88 percent; non-Hodgkin lymphoma, 86 percent; leukemia, 83 percent; neuroblastoma, 74 percent; brain and other nervous system tumors, 71 percent; osteosarcoma, 70 percent; and rhabdomyosarcoma, 68 percent (ACS, 2012). Treatment, which can include any combination of surgery, chemotherapy, and radiation therapy, while often medically successful, also produces long-term and late effects. Approximately two-thirds of children treated for cancer experience at least one late effect, and about a quarter of these are life-threatening (ACS, 2012; Hewitt et al., 2003). These long-term and late effects include damage to the liver; kidney; bladder; heart and lungs; muscles and bones; teeth; and gastrointestinal, endocrine, and immune systems, as well as the threat of secondary malignancies. They also include neurocognitive and psychological effects, which involve learning issues, social difficulties, behavioral adjustment issues, and educational and vocational difficulties (Hewitt et al., 2003). For young female lymphoblastic leukemia survivors, obesity due to cranial radiation is a particular problem (Hewitt et al., 2003). These physically challenging aftereffects lead to difficulties in other areas related to young people's social, psychological, and socioeconomic development.

DEVELOPMENTAL AND SOCIAL CHALLENGES

Individuals encounter several opportunities to achieve developmental milestones as they progress through the various stages of the life span. Unfortunately, such opportunities are often painfully complicated for survivors of pediatric cancers. Though the cancer itself may disappear, the ramifications of such a diagnosis may not. Much of the literature on child and adolescent cancer survivors suggests that the long-term effects and limitations of childhood cancer and its treatment are repeatedly realized in new and different ways as survivors mature into adults (Rourke, Stuber, Hobbie, & Kazak, 1999). These effects may interfere with the successful resolution of major life events such as completing school, beginning to assert oneself in the workforce, leaving the nest and living independently, forming interpersonal relationships, and starting a family. Compared to their peers, it may be more difficult for survivors of childhood cancers to meet the challenges of each new phase and successfully move forward.

Adolescence

Adolescence is a time during which the development of positive interpersonal relationships at school and during extracurricular activities is critically important. Many survivors of childhood cancers are at a disadvantage because they do not fully participate in such activities. Stam, Grootenhuis, and Last (2005) administered a Course of Life questionnaire to 353 Dutch survivors of childhood cancer and 508 peers without a history of cancer, all between the ages of 18 and 30. The authors found that, when compared to the control group, the survivor group less often had at least one year of membership in a sports club in primary school (73.3% vs. 84.2%) and in secondary school (61.2% vs. 73.6%). Similarly, Pendley, Dahlquist, and Dreyer (1997) examined differences in activity level between a sample of 21 adolescent cancer survivors (12 male, 9 female) and a healthy control group. The authors found that survivors reported participating in less than half the amount of peer activities than the control group. Without access to these arenas, social development may be hampered, as is demonstrated in a project using data from the Childhood Cancer Survivor Study to investigate social outcomes for adolescents who had battled cancer earlier in life. Based on this sample of 2,979 survivors and 649 siblings, the authors found that survivors fared worse in all measured social domains. Particularly, survivors were 1.4 to 1.7 times more likely than the sibling group to demonstrate social difficulties (Schultz et al., 2007).

Further research suggests that female survivors of childhood cancer, in particular, are at a severe disadvantage with regard to developing social relationships during this stage of life, given the preoccupation that many adolescent females have with body image and physical appearance. Negative body image, possibly due to physical disfigurement from diagnosis or treatment, has serious implications for social adjustment (Pendley et al., 1997) and affects female survivors' ability to fit in among peers.

When it comes to barriers to successful social adjustment in adolescence, the disparities between males and females are not limited to survivors; these differences even begin to emerge in adolescents who are still battling disease or recently completed treatment. In a study comparing 349 healthy adolescents to 168 adolescents with chronic diseases, researchers found that females conveyed lower self-esteem than males in both healthy and diseased groups and that the difference between male and female reports of self-esteem were greatest when the disease was a type of cancer (Kellerman, Zelter, Ellenberg, Dash, & Rigler, 1980). In another study, researchers examined a sample of 752 patients 12 months after diagnosis. The authors found that younger survivors and female survivors reported higher numbers of problems (females' mean = 10.4, males' mean = 9.8). Females reported 420 problems, whereas males reported 291 problems. Younger patients reported 3 or more problems on average than older patients (Baker, Denniston, Smith, & West, 2005).

Young Adulthood

As adolescence gives way to young adulthood, cancer survivors are confronted with a whole new set of challenges for which they may be ill prepared. If survivors were unable to form successful friendships with peers during adolescence, then they may find it more difficult to achieve intimacy and find the person they intend to spend the rest of their lives with. In their study comparing 102 survivors of acute lymphoblastic leukemia and Wilm's tumor, between the ages of 19 and 30, to 102 unrelated healthy controls, researchers found that 36 percent of survivors compared with 9 percent of controls showed avoidant functioning in relationships, indicating that the survivors' relationships were shorter in length and characterized by lack of involvement and confiding (Mackie, Hill, Kondryn, & McNally, 2000). Relationships conceived of poor quality are not as stable as those borne out of years of practice with social encounters.

It is no surprise, then, that the research suggests that marriage rates for survivors of childhood cancers are lower than those of control groups. For example, Byrne et al. (1989) conducted a study of long-term survivors of childhood and adolescent cancers compared to sibling controls and found that not only were survivors of both genders less likely to be married than the control group, but also the average length of time of survivors' marriages was shorter than those of controls. Similar results were found in a sample of survivors with a mean age of diagnosis at age 7 and assessment at age 26, culled from 25 oncology centers throughout the United States and Canada. The researchers found that less than half (32%) of their sample was married or living as married, 6 percent were divorced or separated, and 62 percent had never been married. Comparing this to the general population, the authors concluded that their sample was less likely to marry (Rauck, Green, Yasui, Mertens, & Robison, 1999). In general, then, survivors of childhood cancers seem to be more often single than do individuals without a history of cancer.

The research also seems to suggest that when looking at all women cross-sectionally, female survivors of childhood cancers fare worse in terms of marriage than do female controls or the general female population. One study analyzed marriage rates of female survivors of childhood cancers and controls and found that female survivors were less often married and more often living with their parents than female controls, 39 percent versus 46.6 percent, and 35.8 percent versus 29.4 percent, respectively (Stam et al., 2005). In another study comparing female cancer survivors to females of the general population in England and Wales, the authors found that in every age group there was a greater percentage of married women in the general population than in the survivor group. The difference was most stark in the age group 30–34 years old, where 53.4 percent of survivors were ever married compared to 63.1 percent of women in the general population. Even much later in life, in the age group 45–49 years old, only 80.2 percent of the survivors were ever married compared to 90.5 percent of the women in the general population (Frobisher, Lancashire, Winter, Jenkinson, & Hawkins, 2007).

Despite the bleak picture these studies paint, some studies show that with regard to marriage, females may actually be at an advantage over male cancer survivors. In one study comparing a sample of young adult survivors of childhood cancer diagnosed before age 18 with a group of healthy controls using a structured self-report questionnaire, the authors found that survivors of both genders, especially men, were less likely to marry and more likely to be living with their parents than were the men in the healthy comparison group (Langeveld et al., 2003). In a similar study comparing 1,237 survivors of malignant neoplasms diagnosed between 0 and 14 years old to the general population in the Piedmont region of Italy, the authors found that both male and female survivors demonstrated a marriage deficit, though the deficit was much higher in men than in women, 32 percent versus 18 percent (Dama et al., 2009).

Adulthood

Survivors of childhood cancers will soon find themselves in a world where their peers are not only married, but are also taking the next step into adulthood: starting families of their own. Although their diagnosis and treatment during their first decade of life may be a distant memory, cancer survivors in their late 20s and early 30s may experience the negative effects all over again when they try to conceive. Indeed, for survivors of childhood cancer, there are significant worries and fears that accompany what most people consider to be a joyous time in their lives. In one study, the researchers administered a questionnaire to 283 survivors free of disease from the Cleveland Clinic Foundation Cancer Tumor Registry, with a mean age of diagnosis at 26 years old. They found that of those without children, 76 percent desired having children in the future. However, about 50 percent of the sample expected to have impaired fertility due to their previous diagnoses; 19 percent expressed anxiety that their children would be affected by the treatment they had undergone; and 18 percent of the females were concerned that a pregnancy would lead to a reoccurrence in their disease (Schover, Rybicki, Martin, & Bringelsen, 1999). Similarly, in a pilot survey of 132 young men and women cancer survivors, the researchers found that 17 percent of the women in their sample had unrealistically high levels of anxiety about the potential for pregnancy to cause cancer reoccurrence (Schover, 2005). Regardless of whether or not fertility is actually threatened for this group, the fears and concerns are very much a part of their reality.

Studies confirm that the rates of pregnancy of female survivors of childhood cancers are much lower than those of the general population. Based on data reported to a Finnish cancer registry, the probability of parenthood was reduced among pediatric and adolescent cancer survivors compared to the general population. For women specifically, the cumulative probability of parenthood by the age of 35 for survivors was 38 percent compared to 73 percent for healthy siblings (Madanat et al., 2008).

Much research (Bath et al., 1999; Critchley et al., 1992; Shalet, Beardwell, Morris-Jones, Pearson, & Orrell, 1976; Thomson, Critchley, Kelnar, & Wallace, 2002; Wallace, Shalet, Crowne, Morris-Jones, & Gattamaneni, 1989) demonstrates the negative long-term effect that radiation in particular has on fertility and the health of offspring of both men and women cancer survivors. In one study, researchers administered questionnaires on pregnancy outcomes to 10,483 survivors of childhood cancers; the results showed that female survivors who had received abdominal radiotherapy were three times more likely to deliver pre-term and two times more likely to have low-birth-weight offspring than the general population (Reulen, Zeegers, Hammish, & Wallace, 2009). Similarly, Chiarelli, Marrett, and Darlington (1999) conducted a retrospective cohort design study with data from the Ontario Cancer registry to analyze 719 women who had survived childhood cancer diagnosed before age 20. The authors found that women who had been treated with abdominal pelvic radiation had a fertility deficit of 23 percent in comparison to those who had only had surgery. Based on data from the Childhood Cancer survivor study, researchers found that survivors' children were more likely to be born pre-term than were siblings' children. Furthermore, looking within the survivor group, survivors treated with radiotherapy during childhood had a 50 percent chance of having children born pre-term and a 36.2 percent chance of having children born at low birth weights, compared to those survivors not treated with radiotherapy, who had only a 19.6 percent chance of having children born pre-term and a 7.2 percent chance of children having low birth weight (Signorello et al., 2006).

HEALTH-RELATED BEHAVIOR

Evidence shows that survivors of childhood cancers are prone to cancer recurrence throughout their life span. Using a sample of 1,380 patients treated with radiation for childhood Hodgkin's disease, researchers found that cumulative risk of a second cancer was 7 percent greater in this sample than in the general population at 15 years post-diagnosis, showing an 18-fold increase in risk. Women in this cohort had a risk of breast cancer 75 times greater than the general population, and such risk increased as the dose of radiation they received years earlier increased (Bhatia et al., 1996).

According to the Scottish Intercollegiate Guideline network bulletin, a subsequent malignancy is the leading cause of death in long-term survivors of Hodgkin's disease, especially so for women developing breast cancer. Beaty et al. (1995) reviewed records of 499 Hodgkin's disease patients who were diagnosed at either preadolescence (less than 10 years old) or adolescence (greater than or equal to 10) and treated with both radiation and chemotherapy. The authors found that, at follow-up, 25 patients in the sample had second malignancies, and 3 had third malignancies. Adolescent females emerged as having the greatest risk in the sample, with subsequent malignancies being most common among females, even when breast cancer was removed from the analysis. In another chart review of the records of 885 women treated for Hodgkin's disease in childhood, the researchers found that 25 women in the sample developed invasive breast cancer. Those at the highest risk appeared to be women treated with radiation before 30 years old (Hancock, Tucker, & Hoppe, 1993).

Given this precarious situation, the health behaviors of cancer survivors are critically important. Minimizing risky behavior, such as smoking and drinking, and increasing safe practices, such as screening, physical activity, and eating healthy, may decrease the risk of being diagnosed with a second malignancy. Unfortunately, earlier experiences may affect the way survivors behave; whereas some may feel invincible and engage in risky behaviors they do not believe can hurt them, others may be overly cautious about their behaviors (Childhood Cancer Survivorship Bulletin). Cognitions about their susceptibility to subsequent malignancies may also play a role in behaviors. According to a survey on the opinions of health behaviors of preadolescent and adolescent cancer survivors between the ages of 10 and 18 years old, 78 percent of the sample believed that, compared to their healthy peers, it was "somewhat more" or "a lot more" important for them to practice healthy behaviors, and the majority of the sample believed that their health was within their control (Tyc, Hadley, & Crockett, 2001).

It is not uncommon for newly diagnosed individuals to alter their behaviors immediately or shortly after diagnosis. One study noted the dietary changes of 250 women 12 months after receiving a diagnosis of nonmetastatic breast cancer. The authors found that 41 percent of the sample reported dietary changes within the year, most notably a decrease in the consumption of red meat by 77 percent of the sample and increase in fruit and vegetable intake by 72 percent of the sample. The authors noted that women's behavior changes in the initial months following diagnosis are consistent with the current guidelines for cancer prevention, and they suggested that women appear to be changing their eating behaviors in an effort to prevent cancer progression (Maunsell, Drolet, Brisson, Robert, & Deschenes, 2002).

While the immediate behavior changes are often dramatic in a positive way, the longer-term behavior changes of survivors do not always appear to be so. In fact, the results appear mixed. Using data from the annual health survey on noninstitutionalized civilians to compare smoking in survivors and controls, researchers found that there was a significantly higher rate of smoking for younger cancer survivors (37.7%) compared to a young, noncancer control group (26.2%). In particular, high levels of smoking were seen among women survivors of cervical and uterine cancer (Coups & Ostroff, 2005). On the other hand, Stam et al. (2005) found in their study that alcohol use during secondary school was higher in their control group (27.3%) than in their survivor group (19%). Similarly, they also found that smoking was more common in the control group (39.7%) compared to the cancer group (23.9%). These patterns appeared stable even after secondary school, with alcohol and smoking higher in both control groups compared to survivor groups, 50.1 percent versus 45.3 percent and 48 percent versus 29.7 percent, respectively.

Some research suggests that survivors of childhood cancers are likely to take steps to increase their positive health behaviors. Humpel, Magee, and Jones (2007) found that in their overwhelmingly female (81.4%) sample, 71.7 percent of the survivors reported that they engaged in a sufficient amount of physical activity to meet the recommended guidelines. Similarly, based on a population-based investigation using the National Health Interview Study, researchers found that female cancer survivors were

34 percent and 36 percent more likely to meet the guidelines for mammogram and Pap smear screenings than were controls with no history of cancer (Bellizzi, Rowland, Jeffery, & McNeel, 2005).

EDUCATIONAL AND OCCUPATIONAL ATTAINMENT AND INSURANCE COVERAGE

It goes without saying that medical treatment can result in academic disruptions for young cancer patients who are still in school. Furthermore, in addition to the physical effects, the neurocognitive effects of cancer and cancer treatment on mental processes such as concentration and memory, especially for those with central nervous system (CNS) cancers, can compromise educational attainment (Ellenberg et al., 2009). Educational attainment is related, in turn, to employment level and employment status, even in the absence of blatant employment discrimination (against which there are now some legal protections; IOM & NRC, 2003). Type of employment and employment status are intimately tied to one's identity and sense of worth (Parsons et al., 2012) and are, in turn, related to economic advantage and to having health and life insurance coverage. Access to health insurance is particularly important for cancer survivors, who need follow-up care to treat potential long-term complications of primary treatment and continued surveillance to detect second malignancies (Park et al., 2005). Finally, obtaining life insurance can also be problematic, as a history of cancer may be a disqualifying criterion (IOM & NRC, 2003).

Data from the Childhood Cancer Survivor Study (CCSS), a multi-institution consortium survey that includes the most comprehensively studied cohort of childhood and adolescent cancer survivors (Robinson et al., 2009), provide much evidence related to these educational, occupational, and health insurance outcomes. For instance, one report noted that among survivors who were 25 years of age or older, health-related unemployment was predicted by impaired physical health (Kirchoff, Krull, Ness, Armstrong et al., 2011). Also, for males, problems with somatic distress, task efficiency (ability to complete work or multitask), and memory (ability to remember instructions), and for females, task efficiency problems, were additional predictors of employment status. Furthermore, for females, problems with task efficiency, emotional regulation (becoming easily upset), and memory predicted a lower likelihood of holding professional positions, whereas for males these difficulties were not significant predictors. Importantly, when this model was adjusted for educational achievement and a history of cranial radiation therapy, the associations for females were no longer significant, leading the authors to suggest that these factors could represent potential targets for intervention, such that by addressing educational barriers and late effects of cranial radiation, females' occupational attainment might be improved. When compared with their siblings, adult survivors of childhood cancers also have been found to have higher health-related unemployment, particularly if they are female, and a higher likelihood of being unemployed but seeking work (Kirchoff et al., 2010). Adult survivors of childhood cancer who were employed earned less and were less likely to hold managerial or professional positions compared to their unaffected siblings, and female survivors were less likely to hold these types of positions than male survivors (Kirchoff, Krull, Ness, Park et al., 2011). Compared to unemployed siblings, unemployed survivors had lower education and income and were more likely to have public rather than private health insurance; compared to employed survivors, unemployed survivors had worse physical functioning (Kirchoff et al., 2010).

In another report based upon data from this large cohort that focused just on adult survivors of pediatric bone tumors in the lower extremities or pelvis, level of education was a significant predictor of employment and having health insurance (Nagarajan et al., 2003). For the outcome of being in the workforce, gender was also a significant predictor, with males more likely to be employed than females. One encouraging finding was that 87 percent of the sample reported having health insurance, with females being more likely than males to have coverage. This was attributed to the fact that the female cancer survivors were also more likely to be married, which may have increased their likelihood of having such coverage (through their spouses). Other analyses of data from this study cohort provide evidence for academic risk for many survivors of childhood cancer, especially for those treated for brain tumors, as well as risk for unemployment, especially for females (Gurney et al., 2009). In addition, among those with CNS tumors, degree of impairment was related to risk for low educational attainment and income, and risk for unemployment (Ellenberg et al., 2009).

With respect to access to health insurance for survivors of all types of childhood cancers, the overall data from the CCSS noted that survivors had lower rates of coverage than their unaffected siblings (84 percent vs. 88 percent) and reported more difficulty obtaining this coverage (29 percent vs. 3 percent; Park et al., 2005). Factors associated with not having insurance coverage among the survivors in the study included having been diagnosed at a younger age, having been treated with cranial radiation, being younger, having less education, being of low income, not being married, and being a current smoker. Data from a nationally representative U.S. survey that identified adolescent and young adult cancer survivors indicated that the proportion who were uninsured (21%) was similar to that among those in the sample without a cancer history (23%), and these proportions did not differ significantly after controlling for age, sex, and race (Kirchoff, Lyles, Fluchel, Wright, & Leisenring, 2012). Although they were not less likely to have a medical provider or to have not had any routine medical visits in the past year, survivors were, however, more likely than those without a cancer history to report forgoing medical care due to costs in the past year.

Other studies conducted in the Netherlands, for example, have similarly shown that, compared to individuals with no cancer history, long-term young adult survivors of childhood cancers had lower educational attainment, were more likely to have been enrolled in programs for the learning disabled, and, if female, were less likely to have finished high school or earned an advanced degree (Langeveld et al., 2003). Likewise, survivors were less likely to be employed, had reported some kind of job discrimination, and indicated being denied entrance to the military due to their cancer history. Some of the occupationally relevant disabilities that these long-term survivors reported were visual handicaps, mobility problems, learning difficulties, and extreme fatigue. Other research conducted in that country indicated that, although there were some limitations in terms of developmental milestones, survivors of childhood cancer had attained comparable levels of education as their peers without a history of cancer (Stam et al., 2005). Similarly, a smaller case-control study found less evidence of long-term economic limitations for survivors of childhood cancer several years into adulthood, in general, but did note setbacks in education, employment, and insurance for individuals with histories of CNS cancers in particular (Hays et al., 1992).

In sum, educational, employment, and insurance difficulties have the potential to build upon one another and influence the course of young cancer survivors' adult lives in real, practical, and day-to-day ways, even years after initial cancer treatment. In several research reports, evidence for particular disadvantages for females was noted. As women often reside in lower socioeconomic positions than do males (American Psychological Association, 2012), despite the possibility of holding stronger positions by virtue of the standing of their spouses, this group of cancer survivors appears to be especially vulnerable.

LONG-TERM PSYCHOLOGICAL AND MENTAL FUNCTIONING

Cancer survivors in general are found to cope well with the aftereffects of their illness, although a subset is documented to have poor adjustment (Stanton, 2006); this type of pattern has also been seen in adolescent and young adult cancer survivors (Evan & Zelzer, 2006; Kellerman et al., 1980). Depression, anxiety, and fears of recurrence are common difficulties for cancer survivors, but these may be mitigated by individual difference factors, such as optimism, self-efficacy, emotional intelligence, spirituality, and interpersonal, informational, and tangible social support, that help them cope with the stress and burden of cancer (Andrykowski, Lynkins, & Floyd, 2008). A summary report from the CCSS considered psychological distress, quality of life, life satisfaction, and neurocognitive functioning, and noted elevated rates of compromised health and mental health–related quality of life, and clinically significant rates of emotional distress in comparison to siblings, as well as neurocognitive problems among childhood cancer survivors (Zelzer et al., 2009). Particular problems were noted for females with respect to fatigue, anxiety, and depression, as well as for those who were low income, unemployed, and experiencing physical late effects of treatment. In another analysis of data from this study, importantly, poorer emotional functioning was found to be related to lower educational and income attainment and a lower likelihood of marrying in childhood cancer survivors (Gurney et al., 2009). In another, smaller study of adolescent and young adult survivors of pediatric cancer, however, psychological indices such as distress and health-related quality of life were found to be similar to those of controls (Kazak et al., 2010).

More recently, coping with a life-threatening illness has come to be recognized as an experience sufficiently horrifying and intense to have the potential to lead to post-traumatic stress disorder (PTSD; American Psychiatric Association, 1994; IOM & NRC, 2003). For those diagnosed with and treated for cancer at a young age, the traumatic aspects of their illness are particularly relevant, as their treatment can involve painful procedures, such as bone marrow biopsies, and frightening experiences such as separation from parents (Stuber et al., 2011). Although varying diagnostic criteria have been applied in the pediatric oncology literature, typical PTSD symptoms include increased arousal, avoidance of reminders (e.g., the smells, sights, or places associated with treatment) of the traumatic event, and involuntarily reexperiencing the event, especially in the presence of reminders (Stuber et al., 2011). The documented rates of post-traumatic stress in adults who were treated for cancer at a younger age are striking. For instance, one study of adults aged 18–40 years who had been treated for cancer as children found that 21 percent met formal American Psychiatric Association PTSD diagnostic criteria determined by clinical interview at some point since completing their treatment (Hobbie et al., 2000). Although being diagnosed was not predicted by the intensity of their medical treatment, those meeting criteria for PTSD also scored significantly higher than those who did not meet criteria on all subscales of distress measured by the Brief Symptom Inventory. Similarly, among another sample of adult survivors of childhood cancer that used a self-report instrument to assess post-traumatic stress symptoms, 13 percent evidenced scores indicative of possible PTSD (Lee & Santacroce, 2007). A study of adolescent and young adult survivors of childhood cancer (at least five years post diagnosis) found self-reported levels of post-traumatic stress symptoms of reexperiencing, avoidance, and arousal to be similar to those of controls (Kazak et al., 2010). However, among the survivors those diagnosed in adolescence had higher levels of post-traumatic symptoms than did those diagnosed as school-age children, suggesting that this time of transition may be one in which young cancer patients are particularly vulnerable. A post-traumatic response framework fits well with the common psychological symptoms experienced by young cancer survivors and can help explain common findings of distressing symptoms persisting against a background of largely adaptive functioning (Rourke et al., 1999).

An alternative notion is that traumatic events, including life-threatening illness, can lead to growth, in the form of changes in the perception of oneself, closer relationships with others, and a more expansive philosophy of life (Tedeschi & Calhoun, 1996). Some research has documented positive psychological outcomes for young adult survivors of pediatric cancer (Elkin, Phipps, Mulhern, & Fairclough, 1997; Zebrack et al., 2012). However, reports of post-traumatic growth following cancer have also been found to be subject to bias in recall of autobiographic memory (Ransom, Sheldon, & Jacobsen, 2008).

Interventions to assist long-term survivors of cancer at younger ages are productively aimed at helping them cope with the uncertainty accompanying the possibility of late-effects manifests. For instance, uncertainty may surround the issues of what kind of late effects are likely to occur, their severity, how they will impact quality of life and longevity, and what can be done to control them, and addressing this in tandem with medically supervised follow-up may be particularly helpful (Santacroce, Asmus, Kadan-Lottick, & Grey, 2010). Many major medical centers now offer programs of integrated medical and psychological follow-up care, such as the Adult Long-Term Follow-Up Program, that provide services related to dental and sexual health, integrative medicine, speech and hearing, nutrition, smoking cessation, and physical rehabilitation, as well as informational resources (Memorial Sloan-Kettering Cancer Center, 2010). Also, many organizations offer resources, support, and advocacy, such as the National Childhood Cancer Society (http://www.beyondthecure.org/), which provides financial, emotional, and educational resources; Stupid Cancer (the I'm Too Young for This! Cancer Foundation; http://stupidcancer .com/), which supports and empowers young adults with cancer; and the National Collegiate Cancer Foundation (http://www.collegiatecancer .org/), which assists young adults in pursuing higher education and coping with the transition from cancer patient to cancer survivor.

GOING FORWARD: COPING WITH THE "NEW NORMAL" AND FUTURE RESEARCH DIRECTIONS

Even after treatment is over, a person with cancer still continues to be affected by the disease (Kyngäs et al., 2000; Woodgate, 2006). For younger cancer patients in particular, it is critical to consider this long-term impact. Many families maintain that their lives and future plans were forever changed by childhood cancer (Woodgate, 2006). Many cancer survivors are not prepared for the ongoing physical, psychological, social, and financial concerns that result (Alfano & Rowland, 2006), and this is even more pronounced for those treated for cancer at a young age. Further-more, there is a lack of knowledge regarding long-term and late effects and often survivors only discover these much later, and on their own (Ben-Ari, 2011). Long-term and late effects that affect females dispropor-tionately, such as disruptions to fertility, mean that women will have a more challenging time adjusting to their ensuing altered reality, often re-ferred to as the "new normal" (Silk, 2011; James, 2012).

While the concept of the "new normal" of long-term cancer survivor-ship is becoming better understood in the research community, most of the literature found on the topic is from narratives and anecdotes of survi-vors and their families directly (Costanzo et al., 2007). The "new normal" is a concept commonly understood within the cancer community and by treatment teams; however, there is still a need for clinical and empirical research on this emerging topic.

Some of the methodological challenges of such future research and for the research summarized in this chapter include self-selection of research participants (a particular difficulty for the CCSS sample) among a group of people who may want to put the experience of cancer behind them; appropriate selection of comparison groups; selection of assessment instruments appropriate to the experience of pediatric, adolescent, and young adult cancers that can measure potentially subtle but important effects; and an emphasis on self-report measures (see Patenaude & Kupst, 2005). One encouraging ongoing research initiative includes the NIH-funded Oncofertility Consortium's Fertility Research Study (FIRST), which aims to better understand, assess, and preserve fertility among adolescent and young adult cancer survivors (Robinson, 2012). Among this group, despite the challenges of approaching patients at a sensitive time in their treatment, accessibility through social media has aided in recruitment. Such initiatives begin to address the gaps in knowledge re-garding remedies for some of the late and long-term effects of cancer treat-ment at a young age and offer hope for coping more effectively through adulthood as a survivor.

REFERENCES

Alfano, C. M., and Rowland, J. H. (2006). Recovery issues in cancer survivorship: A new challenge for supportive care. *The Cancer Journal 12*, 432–443.

American Cancer Society [ACS]. (2012). *Cancer Facts & Figures 2012*. Atlanta: American Cancer Society.

American Psychiatric Association. (1994). *Diagnostic and statistical manual, IV*.

American Psychological Association. (2012). Fact sheet: Women & socioeconomic status. Retrieved from http://www.apa.org/pi/ses/resources/publications/factsheet-women.aspx.

Andrykowski, M. A., Lynkins, E., & Floyd, A. (2008). Psychological health in cancer survivors. *Seminars in Oncology Nursing, 24*, 193–201. doi:10.1016/j.soncn.2008.05.007.

Baker, F., Denniston, M., Smith, T., & West, M. (2005). Adult cancer survivors: How are they faring? *Cancer, 104*, 2565–2576. doi:10.1002/cncr.21488.

Bath, L. E., Critchley, H. O. D., Chambers, S. E., Anderson, R. A., Kelnar, C., & Wallace, H. (1999). Ovarian and uterine characteristics after total body irradiation in childhood and adolescence: Response to sex steroid replacement. *British Journal of Obstetrics and Gynecology, 106*, 1265–1272.

Beaty, O., Hudson, M. M., Greenwald, C., Luo, X., Fang, L., Williams, J. A., . . . & Pratt, C. B. (1995). Subsequent malignancies in children and adolescents after treatment for Hodgkin's disease. *Journal of Clinical Oncology, 13*, 603–609.

Bellizzi, K. M., Rowland, J. H., Jeffery, D. D., & McNeel, T. (2005). Health behaviors of cancer survivors: Examining opportunities for cancer control intervention. *Journal of Clinical Oncology, 23*, 8884–8893. doi:10.1200/JCO.2005.02.2343.

Ben-Ari, E. (2011). For many young cancer survivors, late effects pose lasting problems. *NCI Cancer Bulletin, Special Issue: Adolescents and Young Adult Cancer 8*.

Bhatia, S., Robinson, L. L., Oberlin, O., Greenberg, M., Bunin, G., Fossati-Bellant, F., . . . & Meadows, A. T. (1996). Breast cancer and other second neoplasms after childhood Hodgkin's disease. *New England Journal of Medicine, 334*, 745–751. doi:10.1056/NEJM199603213341201.

Byrne, J., Fears, T. R., Steinhorn, S. C., Mulvihill, J. J., Connelly, R. R., Austin, D. F., . . . & Teta, M. J. (1989). Marriage and divorce after childhood and adolescent cancer. *The Journal of the American Medical Association, 262*, 2693–2699. doi:10.1001/jama.1989.03430190077035.

Chiarelli, A. M., Marrett, L. D., & Darlington, G. (1999). Early menopause and infertility in females after treatment for childhood cancer diagnosed in 1964–1988 in Ontario, Canada. *American Journal of Epidemiology, 150*, 245–254.

Costanzo, E. S., Lutgendorf, S. K., Mattes, M. L., Trehan, S., Robinson, C. B., Terfik, F., & Roman, S. L. (2007). Adjusting to life after treatment: Distress and quality of life following treatment for breast cancer. *British Journal of Cancer 97*, 1625–1631. doi: 10.1038/sj.bjc.6604091.

Coups, E. J., & Ostroff, J. S. (2005). A population-based estimate of the prevalence of behavioral risk factors among adult cancer survivors and noncancer controls. *Preventive Medicine, 40*, 702–711. doi:10.1016/j.ypmed.2004.09.011.

Critchley, H. O. D., Wallace, W. H. B., Shalet, S. M., Mamtora, H., Higginson, J., & Anderson, D. C. (1992). Abdominal irradiation in childhood: The potential for pregnancy. *British Journal of Obstetrics and Gynecology, 99*, 392–394.

Dama, E., Maule, M., Mosso, M., Alessi, D., Ghisleni, M., Pivetta, E., . . . & Merletti, F. (2009). Life after childhood cancer: Marriage and offspring in adult long-term survivors—a population-based study in the Piedmont region, Italy. *European Journal of Cancer Prevention, 18*, 425–430. doi:10.1097/CEJ.0b013e3283307770.

Elkin, T. D., Phipps, S., Mulhern, R. K., & Fairclough, D. (1997). Psychological functioning of adolescent and young adult survivors of pediatric malignancy. *Medical and Pediatric Oncology, 29,* 582–588. doi:10.1002/(SICI)1096-911X (199712)29:6<582::AID-MPO13>3.0.CO;2-8.

Ellenberg, L., Lui, Q., Gioia, G., Yasui, Y., Packer, R. J., Mertens, A., . . . & Zelzer, L. K. (2009). Neurocognitive status of long-term survivors of childhood CNS malignancies: A report from the Childhood Cancer Survivor Study. *Neuropsychology, 23,* 705–717. doi: 10.1037/a0016674.

Evan, E. E., & Zelzer, L. K. (2006). Psychosocial dimensions of cancer in adolescents and young adults. *Cancer, 107,* 1663–1671. doi:10.1002/cncr.22107.

Frobisher, C., Lancashire, E. R., Winter, D. L., Jenkinson, H. C., & Hawkins, M. M. (2007). Long-term population-based marriage rates among adult survivors of childhood cancer in Britain. *International Journal of Cancer, 121,* 846–855. doi:10.1002/ijc.22742.

Gurney, J. G., Krull, K. R., Kadan-Lottick, N., Nicholson, H. S., Nathan, P. C., Zebrack, B., . . . & Ness, K. K. (2009). Social outcomes in the Childhood Cancer Survivor Study cohort. *Journal of Clinical Oncology, 27,* 2390–2395. doi:10.1200/JCO.2008.21.1458.

Hancock, S. L., Tucker, M. A., & Hoppe, R. T. (1993). Breast cancer after treatment of Hodgkin's disease. *Journal of the National Cancer Institute, 85,* 25–31. doi:10.1093/jnci/85.1.25.

Hays, D. M., Landsverk, J., Sallan, S. E., Hewett, K. D., Patenaude, A. F., Schoonover, D., . . . & Siegel, S. E. (1992). Educational, occupational, and insurance status of childhood cancer survivors in their fourth and fifth decades of life. *Journal of Clinical Oncology, 10,* 1397–1406.

Hewitt, S., Weiner, S. L., & Simone, J. V. (2003). *Childhood cancer survivorship: Improving care and quality of life.* Washington, DC: The National Academies Press.

Hobbie, W. L., Stuber, M., Meeske, K., Wissler, K., Rourke, M. T., Ruccione, K., . . . & Kazak, A. E. (2000). Symptoms of posttraumatic stress in young adult survivors of childhood cancer. *Journal of Clinical Oncology, 18,* 4060–4066.

Humpel, N., Magee, C., & Jones, S. C. (2007). The impact of a cancer diagnosis on the health behaviors of cancer survivors and their family and friends. *Supportive Care in Cancer, 15,* 621–630. doi:10.1007/s00520-006-0207-6.

IOM (Institute of Medicine). (2008). Cancer care for the whole patient: Meeting psychosocial health needs. Adler, N. E., & Page, Ann E. K. (Eds.). Washington, DC: National Academies Press.

IOM and NRC (National Research Council). (2003). *Childhood cancer survivorship: Improving care and quality of life.* Hewitt, M., Weiner, S., & Simone, J. V. (Eds.). Washington, DC: National Academies Press.

James, S. D. (2012, August 23). Cancer rehab helps survivors overcome the new normal. *ABC News.* Retrieved from http://abcnews.go.com/Health/cancer-rehab-helps-survivors-cope-impairments-caused-chemo/story?id =17059912#.UM50GGfF4_J.

Kazak, A. E., DeRosa, B. W., Schwartz, L. A., Hobbie, W., Carlson, C., Ittenbach, R. F., . . . & Ginsberg, J. P. (2010). Psychological outcomes and health beliefs in adolescent and young adult survivors of childhood cancer and controls. *Journal of Clinical Oncology, 28,* 2002–2007. doi: 10.1200/JCO.2009.25.9564.

Kellerman, J., Zelter, L., Ellenberg, L., Dash, J., & Rigler, D. (1980). Psychological effects of illness in adolescence. Anxiety, self-esteem, and perception of control. *Pediatrics, 97,* 126–131.

Kirchoff, A. C., Krull, K. R., Ness, K. K., Armstrong, G. T., Park, E. R., Stovall, M., . . . & Leisenring, W. (2011). Physical, mental, and neurocognitive status and employment outcomes in the Childhood Cancer Survivor Study cohort. *Cancer Epidemiology, Biomarkers, & Prevention, 20,* 1839–1849. doi:10.1158/1055 -9965.EPI-11-0239.

Kirchoff, A. C., Krull, K. R., Ness, K. K., Park, E. R., Oeffinger, K. C., Hudson, M. M., . . . & Leisenring, W. (2011). Occupational outcomes of adult childhood cancer survivors: A report from the Childhood Cancer Survivor Study. *Cancer, 117,* 3033–3044. doi:10.1002/cncr.25867.

Kirchoff, A. C., Leisenring, W., Krull, K. R., Ness, K. K., Friedman, D. L., Armstrong, G. T, . . . & Wickizer, T. (2010). Unemployment among adult survivors of childhood cancer. *Medical Care, 48,* 1015–1025. doi:10.1097/ MLR.0b013e3181eaf880.

Kirchoff, A. C., Lyles, C. R., Fluchel, M., Wright, J., & Leisenring, W. (2012). Limitations in health care access and utilization among long-term survivors of adolescent and young adult cancer. *Cancer, 118,* 5964–5972. doi:10.1002/cncr.27537.

Kyngäs, H., Mikkonen, R., Nousiainen, E. M., Rytilahti, M., Seppänen, P., Vaattovaara, R., and Jämsä, R. (2000). Coping with the onset of cancer: Coping strategies and resources of young people with cancer. *European Journal of Cancer Care 10,* 6–11. doi:10.1046/j.1365-2354.2001.00243.x.

Langeveld, N. E., Ubbink, M. C., Last, B. F., Grootenhuis, M. A., Voûte, P. A., & de Haan, R. J. (2003). Educational, achievement, employment, and living situation in long-term young adult survivors of childhood cancer in the Netherlands. *Psycho-Oncology, 12,* 213–225. doi:10.1002/pon.628.

Lee, Y.-L., & Santacroce, S. J. (2007). Posttramatic stress in long-term young adult survivors of childhood cancer: A questionnaire survey. *International Journal of Nursing Studies, 44,* 1406–1417. doi:10.1016/j.ijnurstu.2006.07.002.

Mackie, E., Hill, J., Kondryn, H., & McNally, R. (2000). Adult psychosocial outcomes in long term survivors of acute lymphoblastic leukemia and Wilms' tumor: A controlled study. *Lancet, 355,* 1310–1314.

Madanat, L. S., Malila, N., Dyba, T., Hakulinen, T., Sankila, R., Boice, J. D., . . . & Lahteenmaki, P. M. (2008). Probability of parenthood after early onset cancer: A population-based study. *International Journal of Cancer, 123,* 2891–2898. doi:10.1002/ijc.23842.

Maunsell, E., Drolet, M., Brisson, J., Robert, J., & Deschenes, L. (2002). Dietary change after breast cancer: Extent, predictors, and relation with psychological distress. *Journal of Clinical Oncology, 20,* 1017–1025.

Memorial Sloan-Kettering Cancer Center. (2010). Living beyond cancer: Adult long-term follow-up program. Retrieved from http://www.mskcc.org/sites/ www.mskcc.org/files/node/6316/documents/adult-long-term-followup.pdf.

Nagarajan, R., Neglia, J. P., Clohisy, D. R., Yasui, Y., Greenberg, M., Hudson, M., . . . & Robinson, L. L. (2003). Education, employment, insurance, and marital status among 694 survivors of pediatric lower extremity bone tumors: A report from the Childhood Cancer Survivor Study. *Cancer, 97,* 2554–2564. doi:10.1002/cncr.11363.

National Association of Social Workers. (2006). *Childhood cancer survivorship: An overview for social workers.* Retrieved from http://www.naswdc.org/practice/ health/cancerflyer0206.pdf.

National Cancer Institute. (2012). Cancer Trends Progress Report—2011–2012 Update. Retrieved from http://progressreport.cancer.gov/doc_detail.asp?pid=1 &did=2011&chid=103&coid=1020&mid=.

Park, E. R., Li, F. P., Liu, Y., Emmons, K. M., Ablin, A., Robinson, L. L., . . . & Mertens, A. C. (2005). Health insurance coverage in survivors of childhood cancer: The childhood cancer survivor study. *Journal of Clinical Oncology, 23,* 9187–9197. doi:10.1200/JCO.2005.01.7418.

Parsons, H. M., Harlan, L. C., Lynch, C. F., Hamilton, A. S., Wu, X.-C., Kato, I., . . . & Keegan, T. H. M. (2012). Impact of cancer on work and education among adolescent and young adult cancer survivors. *Journal of Clinical Oncology, 30,* 2393–2400. doi:10.1200/JCO.2011.39.6333.

Patenaude, A. F., & Kupst, M. J. (2005). Psychosocial functioning in pediatric cancer. *Journal of Pediatric Cancer, 30,* 9–27. doi:10.1093/jpepsy/jsi012.

Pendley, J. S., Dahlquist, L. M., & Dreyer, Z. (1997). Body image and psychosocial adjustment in adolescent cancer survivors. *Journal of Pediatric Psychology, 22,* 29–43.

Ransom, S., Sheldon, K. M., & Jacobsen, P. B. (2008). Actual change and inaccurate recall contribute to posttraumatic growth following radiotherapy. *Journal of Consulting and Clinical Psychology, 76,* 811–819. doi:10.1037/a0013270.

Rauck, A. M., Green, D. M., Yasui, Y., Mertens, A., & Robison, L. L. (1999). Marriage in the survivors of childhood cancer: A preliminary description from the childhood cancer survivor study. *Medical and Pediatric Oncology, 33,* 60–63.

Reulen, R. C., Zeegers, M. P., Hammish, W., & Wallace, B. (2009). Pregnancy outcomes among adult survivors of childhood cancer in the British Childhood Cancer survivor study. *Cancer Epidemiology, Biomarkers, and Prevention, 18,* 2239–2247. doi:10.1158/1055-9965.EPI-09-0287.

Robinson, B. (2012). Spotlight: So others may benefit: Young cancer patients and survivors take part in oncofertility research. *NCI Cancer Bulletin, 9*(12), 4. Retrieved from http://www.cancer.gov/ncicancerbulletin/062612/page4.

Robinson, L. R., Armstrong, G. T., Boice, J. D., Chow, E. J., Davies, S. M., Donaldson, S. S., . . . & Zelzer, L. K. (2009). The Childhood Cancer Survivor Study: A National Cancer Institute-supported resource for outcome and intervention research. *Journal of Clinical Oncology, 27,* 2308–2318. doi:10.1200/ JCO.2009.22.3339.

Rourke, M. T., Stuber, M. L., Hobbie, W. L., & Kazak, A. E. (1999). Posttraumatic stress disorder: Understanding the psychosocial impact of surviving childhood cancer into young adulthood. *Journal of Pediatric Oncology Nursing, 16,* 126–135. doi:10.1177/104345429901600303.

Santacroce, S. J., Asmus, K., Kadan-Lottick, N., & Grey, M. (2010). Feasibility and preliminary outcomes from a pilot study of coping skills training for adolescent–young adult survivors of childhood cancer and their parents. *Journal of Pediatric Oncology Nursing, 27,* 10–20. doi:10.1177/1043454209340325.

Schover, L. R. (2005). Motivation for parenthood after cancer: A review. *Journal of the National Cancer Institute Monographs, 34,* 2–5. doi:10.1093/jncimonographs/lgi010.

Schover, L. R., Rybicki, L. A., Martin, B. A., & Bringelsen, K. A. (1999). Having children after cancer: A pilot survey of survivors' attitudes and experiences. *Cancer, 86,* 697–709.

Schultz, K. P., Ness, K. K., Whitton, J., Recklitis, C., Zebrack, B., Robison, L. L., . . . & Mertens, C. (2007). Behavioral and social outcomes in adolescent survivors of childhood cancer: A report from the childhood cancer survivor study. *Journal of Clinical Oncology, 25,* 3649–3656. doi:10.1200/JCO.2006.09.2486.

Scottish Intercollegiate Guidelines Network. (2004). *Long-term follow-up of survivors of childhood cancer: A national clinical guideline.* Retrieved from http://www .sign.ac.uk/pdf/sign76.pdf.

Shalet, S. M., Beardwell, C. G., Morris-Jones, P. H., Pearson, D., & Orrell, D. H. (1976). Ovarian failure following abdominal irradiation in childhood. *British Journal of Cancer, 33,* 655–658.

Signorello, L. B., Cohen, S. S., Bosetti, C., Stovall, M., Kasper, C. E., Weathers, R. E., . . . & Boice, J. D. (2006). Female survivors of childhood cancer: Pre-term birth and low birth weight among their children. *Journal of the National Cancer Institute, 98,* 1453–1461. doi:10.1093/jnci/djj394.

Silk, J. (2011, November 9). The new normal: Life lived with cancer. [Web log comment]. Retrieved from http://www.huffingtonpost.com/judy-silk/life-with -cancer_b_1082971.htmlv.

Stam, H., Grootenhuis, M. A., & Last, B. F. (2005). The course of life of survivors of childhood cancer. *Psycho-Oncology, 14,* 227–238. doi: 10.1002/pon.839.

Stanton, A. L. (2006). Psychosocial concerns and interventions for cancer survivors. *Journal of Clinical Oncology, 24,* 5132–5137. doi:10.1200/JCO.2006.06.8775.

Stein, K. D., Syrjala, K. L., & Andrykowski, M. A. (2008). Physical and psychological long-term and late effects of cancer. *Cancer, 112*(Suppl), 2577–2592. doi: 10.1002/cncr.23448.

Stuber, M. L., Meeske, K. A., Leisenring, W., Stratton, K., Zelzer, L. K., Dawson, K., . . . & Krull, K. R. (2011). Defining medical posttraumatic stress among young adult survivors in the Childhood Cancer Survivor study. *General Hospital Psychiatry, 33,* 347–353. doi: 10.1016/j.genhosppsych.2011.03.015.

Tedeschi, R. G., & Calhoun, L. G. (1996). The Posttraumatic Growth Inventory: Measuring the positive legacy of trauma. *Journal of Traumatic Stress, 9,* 455– 471. doi: 10.1002/jts.2490090305.

Thomson, A. B., Critchley, H. O. D., Kelnar, C. J. H., & Wallace, W. H. B. (2002). Late reproductive sequelae following treatment of childhood cancer and options for fertility preservation. *Best Practice and Research Clinical Endocrinology and Metabolism, 16,* 311–334. doi:10.1053/beem.2002.0200.

Travis, L. B., Hill, D. A., Dores, G. M., Gospordarowicz, M., van Leeuwen, F. E., Holowaty, E., ... & Gilbert, E. (2003). Breast cancer following radiotherapy and chemotherapy among young women with Hodgkin's disease. *JAMA, 290,* 465–475.

Tyc, V. L., Hadley, W., & Crockett, G. (2001). Prediction of health behaviors in pediatric cancer survivors. *Medical and Pediatric Oncology, 37,* 42–46. Retrieved from http://www.ncbi.nlm.nih.gov/pubmed/11466722.

Wallace, W. H., Shalet, S. M., Crowne, E. C., Morris-Jones, P. H., & Gattamaneni, H. R. (1989). Ovarian failure following abdominal irradiation in childhood: Natural history and prognosis. *Clinical Oncology, 1,* 75–79.

Woodgate, R. L. (2006). Life is never the same: Childhood cancer narratives. *European Journal of Cancer Care 15,* 8–18. doi:10.1111/j.1365-2354.2005.00614.x.

Yang, Y. (2008). Trends in U.S. adult chronic disease mortality, 1960–1999: Age, period, and cohort variations. *Demography, 45*(2), 387–416. doi: 10.1353/dem.0.0000.

Zebrack, B. J., Stuber, M. L., Meeske, K. A., Phipps, S., Krull, K. R., Liu, Q., ... & Zeltzer, L. K. (2012). Perceived positive impact of cancer among long-term survivors of childhood cancer: A report from the Childhood Cancer Survivor Study. *Psycho-Oncology, 21,* 630–639. doi: 10.1002/pon.1959.

Zelzer, L. K., Recklitis, C., Buchbinder, D., Zebrack, B., Casillas, J., Tsao, J. C. I., ... & Krull, K. (2009). Psychological status in childhood cancer survivors: A report from the Childhood Cancer Survivor Study. *Journal of Clinical Oncology, 27,* 2396–2404. doi: 10.1200/JCO.2008.21.1433.

Chapter 10

Impact of Psychosocial Factors on Health Outcomes of Cancer in Women

Anna-Lena Lopez and Phyllis Butow

INTRODUCTION

Improvements in medical treatments have enhanced cancer survival rates. However, the observation that cancer patients who have similar tumor characteristics at the time of diagnosis may go on to experience different overall survival duration or time to relapse suggests that other variables may also influence outcome (Falagas et al., 2007). A large body of literature has explored the question of whether psychosocial factors may influence the clinical course of cancer; however, it has produced contradictory findings.

The majority of such studies have focused on women, and in particular, the breast cancer patient population. Psychosocial variables are an important consideration in women's adjustment to cancer. Female cancer patients are more likely to report being affected by psychosocial factors such as distress and unmet needs, and are more likely to seek help for these than male cancer patients (Keller & Henrich, 1999; Fife, Kennedy, & Robinson, 1994). The psychosocial variables commonly thought to influence adjustment to cancer, and therefore cancer outcome, include coping strategies, optimism, emotional responses, and social support.

This chapter will firstly consider possible mechanisms that may explain a role for psychosocial factors in the clinical course of cancer. Second, it will examine evidence garnered from population-based studies and bio-behavioral research on the role of psychosocial factors in cancer outcome. Finally, if psychosocial variables have a role in influencing cancer outcome, then it is plausible that altering psychosocial responses or experiences may also have an impact on cancer outcome. Therefore, this chapter will also consider the impact of psychosocial interventions on cancer survival.

PSYCHOSOCIAL FACTORS AND CANCER OUTCOME: POTENTIAL MEDIATING PATHWAYS

The mechanisms that may underlie a potential link between psychosocial factors and cancer outcome are unclear. However, three potential mechanisms have been proposed: (a) the neuroendocrine and immune pathway (e.g., Andersen et al., 2004); (b) the behavioral pathway (e.g., Chida, Hamer, Wardle, & Steptoe, 2008); and (c) social support pathway (e.g., Cohen, 2004).

Neuroendocrine and Immune Pathway

Psychosocial factors and psychosocial interventions may influence tumor cell biology and immune function, and therefore cancer outcome, through pathways involving the neuroendocrine and immune systems (Andersen et al., 2004; Antoni et al., 2006; Antoni & Lutgendorf, 2007). Two neuroendocrine systems, the sympathetic-adrenal medullary system and the hypothalamic-pituitary-adrenocortical (HPA) axis, are hypothesised to be reactive to psychological stress and affect immune system activity (Antoni & Lutgendorf, 2007; Institute of Medicine [IOM], 2008). Under normal stress reactions, the sympathetic nervous system (SNS) stimulates the adrenal medulla to excrete catecholamine hormones (e.g., epinephrine). Simultaneously, the HPA axis activates the adrenal gland to release glucocorticoid hormones (e.g., cortisol). The release of catecholamines and glucocorticoids under challenging conditions is adaptive and prepares an individual to take action (fight or flight). However, under chronic stress conditions, prolonged exposure to catecholamine and glucocorticoids may dysregulate cellular processes involved in cell replication, repair, growth, metabolism, and gene expression (Antoni & Lutgendorf, 2007; IOM, 2008; McGregor & Antoni, 2009). Prolonged stress responses have also been shown to suppress immune activity, such as in immuno-surveillance (Antoni et al., 2006), T lymphocyte (T-cell) proliferation (Andersen et al., 2004), and natural killer cell cytotoxicity (NKCC) (Lutgendorf et al., 2005). Stressors associated with altered neuroendocrine activity include depression, chronic sleep disturbance, reduced social support, stress, anxiety, bereavement, and post-traumatic stress disorder (Antoni et al., 2006). Many of these stressors are common responses to the cancer experience.

There is some support for an association between psychosocial variables and immune activity in cancer patients (e.g., McGregor & Antoni, 2009). Lutgendorf et al. (2005) found that ovarian cancer patients who reported high levels of social support had elevated levels of NKCC, while patients who reported high levels of distress had low levels of NKCC. Social support is also associated with lower serum levels of vascular endothelial growth factor (which promotes angiogenesis [vascularization] of tumors) in ovarian cancer patients (Lutgendorf et al., 2002). Sleep disruption has also been found to be associated with increased secretion of cortisol and pro-inflammatory cytokines in patients with metastatic colorectal cancer (Antoni et al., 2006). Pro-inflammatory cytokines may have a role in the development and survival of tumor cells by altering several physiological processes that result in damage to DNA or obstruction of DNA repair, deactivation of tumor-suppressor genes, production of growth factors, and promotion of angiogenesis (Antoni et al., 2006). (For a detailed explanation of neuroendocrine and immune processes in tumor biology see Antoni et al., 2006.)

Behavioral Pathway

Psychosocial factors may impact cancer outcome by influencing patient behavior. Negative psychological factors such as anxiety, depression, and poor social support may promote maladaptive or high-risk behaviors (such as smoking, excessive alcohol consumption, sleep disturbance, poor dietary intake, reduced physical activity, and poor treatment adherence), which may in turn compromise health outcomes (Chida et al., 2008). Consequently, facilitating health-enhancing behaviors (e.g., improvements to dietary habits and physical activity, uptake of screening and follow-up services, medical treatment adherence, reduction in such health-depleting behaviors as smoking and excessive sun exposure) may influence cancer outcome by optimizing health and medical care (Andersen et al., 2004; Coyne, Hanisch, & Palmer, 2007).

Social Support Pathway

Social support may beneficially influence cancer outcome in two ways: (a) the main effect hypothesis (Cohen, 2004); and (b) the stress-buffering hypothesis (Cohen, 2004). According to the main effect hypothesis, perceived social support, social network membership, and social interaction have a direct influence on health by promoting positive cognitions, emotions, and behaviors.

The stress-buffering hypothesis posits that social network membership, interaction, and support provide an individual with helpful coping resources, such as information and emotional and practical support, which help to lessen the impact of stressful events and protect individuals from, or reduce the effects of, anxiety, depression, and psychological distress (IOM, 2008). Through these pathways, social support may improve depression and reduce distress, encourage the adoption of health-enhancing behaviors (such as uptake of screening and treatment adherence) through peer support, and improve immune function and resistance to infection by alleviating stress responses (Beasley et al., 2010; Smedslund & Ringdal, 2004). The research literature on the impact of social support on cancer outcome is explored in greater detail in the following section.

SPECIFIC PSYCHOSOCIAL FACTORS IMPLICATED IN CANCER OUTCOME

The association between psychosocial factors and cancer outcome is both contentious and inconsistent. Psychosocial factors thought to influence cancer outcome include coping style (e.g., fighting spirit, helplessness/hopelessness) (Greer, Morris, & Pettingale, 1979), optimism (Allison, Guichard, Fung, & Gilain, 2003), or a perception that the aim of treatment is cure (Brown, Butow, Culjak, Coates, & Dunn, 2000; Butow, Coates, & Dunn, 1999); emotional reactions (e.g., depression, anxiety) (Spiegel & Giese-Davis, 2003); and social support (Pinquart & Duberstein, 2010). While these constructs are interrelated (e.g., individuals who are depressed will likely exhibit coping styles that are characteristic of helplessness/hopelessness), they are each considered separately in this section for clarity.

Coping Style

Coping is defined here as the approach that characterizes an individual's behavioral and attitudinal response to his or her cancer experience. Several studies have investigated the impact of psychological coping styles on cancer survival and recurrence; however, they have produced inconsistent findings. The coping styles most commonly investigated in this context include fighting spirit, helplessness/hopelessness, and denial/avoidance. Other coping styles that have been investigated include acceptance and fatalism, anger, anxious coping/anxious preoccupation, depressive coping, active or problem-focused coping, emotional suppression, and emotional-focused coping (Falagas et al., 2007; Petticrew, Bell, & Hunter, 2002; Greer, 1991).

Fighting Spirit

A fighting-spirit coping style is defined by a conscious effort to "fight" the cancer and improve outcomes (Greer, 1991). It is characterized by proactive problem-solving and help-seeking behaviors, and by active in-volvement in treatment decisions (Greer, 1991). In a systematic review that evaluated the impact of psychological coping style on cancer outcome, Pet-ticrew, Bell, and Hunter (2002) found that of the 10 studies investigating an association between fighting spirit and survival, 2 small studies (n<125) provided supporting evidence. Of 4 studies that investigated the associa-tion between fighting spirit and recurrence, 3 studies (n<125) found that coping characterized by a fighting spirit was associated with a reduced risk of recurrence. However the fourth and largest study (n=578) found no evi-dence of a survival advantage (Watson, Haviland, Greer, Davidson, & Bliss, 1999; Watson, Homewood, Haviland, & Bliss, 2005). A more recent systematic review on the impact of psychosocial factors on breast cancer outcome found similar contradictory findings (Falagas et al., 2007).

Helplessness/Hopelessness

A helplessness/hopelessness coping mind-set is characterized by re-duced hope for the future and the belief that one is unable to exert influ-ence over one's circumstances (Watson et al., 2005). A coping style characterized by helplessness/hopelessness is characteristic of individuals with depression and is thought to hinder individuals from engaging in proactive behaviors that may enhance their health (e.g., treatment adher-ence, lifestyle improvements, seeking support) and ultimately influence health outcomes. Nevertheless, evidence for an association between a help-lessness/hopelessness coping style and cancer outcome has been mixed. In their systematic review, Falagas and colleagues (2007) found that of the eight studies investigating the efficacy of a coping style characterized by helplessness/hopelessness on survival, one study showed evidence for a negative association between survival and a helplessness/hopelessness coping style, three studies showed evidence for higher recurrence rates as-sociated with this coping style, and four studies found no evidence of an association between this coping style and survival. Petticrew and col-leagues (2002) found similar contradictory results in their review.

Denial/Avoidant Coping

Denial or avoidant-based coping is characterized by minimizing or down-playing the seriousness of a situation and avoiding or suppressing related stressful thoughts or information (Greer, 1991). Several studies have investi-gated the association between these coping styles and cancer outcomes and have yielded mixed results. Petticrew, Bell, and Hunter (2002) found that of 10 studies investigating the association between avoidant coping and cancer survival, none provided evidence of any association. Of the 5 studies that investigated the association between denial as a coping strategy and cancer outcome, 1 small study reported an association with reduced survival. Eight studies included in the review investigated the association between denial/avoidant coping and cancer recurrence, 1 of which showed an association with an increase in risk of recurrence in patients with breast cancer.

A later review (Falagas et al., 2007) found similar contradictory results in the breast cancer population. Of the five studies investigating the association between denial/avoidance and survival and recurrence, one showed that utilizing this coping strategy provided a survival advantage, while another found this coping style to be associated with an increased risk of mortality and recurrence. Two studies showed no association with survival or recurrence.

While very few studies have reported results in the direction opposite to that hypothesized, overall, there is a lack of strong evidence to support an association between psychological coping style and cancer survival or recurrence. In their systematic review, Petticrew and colleagues (2002) found that most studies reporting a positive association between coping style and cancer outcome were small in size, and few had made appropriate adjustments for known prognostic indicators. Additionally, interpretation of studies is made more difficult by the inconsistent use of terms to describe constructs related to psychological coping, and the use of subjective categorization of coping style in some studies.

Optimism and Perceived Aim of Treatment

Optimism

Dispositional optimism is defined by generalized positive or favorable expectations for future outcomes (Segerstrom, 2005). Cultural beliefs about the interaction between the mind and body perpetuate widely held views that personality traits such as optimism can enhance psychological adjustment to illness, including cancer, and also prolong survival (Ranchor, Sanderman, & Coyne, 2010). Consequently, cancer patients are often encouraged to be optimistic or to think positively about their diagnosis and cancer experience (Rittenberg, 1995).

Several pathways may explain a role for optimism in cancer outcome. An optimistic or positive attitude may have a direct influence on the neuroendocrine or immune pathways (Segerstrom, 2005). Alternatively, optimists are more likely to engage proactively in activities that can lead to the termination of a challenging situation, such as acquiring information about their disease and treatment options to make better treatment decisions, engaging in health-enhancing behaviors, and seeking support when needed (Schofield et al., 2004; Butow et al., 1999).

Despite its popularity, evidence for an influence of optimism or a positive attitude on cancer outcome is scarce. To our knowledge, there has been no review specifically examining the association between optimism and cancer survival to date. A recent meta-analytic review by Chida and Steptoe (2008) examined the relationship between positive psychological well-being and survival in healthy populations and patient populations with chronic illness. Of the 28 studies of chronic illness populations included in the review, 6 examined cancer. Chida and Steptoe (2008) defined positive psychological well-being broadly to include optimism, vitality, positive mood, joy, happiness, vigor, energy, sense of humor, life satisfaction, hopefulness, and emotional well-being. The authors concluded that psychological well-being was related to better survival outcomes in both healthy and chronic disease populations. However, subanalyses indicated null results for a relationship between positive psychological well-being and cancer survival. Additionally, as subanalyses were not conducted for individual constructs, it is difficult to disentangle the role of optimism alone. This meta-analysis has several limitations. First, several study samples were counted more than once (e.g., see Coyne & Tennen, 2010). Second, heterogeneous variables were combined to define "positive psychological well-being." Third, as acknowledged by the authors, various measures were used to assess the different constructs included in the definition of positive psychological well-being, and even the same constructs were assessed using different measures in different studies (Chida & Steptoe, 2008). Fourth, the analyses included a heterogeneous sample of patient and nonpatient populations. Fifth, the authors reported a positive result publication bias in the literature (Chida & Steptoe, 2008).

Another recent meta-analysis investigated the association between optimism and physical health outcomes (Rasmusssen, Scheier, & Greenhouse, 2009). Only studies that used specific measures of optimism were included. Healthy population samples as well as patient samples with various acute and chronic medical conditions, including cancer, were examined. Physical health outcomes were broadly defined to comprise an aggregate of various physical outcome variables, including survival, mortality, cardiovascular outcomes, physiological markers, immune function, physical symptoms (e.g., fatigue, pain, and influenza symptoms), perceived health, and pregnancy outcomes (e.g., birth weight, pregnancy loss). The authors concluded that the overall analysis of effect sizes provided strong support for a relationship between optimism and physical health outcomes. Subanalyses indicated that optimism was associated with survival, and that optimism was significantly related to cancer health outcomes (e.g., survival, lymph node status, pain, fatigue, physical functioning, and cancer antigen markers) in cross-sectional and longitudinal studies (n=14) but not in prospective studies (n=4). This meta-analysis has several limitations that make it difficult to interpret the results. First, several samples included in the analyses were counted multiple times. Second, as acknowledged by the authors, the majority of studies included in the analyses did not control for prognostic indicators (Rasmussen et al., 2009). Third, the operational definition of physical health outcomes in this meta-analysis comprised an aggregate of highly dissimilar variables (e.g., survival, influenza symptoms, gestational age, perceived health, and biological markers). Fourth, the sample population was heterogeneous; it included both nonpatient samples and patient samples with diverse medical conditions.

A small number of studies have assessed the associations between optimism and cancer survival. The following studies are evaluated here because they investigated relatively homogeneous cancer types; utilized the same reliable and validated measure of optimism, the Life Orientation Test (LOT) (Scheier & Carver, 1985); and adjusted for prognostic variables in their analyses. One study found that optimism was associated with improved survival status one year post-diagnosis in head and neck cancer patients (Allison et al., 2003). However, this study was small (n=101) and underpowered (the number of relevant events, in this case death, was 45) and used multivariate analyses that were unsuitable for the number of deaths being explained (Coyne, Tennen, & Ranchor, 2010). Another study found no association between pretreatment optimism scores and cancer survival in patients with lung cancer (Schofield et al., 2004). This study had several strengths: the study was large (n=179) with a large number of deaths (n=171) by the closeout date; the participants had a single type of cancer; and the patients were involved in a multicenter radiotherapy clinical trial, which provided some standardization of treatment. Similarly, a recent study found that neither hope nor optimism were associated with survival or recurrence in metastatic colorectal cancer patients (n=421) who were participating in a chemotherapy clinical trial (Schofield et al., 2010).

Associations between dispositional optimism or positive attitude and cancer outcomes remain to be clearly defined (Segerstrom, 2005). Several factors complicate the interpretation of findings in this area. First, studies have used different operational definitions of optimism, which have included such associated constructs as positive coping, fighting spirit (Coyne & Tennen, 2010), and extroversion (Ranchor et al., 2010), and such aggregated constructs as positive emotional well-being, which includes quality-of-life variables and positive affect (Chida & Steptoe, 2008; Coyne, Pajak et al., 2007). Second, while most studies have used the LOT to measure optimism (Rasmussen et al., 2009), some studies have used measures of quality of life (Coyne, Pajak et al., 2007), and personality assessment inventories (Rasmussen et al., 2009). Third, in samples that are small, the number of relevant events (deaths) is invariably smaller, which makes statistical control of confounding patient, disease, and treatment variables less effective (Coyne, Pajak et al., 2007). Fourth, inclusion of heterogeneous disease types or medical conditions in statistical analyses may make it difficult to control for the influence of different biological processes involved in health outcomes.

Perceived Aim of Treatment

Perceived aim of treatment may be related to an optimistic coping style. As with most of the research on the impact of psychosocial factors on cancer outcome, the findings have been inconsistent. In a series of studies in breast cancer and melanoma, Butow and colleagues found that the perception of the treatment aim was not prognostic of survival duration in metastatic breast cancer patients (Butow, Coates & Dunn, 2000) or early-stage melanoma patients (Brown et al., 2000), but it was for metastatic melanoma patients (Butow et al., 1999). In addition, early-stage melanoma patients who believed that the intention of treatment was cure experienced a longer interval before relapse (Brown et al., 2000). The authors proposed that one reason for these inconsistent findings may be that the expectations for treatment outcome may be unstable over time and influenced by disease progression. However, as this variable was measured at baseline only, this conclusion could not be substantiated. Moreover, it is difficult to determine the extent to which treatment expectations are based on other influencing factors, such as coping style or prognostic information provided by the treating physician (Brown et al., 2000).

Emotional Response

Emotional response (or expression or reaction) refers to the emotional content of the psychological response to an individual's cancer experience and commonly includes depression and anxiety. Up to 30 percent of women diagnosed with breast cancer will experience symptoms of depression or anxiety within the first year following their diagnosis (Edwards, Hulbert-Williams, & Neal, 2008), and up to 23 percent of women diagnosed with gynecological cancer will go on to experience depression (Massie, 2004). Depression and anxiety may make it more difficult to cope with the challenges inherent in receiving a cancer diagnosis and its treatment; however, the question of whether they can also influence disease outcome remains contentious.

Depression

Several early studies reported links between depression and increased risk of cancer mortality (e.g., Spiegel & Giese-Davis, 2003). However, the studies that showed affirmative results typically used smaller samples and shorter follow-up periods than did the studies that produced null results. In a recent systematic review, Falagas and colleagues (2007) found mixed results. Of 15 studies that investigated the impact of depression on cancer outcome, 1 study reported that depression had an advantageous effect on survival, while 4 were associated with increased risk of mortality. Nine studies reported no association with survival.

Investigating the impact of depression on cancer outcome is further complicated by several other factors. First, it is difficult to separate depressive symptoms from manifestations of the biological processes of cancer. Symptoms of depression (emotional and cognitive disturbances, weight fluctuations, sleep disruption, fatigue) may be confused with symptoms of cancer or the side effects of cancer treatments. Conversely, symptoms of the disease and treatment side effects may imitate symptoms of depression (Spiegel & Giese-Davis, 2003). This makes it difficult to ascertain whether the depression exerts a separate influence on outcome above that of the disease. Second, depression may influence an individual's coping style (e.g., helplessness/hopelessness), which in turn may adversely affect adherence to medical treatment and screening, consequently affecting cancer outcome. Third, biological processes associated with depression may also dysregulate endocrine and immune activity via stress mechanisms involving the HPA and cortisol activity, which may ultimately influence tumor activity (Antoni et al., 2006; Spiegel & Giese-Davis, 2003). Finally, tumor activity may produce symptoms of depression whereby the severity of depression may indicate faster disease progression (Spiegel & Giese-Davis, 2003).

Anxiety/Worry

Evidence of an association between anxiety and cancer outcome has been equally diverse. Falagas et al. (2007) identified 11 studies that investigated the association between anxiety and cancer outcome. Of these studies 1 reported that anxiety was associated with an increased risk of mortality, 1 found an association between anxiety and an increased risk of recurrence, and 9 found no association between anxiety and cancer outcome. Interestingly, Brown et al. (2000) found that different targets of worry produced different survival outcomes. In their prospective investigation of early-stage melanoma patients, concern about the disease was associated with longer time to relapse and overall survival duration. However, worrying about the impact of the cancer on family members was found to have a negative influence on survival duration. The authors suggested that the negative impact of family concern may be mediated by coping style and/or disease progression, whereby those who worry about their families may typically focus their resources on family rather than on themselves, or alternatively, patients with symptoms of progressive disease may show more concern about their families.

Overall, the research investigating an association between emotional response and cancer outcome is at best inconclusive. Methodological limitations in study design and the measurement of constructs such as depression and anxiety, as well as difficulty in disentangling the multidirectional influence of emotional response, biological processes, and tumor activity, have made it difficult to identify any impact that depression or anxiety may have on the biological course of cancer.

Social Support

The construct of social support takes into account the multiple dimensions of social connectedness, including the structural and functional aspects of the various relationships that exist between an individual and his or her family, friends, and community (social networks), as well as the depth and extensiveness of these relationships (social integration) (IOM, 2008). Kayser, Sormanti, and Strainchamps (1999) utilized relational theory as a guiding framework to understand women's adjustment to cancer and proposed that women's coping abilities are developed and tempered within the context of social interactions.

There is evidence to suggest that a lack of social support can have detrimental effects on outcomes, including mortality, for a variety of illnesses (Beasley et al., 2010; IOM, 2008), including cancer. A large number of studies have investigated the impact of social support on outcomes of cancer in women but have produced mixed results. In their systematic review that evaluated the effect of psychosocial factors on breast cancer outcome, Falagas et al. (2007) found that of the nine studies investigating the impact of social support, three studies provided evidence of a positive impact on survival using one or more index of social support, while five failed to show any association, and one showed mixed support. A possible explanation for the lack of association between social support and cancer outcome may be the relatively small sample size in these studies (< 250), which may not have provided enough power to detect relationships. An alternative explanation is that there is no association.

A later meta-analysis of 126 studies (various cancer types included) assessing the association between psychosocial factors and cancer survival found that poor social support was not associated with cancer outcome (Chida et al., 2008). However, the authors proposed that the results reflected the small number of social support studies included in their meta-analysis.

Pinquart and Duberstein (2010) conducted a meta-analysis of 87 studies (various cancer types) that investigated the associations between social support and cancer outcomes. They found that high perceived social support, larger social networks, and being married were associated with reduced risk of mortality. Interestingly these relationships varied by cancer site, with stronger associations for network size observed in studies of breast cancer.

Beasley et al. (2010) investigated the impact of social networks on survival in a large population-based cohort of invasive breast cancer survivors in the United States. In particular, the study assessed marital status; the frequency of contact with and number of close friends, relatives, or confidants; frequency of attending religious activities; and involvement in community activities. Of the 4,589 participants, a total of 552 died at follow-up, 146 from breast cancer. The results showed no significant trends for breast cancer–specific survival. The size of an individual's social networks and the number of frequent social contacts (defined as at least once per month) were not related to overall or breast cancer–specific survival. Neither did marital status nor the number and frequency of contacts with close friends, relatives, or confidants have an impact on overall or breast cancer–specific survival. However, social connectedness (a composite measure combining the number of contacts and frequency of social activities) was associated with overall survival. Additionally, greater involvement in religious or community activities was associated with improved overall survival. Past or present participation in a cancer support group had no impact on breast cancer survival.

Overall, studies that have investigated the impact of social support on outcomes of cancer in women have produced mixed results. One explanation for these mixed results may be the emphasis on measuring the quantity of support rather than the quality of support, whereas the latter may be more influential. For example, Weihs, Enright, and Simmens (2008) found that, in a group of 90 breast cancer patients, marital confiding and close relationships were associated with increased survival duration.

In summary there is inconclusive evidence that psychosocial factors influence survival duration or time to relapse in women with cancer. Methodological limitations in research design have made it difficult to interpret results. For instance, constructs have been variously defined and measured, making it difficult to compare the results of studies investigating the impact of similar constructs. Results from small or mixed cancer samples may produce spurious results, as it is difficult to control confounding variables in such samples. Additionally, variations in the follow-up duration of different studies make it difficult to compare results. Nevertheless, results in the opposite direction to those hypothesised are very rare. Given the mixed samples and measures utilized to date, further fine-grained research to explore more specifically the contexts and characteristics of psychosocial variables that might influence cancer outcomes in women is warranted.

THE IMPACT OF PSYCHOLOGICAL INTERVENTIONS ON CANCER OUTCOMES

Psychosocial interventions improve quality of life and well-being in cancer patients (Kissane et al., 2007; Chow, Tsao, & Harth, 2004; Luecken & Compas, 2002); however, the hypothesis that psychological interventions may influence the biological course of cancer is a controversial one. It is based on the premise that if psychological factors can exert influence on the clinical course of cancer, then psychological interventions may have the ability to modify cancer outcome by modifying psychological factors of interest. This hypothesis has received additional support from evidence of changes in immune activity following psychosocial interventions (Andersen et al., 2004).

However, available evidence has failed to consistently demonstrate the survival benefit of psychological interventions, creating uncertainty about the potential of these interventions to influence cancer outcome.

Two early and influential randomized controlled trials investigating the impact of psychosocial interventions on cancer outcome in women with metastatic breast cancer (Spiegel, Bloom, Kraemer, & Gottheil, 1989; n=86) and patients with malignant melanoma (Fawzy et al., 1993; n=68) found that supportive and psychoeducational group therapy, respectively, had a beneficial influence on cancer survival. However, these studies have been criticized for methodological limitations, including small sample sizes and failure to specify survival as an a priori primary end point (Coyne, Stefanek, & Palmer, 2007).

A recent Cochrane review found that subsequent randomized controlled trials of psychosocial interventions in metastatic breast cancer populations have not demonstrated similar beneficial results on cancer survival (Edwards et al., 2008). Null results were found in four out of five randomized controlled trials (the above Spiegel et al. [1989] study was the one affirmative study in the review) that investigated the impact of group cognitive behavioral therapy (Edelman, Lemon, Bell, & Kidman, 1999), supportive-expressive group therapy (Goodwin et al., 2001; Classen et al., 2001), and group supportive plus cognitive behavior therapy (Cunningham et al., 1998) on cancer outcome. However, these interventions provided evidence of short-term psychological benefits, such as reduced distress (Edwards et al., 2008).

In a more recent randomized controlled trial, Kissane et al. (2007) found that supportive-expressive group therapy (SEGT) that included components on improving relationships, creating support networks, and enhancing coping and relaxation skills did not prolong survival duration in women with metastatic breast cancer. However, SEGT appeared to have a beneficial impact on psychosocial well-being with improvements in current cases of clinical depression and prevention of the onset of new cases. Additionally, the results showed an association between SEGT and enhanced adherence to hormone and chemotherapy treatment regimens.

Smedslund and Ringdal (2004) and Chow, Tsao, and Harth (2004) conducted separate meta-analyses of the effects of psychosocial interventions on survival in various cancer populations. Both meta-analyses found no supporting evidence for a treatment effect on overall survival. Furthermore, both research groups performed separate analyses of the effect of group interventions on women with breast cancer, and both failed to find a treatment effect on survival. These results are consistent with results reported in the metastatic breast cancer population.

Several studies have demonstrated changes in neuroendocrine and immune function in cancer patients following participation in psychosocial interventions, adding weight to the argument for a role for psychosocial factors in cancer outcome. In a recent review of randomized controlled trials that investigated the association between psychosocial interventions and biological variables in nonmetastatic breast cancer patients, McGregor and Antoni (2009) found that improvements in psychological adaptation (e.g., decreased depression and anxiety, improved quality of life, improvements in sleep) were associated with parallel changes in neuroendocrine and cellular immune responses, such as reductions in afternoon serum cortisol (one study), increases in lymphocyte proliferative responses (three studies), and increases in T-helper lymphocyte (TH1) cytokine production (of in vitro interferon gamma [IFN-γ] and interleukin-1 beta [IL-1β]; one study). All interventions were provided in a group setting and were based on cognitive behavioral therapy techniques, most of which included components of stress management, health education (e.g., regarding sleep hygiene), relaxation training, and coping skills. While these trials did not measure cancer survival or recurrence, the results provide correlational support for a neuroendocrine and immune pathway that may be in part influenced by such psychosocial factors as social support, psychological distress, and health behaviors. Nevertheless, caution is required in interpreting these results because changes in immune activity following psychosocial interventions will likely be moderated by underlying biological or disease-related activity and/or medical treatment (Miller & Cohen, 2001). Furthermore, cancer treatments may also have deleterious effects on the neuroendocrine and immune systems, which may affect disease activity; thus, unless disease and treatment variables are controlled for, spurious results may be obtained.

Given the multiple psychosocial variables (personality, coping style, current and past life events, emotional reaction, quality of life, social support) that contribute to patients' responses to their cancer diagnoses, and the variations in the amount of influence each of these variables may exert on their responses, these inconsistent results relating to the efficacy of psychosocial interventions may not be surprising. Additionally, the small number of trials and small trial sizes, as well as heterogeneity of study designs, intervention protocols, disease types and stages, outcome measures, and treatment and follow-up duration, may contribute to the current inconsistent findings. Nevertheless, one consistent finding in this literature is that psychosocial interventions that specify survival as an a priori primary end point (e.g., Edelman et al., 1999; Goodwin et al., 2001; Cunningham et al., 1998; Kissane et al., 2007) and are controlled for medical treatment effects have not found an association with survival (Coyne, Stefanek, & Palmer, 2007).

In summary, given the methodological limitations and contradictory findings, there is insufficient evidence to suggest that psychosocial interventions improve overall cancer survival. To assert that psychosocial interventions will improve survival duration is problematic, especially if it provides false hope of longer life following a cancer diagnosis (Coyne, Hanisch, & Palmer, 2007). Nevertheless, this research suggests that psychosocial interventions may help reduce distress and improve the quality of life of cancer patients.

CONCLUSION

An assessment of the literature highlights a lack of strong evidence that coping style, optimism, emotional response, or social support can alter the biological course of cancer in order to influence survival duration or time to relapse in women with cancer. Similarly, there is insufficient evidence to suggest that psychosocial interventions can alter cancer outcomes. However, several studies have demonstrated changes in neuroendocrine and immune parameters in cancer patients following participation in psychosocial interventions, adding weight to the argument for a role for psychosocial factors in cancer outcome. However, these have been correlational studies; thus, conclusions regarding causal relationships cannot be drawn.

Methodological limitations in the research design of many of the studies in this area may have contributed to the contradictory findings. First, small sample sizes invariably contain an even smaller number of relevant events (deaths) to submit to statistical analyses (Coyne, Pajak et al., 2007). Additionally, in samples that are small, statistical controls are less effective, and outcomes may be determined by the anomalous results of a few participants (Coyne, Pajak et al., 2007). Second, heterogeneity within samples with regard to cancer type, stage, and grade may obscure the influence of tumor type–specific biological processes on outcomes (Schofield et al., 2004). Third, failure to control for prognostic indicators such as cancer type, stage of disease, grade, treatment variables, and patient variables using statistical methods or by sampling may produce spurious results (Schofield et al., 2004). Finally, variability in the definitions, categorization, and measurement of constructs; follow-up duration; study/treatment protocols; covariates included in analyses; and type of analyses conducted makes it difficult to compare and interpret results (Coyne, Pajak et al., 2007; Schofield et al., 2004).

The expectation that cancer patients should adopt particular coping styles, or maintain an optimistic or positive attitude while challenged with a serious and life-threatening illness as well as physically and emotionally demanding medical treatments and side effects, may have damaging consequences. First, imposing changes to the way an individual inherently copes with or responds to a cancer diagnosis or any stressful situation introduces an additional burden. Second, it may make it hard for patients to admit that they have concerns or are experiencing difficulties coping with their cancer experiences. Consequently, it may be difficult for them to talk about their concerns, or to seek help or support (Rittenberg, 1995). Third, it may produce unrealistic expectations of survival outcomes that may result in guilt, self-blame, and intense disappointment when outcomes do not match expectations (Rittenberg, 1995).

Nevertheless, while current evidence does not support a role for psychosocial processes in altering the clinical course of cancer, psychological interventions have shown some benefits in reducing distress (Edwards et al., 2008), treating current depression, and preventing the onset of new cases, and in improving quality of life and adherence to medical treatment (Kissane et al., 2007). Psychological interventions, provided in conjunction with medical treatment as part of a multidimensional treatment intervention, may improve the overall experience of cancer patients.

REFERENCES

Allison, P. J., Guichard, C., Fung, K., & Gilain, L. (2003). Dispositional optimism predicts survival status 1 year after diagnosis in head and neck cancer patients. *Journal of Clinical Oncology, 21*, 543–548.

Andersen, B. L., Farrar, W. G., Golden-Kreutz, D. M., Glaser, R., Emery, C. F., Crespin, T. R., Shapiro, C. L., & Carson, W. E. (2004). Psychological, behavioural, and immune changes after a psychological intervention: A clinical trial. *Journal of Clinical Oncology, 223*, 570–580.

Antoni, M. H., & Lutgendorf, S. (2007). Psychosocial factors and disease progression in cancer. *Current Directions in Psychological Science, 16*, 42–46.

Antoni, M. H., Lutgendorf, S. K., Cole, S.W., Dhabhar, F. S., Sephton, S. E., McDonald, P. G., Stefanek, M., & Sood, A. K. (2006). The influence of bio-behavioural factors on tumour biology: Pathways and mechanisms. *Nature Reviews Cancer, 6*, 240–248.

Beasley, J. M., Newcomb, P. A., Trentham-Dietz, A., Hampton, J. M., Ceballos, R. M., Titus-Ernstoff, L., Egan, K. M., & Holmes, M. (2010). Social networks and survival after breast cancer diagnosis. *Journal of Cancer Survivorship, 4*, 372–380.

Brown., J. E., Butow, P. N., Culjak, G., Coates, A. S., & Dunn, S. M. (2000). Psychosocial predictors of outcome: Time to relapse and survival in patients with early stage melanoma. *British Journal of Cancer, 83*, 1448–1453.

Butow, P. N., Coates, A. S., & Dunn, S. M. (1999). Psychosocial predictors of survival in metastatic melanoma. *Journal of Clinical Oncology, 17*, 2256–2263.

Butow, P. N., Coates, A. S., & Dunn, S. M. (2000). Psychosocial predictors of survival: Metastatic breast cancer. *Annals of Oncology, 11*, 469–474.

Chida, Y., Hamer, M., Wardle, J., & Steptoe, A. (2008). Do stress-related psychosocial factors contribute to cancer incidence and survival? *Nature Clinical Practice Oncology, 5*, 466–475.

Chida, Y., & Steptoe, A. (2008). Positive psychological well-being and mortality: A quantitative review of prospective observational studies. *Psychosomatic Medicine, 70*, 741–756.

Chow, E., Tsao, M. N., & Harth, T. (2004). Does psychological intervention improve survival in cancer? A meta-analysis. *Palliative Medicine, 18*, 25–31.

Classen, C., Butler, L., Koopman, C., Miller, E., DiMiceli, S., Giese-Davis, J., Fobair, P., Carlson, R., Kraemer, H., & Spiegel, D. (2001). Supportive-expressive group therapy and distress in patients with metastatic breast cancer. *Archieves of General Psychiatry, 58*, 494–501.

Cohen, S. (2004). Social relationships and health. *American Psychologist, 59*, 676–684.

Coyne, J. C., Hanisch, L. J., & Palmer, S. C. (2007). Psychotherapy does not promote survival: Now what? *Psycho-Oncology, 16*, 1050–1052.

Coyne, J. C., Pajak, T. F., Harris, J., Konski, A., Movsas, B., Ang, K., & Bruner D. W. (2007). *Cancer, 110*, 2568–2575.

Coyne, J. C., Stefanek, M., & Palmer, S. C. (2007). Psychotherapy and survival in cancer: The conflict between hope and evidence. *Psychological Bulletin, 133*, 367–394.

Coyne, J. C., & Tennen, H. (2010). Positive psychology in cancer care: Bad science, exaggerated claims, and unproven medicine. *Annals of Behavioral Medicine, 39*, 16–26.

Coyne, J. C., Tennen, H., & Ranchor, A. V. (2010). Positive psychology in cancer care: A story line resistant to evidence. *Annals of Behavioral Medicine, 39*, 35–42.

Cunningham, A., Edmonds, C., Jenkins, G., Pollack, H., Lockwood, G., & Warr, D. (1998). A randomized controlled trial of the effects of group psychological therapy on survival in women with metastatic breast cancer. *Psycho-Oncology, 7*, 508–517.

Edelman, S., Lemon, J., Bell, D. R., & Kidman, A. D. (1999). Effects of group CBT on the survival time of patients with metastatic breast cancer. *Psycho-Oncology, 8*, 474–481.

Edwards, A. G. K., Hulbert-Williams, N., & Neal, R. D. (2008). Psychological interventions for women with metastatic breast cancer. *Cochrane Database of Systematic Reviews, 3*. doi: 10.1002/14651858.CD004253.pub3.

Falagas, M. E., Zarkadoulia, E. A., Ioannidou, E. N., Peppas, P., Christodoulou, C., & Rafailidis, I. (2007). The effect of psychosocial factors on breast cancer outcome: A systematic review. *Breast Cancer Research, 9*, R44.

Fawzy, F. I., Fawzy, N. W., Hyun, C. S., Elashoff, R., Guthrie, D., Fahey, J. L., & Morton, D. (1993). Malignant melanoma: Effects of an early structured psychiatric intervention, coping, and affective state on recurrence and survival 6 years later. *Archives of General Psychiatry, 50*, 681–689.

Fife, B. L., Kennedy, V. N., & Robinson, L. (1994). Gender and adjustment to cancer. *Journal of Psychosocial Oncology, 12*, 1–2.

Goodwin, P. J., Leszcz, M., Ennis, M., Koopman, J., Vincent, L., Guther, H., Drysdale, E., Hundleby, M., Chochinov, H., Navarro, M., Speca, M., & Hunter, J. (2001). The effect of group psychological support on survival in metastatic breast cancer. *New England Journal of Medicine, 345*, 1719–1726.

Greer, S. (1991). Psychological responses to cancer and survival. *Psychological Medicine, 21,* 43–49.

Greer, S., Morris, T., & Pettingale, K. W. (1979). Psychological response to breast cancer: Effect on outcome. *Lancet, 314,* 785–787.

Institute of Medicine (IOM). (2008). *Cancer care for the whole patient: Meeting psychosocial health needs.* Adler, Nancy E., & Page, Ann E. K. (Eds.). Washington, DC: The National Academies Press.

Kayser, K., Sormanti, M., & Strainchamps, E. (1999). Women coping with cancer: The influence of relationship factors on psychosocial adjustment. *Psychology of Women Quarterly, 24,* 725–739.

Keller, M., & Henrich, G. (1999). Illness-related distress: Does it mean the same for men and women? *Acta Oncologica, 38,* 747–755.

Kissane, D. W., Grabsch, B., Clarke, D. M., Smith, G. C., Love, A. W., Bloch, S., Snyder, R. D., & Li, Y. (2007). Supportive-expression group therapy for women with metastatic breast cancer: Survival and psychosocial outcome from a randomized controlled trial. *Psycho-Oncology, 16,* 277–286.

Luecken, L. J., & Compas, B. E. (2002). Stress, coping, and immune function in breast cancer. *Annals of Behavioral Medicine, 24,* 336–344.

Lutgendorf, S. K., Johnsen, E. L., Cooper, B., Sorosky, J. I., Buller, R. E., & Sood, A. K. (2002). Vascular endothelial growth factor and social support in patients with ovarian cancer. *Cancer, 95,* 808–815.

Lutgendorf, S. K., Sood, A. K., Anderson, B., McGinn S., Maiseri, H., Dao, M., Sorosky, J. I., De Geest, K., Ritchie, J., & Lubaroff, D. M. (2005). Social support, psychological distress, and natural killer cell activity in ovarian cancer. *Journal of Clinical Oncology, 23,* 7105–7113.

Massie, M. J. (2004). Prevalence of depression in patients with cancer. *Journal of the National Cancer Institute Monographs, 32,* 57–71.

McGregor, B. A., & Antoni, M. H. (2009). Psychological intervention and health outcomes among women treated for breast cancer: A review of stress pathways and biological mediators. *Brain, Behavior, and Immunity, 23,* 159–166.

Miller, G. E., & Cohen, S. (2001). Psychological interventions and the immune system: A meta-analytic review and critique. *Health Psychology, 20,* 47–63.

Petticrew, M., Bell, R., & Hunter, D. (2002). Influence of psychological coping on survival and recurrence in people with cancer: Systematic review. *British Medical Journal, 325,* 1–10.

Pinquart, M., & Duberstein, P. R. (2010). Associations of social networks with cancer mortality: A meta-analysis. *Critical Reviews in Oncology/Hematology, 75,* 122–137.

Ranchor, A. V., Sanderman, R., & Coyne, J. C. (2010). Invited commentary: Personality as a causal factor in cancer risk and mortality—time to retire a hypothesis? *American Journal of Epidemiology, 172,* 386–388.

Rasmussen, H. N., Scheier, M. F., & Greenhouse, J. B. (2009). Optimism and physical health: A meta-analytic review. *Annals of Behavioral Medicine, 37,* 239–256.

Rittenberg, C. (1995). Positive thinking: An unfair burden for cancer patients? *Support Care Cancer, 3*, 37–39.

Scheier, M. F., & Carver, C. S. (1985). Optimism, coping, and health: Assessment and implications of generalised outcome expectancies. *Health Psychology, 4*, 219–247.

Schofield, P., Ball, D., Smith, J. G., Borland, R., O'Brien, P., Davis, S., Olver, I., Ryan, G., & Joseph, D. (2004). Optimism and survival in lung carcinoma patients. *Cancer, 100*, 1276–1282.

Schofield, P., Stockler, M., Zannino, D., Wong, N., Ransom, D., Moylan, R., Simes, R. J., Price, T. J., Tebbutt, N. C., Jefford, M., & Australasian Gastrointestinal Trials Group. (2010). Hope, optimism, and survival in a randomized trial of first-line chemotherapy for patients with metastatic colorectal cancer [Abstract]. American Society of Clinical Oncology Annual Meeting Proceedings. *Journal of Clinical Oncology, 28*(15s), 9039.

Segerstrom, S. C. (2005). Optimism and immunity: Do positive thoughts always lead to positive effects? *Brain, Behavior, and Immunity, 19*, 195–200.

Smedslund, G., & Ringdal, G. I. (2004). Meta-analysis of the effects of psychosocial interventions on survival time in cancer patients. *Journal of Psychosomatic Research, 57*, 123–131.

Spiegel, D., Bloom, J., Kraemer, H., & Gottheil, E. (1989). Effect of psychosocial treatment on survival of patients with metastatic breast cancer. *The Lancet, 2*, 888–891.

Spiegel, D., & Giese-Davis, J. (2003). Depression and cancer: Mechanisms and disease progression. *Biological Psychiatry, 54*, 269–282.

Watson, M., Haviland, J., Greer, S., Davidson, J., & Bliss, J. M. (1999). Influence of psychological response on survival in breast cancer: A population-based cohort study. *Lancet, 354*, 1331–1336.

Watson, M., Homewood, J., Haviland, J., & Bliss, J. M. (2005). Influence of psychological response on breast cancer survival: 10-year follow-up of a population-based cohort. *European Journal of Cancer, 41*, 1710–1714.

Weihs, K. L, Enright, T. M., & Simmens, S. J. (2008). Close relationships and emotional processing predict decreased mortality in women with breast cancer: Preliminary evidence. *Psychosomatic medicine, 70*, 117–124.

Chapter 11

Meaning Reconstruction in the Wake of Loss: Psychological and Spiritual Adaptation to Bereavement

Laurie A. Burke, Robert A. Neimeyer, and Tina C. Elacqua

Cancerous cell growth was the second leading cause of death in women (22%) in 2009, overshadowed only by heart disease (24%; Centers for Disease Control & Prevention [CDC], 2011). Cancer patients with a terminal diagnosis are subjected to repeated tests, pharmaceuticals, and assessments to aid in prognosis, treatment, and palliation of symptoms. However, for cancer patients who die, evaluations and interventions do not end with the life of the patient, but rather continue in the form of grief assessment and psychotherapy for bereaved family members (e.g., Kissane, Zaider, Li, & Del Guadio, 2012).

Whether by cancer or otherwise, over the course of a lifetime, few individuals are spared from experiencing the loss of a loved one to death. In fact, a single death touches an average of six or more survivors (McDaid, Trowman, Golder, Hawton, & Sowden, 2008), who often find the journey of bereavement to be fraught with physical, psychological, and spiritual stressors. Although the length of bereavement varies, most people find that they are able to adjust to a life without their loved one within a few years. And yet, for a subset of mourners, the journey is both long and arduous—a grief experience that is marked by a protracted, debilitating, sometimes life-threatening (Latham & Prigerson, 2004) response to loss known as *complicated grief* (CG; Prigerson et al., 1995; Shear et al., 2011) or prolonged grief disorder (PGD; Boelen & Prigerson, 2007), often requiring professional counseling (Currier, Neimeyer, & Berman, 2008). Many mourners turn to their religious or spiritual beliefs and activities as a means of coping (Wortmann & Park, 2008), finding them to be a solace when a loved one dies. However, studies show that sometimes the opposite occurs—that bereavement itself can have a detrimental effect on the griever's faith (Burke, Neimeyer, McDevitt-Murphy, Ippolito, & Roberts, 2011; Burke, Neimeyer, Young, Piazza Bonin, & Davis (in press); Neimeyer & Burke, 2011; Shear et al., 2006). Whereas spiritual beliefs, practices, and meaning making can be protective against overall poor health, in some forms they can also be predictive of overall greater distress (Burke & Neimeyer, 2012a). Whether in terms of the lost relationship with a deceased loved one, or a severed or severely compromised relationship with God or one's spiritual community, at the basis of these once-cherished relationships is the common bond of deep emotional attachment and love, and the need to make sense of the losses.

Our goal in this chapter is to review two faces of this work, in the form of a focus on psychological and spiritual struggles in the aftermath of loss, both of which fit within the broad scaffolding of a meaning reconstruction framework. Thus, this chapter outlines empirical findings and theoretical understandings of both spiritual meaning making and spiritual crisis in bereavement, highlighting their significance for the loss of a female loved one to cancer.

WOMEN'S CANCER DEATHS

U.S. statistics for 2007 (the most recent year for which statistics are available) list the following cancers as the most likely to end a woman's life: breast, lung, colon/rectum, uterus, thyroid, non-Hodgkin lymphoma, skin, ovarian, kidney, and pancreas (CDC, 2011). Recent reports also show that although more women are diagnosed with breast cancer (202,964 in 2007) and about 40,598 will die each year from the disease, lung cancer is the leading cause of female cancer deaths, taking the lives of approximately 70,354 women annually. Colorectal cancer is third in the lineup of killers of women, with 26,215 women dying from the disease in 2007. Other gynecological cancers, such as cervical, ovarian, uterine, vaginal, and vulvar cancers together claim the lives of 27,739 U.S. women annually (CDC, 2011). Consequently, based on McDaid et al's (2008) findings, these figures also suggest that each year a significant number of individuals—hundreds of thousands—will grieve the death of a female loved one to cancer.

LOSS OF A LOVED ONE

In that swift second that steals away the life of a cherished loved one, core constructs about the laws of life and death, the order of the universe, and for the religiously inclined, even God's character, can be systemically deconstructed (Neimeyer, 2001). Grieving is the natural, normal, and perhaps even necessary response of humans to loss, but not all grievers respond similarly. In fact, grief-specific distress can be thought of as occurring on a continuum. On one end, for a significant number of grievers who are resilient, the mourning period will produce only transient psychological distress (Bonanno & Kaltman, 2001). Many others experience a good deal of distress (e.g., shock, anguish, sadness) and adjust gradually to a life without their loved over the course of a year or two (Bonanno & Mancini, 2006). On the other end, some grievers suffer from CG—severe, debilitating grief, lasting for many months, years, or even decades. CG signifies a state of unrelenting grief, represented by profound separation distress, psychologically disturbing and intrusive thoughts of the deceased, a sense of emptiness and meaninglessness, trouble accepting the reality of the loss, and difficulty in making a life without the deceased loved one (Holland, Neimeyer, Boelen, & Prigerson, 2009; Prigerson & Jacobs, 2001). While bereavement itself poses an increased risk of early mortality for mourners, especially bereaved spouses (Stroebe, Schut, & Stroebe, 2007), CG in particular has been shown to predict cardiovascular illness (Prigerson et al., 1997), insomnia (Hardison, Neimeyer, & Lichstein, 2005), substance abuse, suicide, immune dysfunction, and impaired quality of life and social functioning (Latham & Prigerson, 2004; Prigerson et al., 2009). Past studies have found that rates of CG in the general bereaved population are approximately 10 percent (Prigerson et al., 2009).

PRIMARY ATTACHMENTS

Bowlby (1969) described the human attachment system as a relational structure that governs the level of desire that an individual has to draw near to primary attachment figures, such as parents or others who provide love, care, and attention. Activation of the attachment system occurs frequently within the context of human relationships; however, loss heightens the arousal of the attachment system when that person, and all that he or she represented in terms of being a place of safety and security, is gone. In their attempt to set criteria for CG as a recognizable disorder, Prigerson and her colleagues (2009; see also Latham & Prigerson, 2004) outlined a set of empirically supported risk factors predictive of CG (e.g., childhood separation anxiety, a close kinship to the deceased, marital supportiveness and dependency), all of which were attachment related. On the other hand, yearning and longing on behalf of the griever to be reunited with the lost one was found by Prigerson's team to be the core symptom of CG. Burke and Neimeyer's (2012b) comprehensive empirical review of CG predictors further confirmed six risk factors for elevated and prolonged grief: low social support, anxious/avoidant/insecure attachment style, discovering or identifying the body (in cases of violent death), being the spouse or parent of the deceased, high predeath marital dependence, and high neuroticism. Thus, both before and after death occurs and grief ensues, the chief factors that govern how well an individual will do in relation to the loss of the loved one appear to be predicated on issues of attachment in the relationship to the deceased.

Although primary attachment figures can have any of several relationships to the survivor (e.g., parent, child, sibling, friend), the love relationship between spouses appears to have distinctive characteristics that warrant deeper exploration. According to Thoits (1995), "the simplest and most powerful measure of social support appears to be whether a person has an intimate, confiding relationship or not (spouse or lover; others less powerfully)" (p. 64). Consistent with theories of attachment, Stroebe, Stroebe, Abakoumkin, and Schut (1996) found that the loss of a partner equated to the loss of a primary attachment figure, and that, rather than providing a buffer, relationships with family and friends could not provide adequate compensation for such a loss. Specifically, they found that the distress incurred through partner loss was experienced as *emotional loneliness*, which was qualitatively different from the *social loneliness* that comes from lack of support from friends and family. In fact, their findings indicated that the only compensation for the loss of a spouse is for the surviving spouse to establish a new intimate relationship. Furthermore, other studies showed that bereaved spouses who suffer the most emotional loneliness tend to be those with high levels of anxious attachment to begin with (van der Houwen et al., 2010), that is, those whose sense of connection to others was tenuous before the loss.

O'Connor et al.'s (2008) study, using functional magnetic resonance imaging (fMRI) to measure grief-generated brain activity in women who lost a mother or sister to breast cancer, found evidence of an addictive quality to complicated grief. While undergoing neuroimaging, women viewed photos of their deceased mother or sister while simultaneously viewing grief-related words stemming from their own previously transcribed narrative report of the loss. Their results showed that whereas all grievers showed neuronal firings in the pain pathways of their brains, only those individuals with CG had activity in the nucleus accumbens (NA), the part of the human brain that governs reward, especially the type of pleasure associated with addiction. And, although activity in the NA was related to self-reported yearning for the lost loved one, there was no association between NA activity levels and time since the loss, age of the griever, or levels of positive or negative affect.

In a similar study, Gündel, O'Connor, Littrell, Fort, and Lane (2003) reported neuroimaging results of women bereaved of a spouse or a parent less than one year earlier. Through the use of fMRI, the women viewed photos of their loved one or a stranger, crossed with a grief-related word or a nonemotive word. Gündel and colleagues found that when the photo of the loved one was coupled with the grief-related word that the following three areas of the brain were activated: the posterior cingulate cortex (PCC), which is believed to respond to emotionally salient stimuli and memories for personal events; the anterior cingulate cortex (ACC), which is linked to attention; and the insula, which is associated with attention to one's bodily state. Discovering *increased* brain activity in the PCC in their study can be juxtaposed with other studies that have shown *decreased* activation in the PCC of depressed individuals, implying that anxiety related to separation distress rather than depression may be a plausible explanation for high activation in grievers. Moreover, finding an association between heightened levels of attention (as measured by increased ACC activity) and visual cues of the women's loved one may indicate a keen sensitivity to the presence of the lost loved one, beyond that of other individuals. Likewise, the activation of the insula indicated that the painful nature of loss seems to require attentional support in terms of one's body. For instance, a frequent report of bereaved individuals is the sensation of a "broken heart" or "pangs of grief," which Gündel and associates illuminated in relation to the insula using neuroimaging techniques. Thus, whether consciously or unconsciously, the love relationship appears to continue in spite of death—to a degree that its physical traces can be observed even in the physiology of the brain.

SPIRITUALITY BEFORE AND AFTER LOSS

Kernohan, Waldron, McAfee, Cochrane, and Hasson's (2007) study with terminally ill patients revealed that their top six spiritual needs were to: (a) have time to think, (b) have hope, (c) deal with unresolved issues, (d) prepare for death, (e) express true feelings without being judged, and (f) speak of important relationships. And yet, although spiritual care is generally considered an essential component of palliative care services that often provides benefits for family members as well as patients (Casarett et al., 2010), research indicates that addressing the spiritual needs of terminally ill patients and their families is fraught with complexity for many health care providers (Ellis & Lloyd-Williams, 2012). Such challenges likely occur because, on the one hand, loss uniquely enables believers to spiritually transpose tragedy into divine providence, God's mercy, or one's appointed destiny (Pargament & Park, 1997), while, on the other hand, it can elicit resentment and doubt toward God, dissatisfaction with the spiritual support received from others, and substantial changes in the bereaved person's spiritual beliefs and behaviors (Burke, Neimeyer, Young et al., in press).

Spiritual Meaning Making

Links have been made between adaptation to bereavement and the common attempt by human beings to make sense of life via spirituality or religion. Stated aptly by Baumeister (1991), "Religion is . . . uniquely capable of offering high-level meaning to human life. [It] may not always be the best way to make life meaningful, but it is probably the most reliable way" (p. 205). Some researchers suggest that being religious might position one better when death occurs and mourning begins. For instance, Park (2005) argued that when an individual has a foundation of spirituality/religion, it provides a ready-made infrastructure for understanding his or her experience. According to Park, approaching life from the premise of faith facilitates a cognitive reframing of the world, which can be especially useful in enduring difficult life trials. Thus, what at first might be seen as a random, cruel catastrophe seemingly has purpose and meaning and is divinely ordained, when contemplated through the lens of faith (Pargament & Park, 1997).

However, although the importance of faith may increase during the mourning period, it may be accompanied by doubt as well as conviction. For example, in relation to the death, some religious individuals struggle with the question of why God allowed their loved ones to die; some question their pre-loss beliefs about God, vacillating between doubt and belief throughout bereavement; and still others wonder why they have been allowed to live when their loved ones have not (Burke, Neimeyer, Young et al., in press; Golsworthy & Coyle, 1999). For some bereaved people, faith was an important resource for making sense of their loss, facilitating an acceptance of the death, and providing reassurance for the future (Smith, 2001). Some grievers report that spirituality put into words for them the invisible, unknowable, and unexplainable parts of life and death, such as where their loved ones went after they died. Parkes (2011) depicted why this is important by expressing some of the confusion experienced by the griever, "'I know where I'm going, and I know who's going with me,' except that when we lose the one we love, we no longer know where we are going or who is going with us" (p. 4).

Participants in faith traditions who received regular, directive teachings on these and other existential matters reported that it not only aided them in the recognition of death as a permanent yet natural part of life, but also inspired hope for reunion with their loved ones (Abrums, 2000). McIntosh, Silver, and Wortman (1993) found that individuals who endorsed faith were more likely to find meaning following loss. In fact, the grief-related meaning making benefits experienced by the participants in Davis and

Nolen-Hoeksema's study were such that those individuals who had spiritual beliefs prior to the death were three times as likely to find meaning afterward as those who did not. Likewise, in response to the death of a child, parents studied by Lichtenthal, Currier, Neimeyer, and Keesee (2010) reported a great deal of spiritual meaning making (e.g., that the death was God's will, and that they would reunite with their children in the afterlife), which was in turn associated with lower levels of complicated grief.

Spiritual Crisis

Without diminishing the protective power of spirituality as a practical tool in bereavement, it is clear that bereavement can, in turn, put one's spiritual resources to the test, sometimes leaving the bereaved feeling spiritually crippled, drained, and purposeless while grieving. It was precisely this that Attig (2001) referred to when he spoke of the dispiriting "spiritual pain" that can follow loss—the kind of pain that leaves life sapped of meaning (p. 37).

Studies show that, just as with the physical loss of a human love relationship to death, breakdown or erosion of one's love relationship with God can elicit a disordered type of grief (Burke et al., 2011; Burke, Neimeyer, Young et al., in press; Neimeyer & Burke, 2011; Shear et al., 2006). Granted, when some people face existential crises, their faith can grow or be strengthened; but, for others, this clearly is not the case. Hill and Pargament's (2008) review of studies on spirituality and mental health supported this notion. As the authors explained, spiritual crisis in the lives of distressed individuals can be the catalyst that makes or breaks their faith. Likewise, the most common results from open-ended questions asked of bereaved parents in Lichtenthal et al.'s (2010) study were expressions of spiritual themes, revealing that it is the love of God and other core spiritual beliefs that are both relied upon and called into question when tragic loss occurs, such as the death of a child.

Shear and colleagues (2006) reported similar findings in their church-based study of the bereavement experiences of 31 African American parishioners. Following the loss of their loved ones, the faith of the grievers in their sample varied greatly from "faith stronger than ever" to "faith seriously shaken," with 19 percent of the participants endorsing some level of negative shift in their faith as a result of the loss. The authors referred to this type of experience as "spiritual grief" (p. 7)—an initial acute and painful spiritual response to unexplained yet important losses allowed by God that seem unfair or untimely—akin to the psychological grief that survivors experience when their human relationships are severed as a result of death. However, according to Shear and her team, the more troublesome variant of this reaction to loss is *complicated spiritual grief* (CSG)—a spiritual crisis in the bereaved individual's relationship with God such that he or she struggles to reestablish spiritual equilibrium following loss, often accompanied by a sense of discord, conflict, and distance from God, and at times with members of one's spiritual community. Although a number of studies have looked at spiritual crisis in distressed or bereaved samples, little is known about spiritual crisis as a *result* of bereavement. However, recent studies indicate that a perceived breakdown in the relationship between spiritually inclined people and God seems to be at its core.

Burke and her associates (2011) conducted a study to examine CSG in a sample of 46 African American homicide survivors. They found that individuals who struggled the most with their grief during bereavement were also the ones who struggled the most in terms of their relationship with God following this horrific form of loss. Specifically, they found that grievers with high levels of CG also wondered what they had done to receive God's punishment, questioned God's love, felt abandoned by the church, and questioned the power of God. With the same sample of grievers, Neimeyer and Burke (2011) established that CG was the strongest predictor of the later development of spiritual crisis following loss, even above other forms of bereavement distress, including post-traumatic stress disorder (PTSD) and depression. Similarly, Burke and Neimeyer's (in press) study with a large, diverse sample of spiritually inclined grievers found that, in addition to replicating previous findings (Burke et al., 2011), grievers who struggled with the loss of their loved ones also simultaneously struggled with feeling angry with or distant from God and from members of their church, felt punished by God for a lack of devotion, wondered whether God had abandoned them, questioned their religious beliefs and faith, and endorsed the notion that the devil made the death occur. Thus, stated differently, it appears that for the grievers in these studies, the anguish over the loss of their relationships to the deceased eventually generalized to a similar anguish in terms of their loss of relationship to God and/or their church community.

Bereaved Christians in Burke, Neimeyer, Young et al.'s (in press) diverse sample responded to open-ended questions designed to encourage them to think about how they felt during the times when they struggled most deeply with the loss of their loved ones and, specifically, to describe how the loss challenged their relationship with God. The following examples illustrate their struggle:

> My problem was that, I would go back to the scripture where it states, "All things work together for the good of me," and I couldn't understand how, how can this be good for me? You know, this is terrible! This is awful! How can this be good for me?
>
> [I felt] challenged, because all my life I have heard of how good and loving God is. Why pray to God if the people I love will not be spared, but [instead] still die.

[I felt] confused. Why would the God that I love and honor allow this to happen to me!

My part was to try and comfort my [young] children. I often received the question, "If God loved us why did he take Grandma?"

Other bereaved individuals expressed mixed emotions:

I despised God for taking away the person I loved most in the world. Yet, when I finished screaming at Him, I felt more acceptance from Him than I would have ever anticipated. My sense of His goodness not being limited to my finite understanding became greatly strengthened.

At first, I was challenged and angry by the way she left the world. My heart aches every day since she has left. But, I still love God.

Naturally, the death of a primary attachment figure can give rise to a myriad of spiritually oriented questions. Questions that are seemingly left unanswered by God or insufficiently so, or ones perceived by the bereaved person to be pointless to even ask, can add further anguish to an already protracted and embittered bereavement, leaving them vulnerable to subsequent losses—of relationship with God or confidence in His ability or concern to protect and love them. God still exists, but remotely. Although God's existence might not be questioned, His power or love might be, particularly following abject loss of a cherished loved one. As opposed to one's pre-bereavement way of thinking, this suggests a shift in one's view of God, which in attachment terms is modeled on the neglectful parent, who is powerless or uninterested in offering us security in the face of life's most difficult trials. This pattern likewise manifests itself in the survivor feeling alone even while surrounded by a community of fellow believers.

These studies underscore the value of recognizing the spiritual processes of people who have experienced a traumatizing loss. Research indicates that clergy, mental health professionals, and other professionals assisting the survivor should not assume that high levels of pre-loss faith or one's usual spiritual activities (e.g., church attendance, prayer, Bible reading, worship) or engagement with fellow churchgoers will act as a panacea or buffer against a crisis of faith (Burke & Neimeyer, in press; Burke et al., 2011; Burke, Neimeyer, Young et al., in press; Thompson & Vardaman, 1997), especially in bereaved individuals who are also struggling to accept and adjust to the loss of a loved one. In fact, those in the helping professions are called on to creatively facilitate psychological accommodation and spiritual progress in grievers who struggle spiritually as a result of loss. However, understanding the foundation of the distress—that spiritual distress in bereavement is directly related to the loss of the loved one, rather than to symptoms of depression or PTSD per se—can guide those who work with

grievers as they search for meaning (Coleman & Neimeyer, 2010) and attempt to make spiritual sense of their loss (Lichtenthal et al., 2010; Pargament,
Koenig, & Perez, 2000; Stein et al., 2009).

Perhaps the essence of CSG was summed up by C.S. Lewis (1961), lay
theologian and Christian apologist, who not only expressed his despond-
ency at the loss of his love relationship with his wife, Joy, who died following
a short bout with cancer, but also openly expressed his despair in relation to
the felt loss of his love relationship with God.

> Meanwhile, where is God? [When things are going right, He is right
> there, with open arms]. But go to him when your need is desperate,
> when all other help is vain, and what do you find? A door slammed
> in your face, and a sound of bolting and double bolting on the inside.
> After that, silence. Why is He so present a commander in our time of
> prosperity and so very absent a help in time of trouble? (pp. 5-6)

One reason to highlight what happens when spiritual coping mechanisms
go awry as a result of bereavement is that the psychological literature is
nearly silent on the topic (Hays & Hendrix, 2008), both in terms of recognizing it and treating it. In fact, to our knowledge, there is nothing in the way of
a specialized intervention available to specifically target bereavement-
induced spiritual crisis. It is to this topic we now turn, offering some suggestions about the treatment of both bereavement distress and concomitant
spiritual struggles.

ASSISTING SUFFERERS OF COMPLICATED GRIEF

Family-Focused Grief Therapy

A growing body of literature suggests that grief therapy, often a limited
resource for many bereaved individuals, should be channeled toward those
most in need, such as high-risk cancer caregivers, burdened by caring for
their terminally ill loved one (Harding & Higginson, 2003), and individuals
suffering from CG (Currier et al., 2008). Research also underscores the psychosocial challenges of being a family member of someone with cancer, and
the special burden of cancer-related loss on families. To address this,
Kissane, Lichtenthal, and Zaider (2008) conducted a randomized controlled
trial of an effective grief intervention for family members bereaved by
cancer-related deaths. Their treatment emphasized the benefits of interven-
ing clinically with the family prior to the death, before the cancer patient
dies, and then again afterward; because, although individual family
members may grieve differently, they do so interactively as a unit, as well.
Overall, they found that families receiving therapy were less distressed at
13 months compared to controls. And families who were most distressed at

baseline showed even greater improvement in terms of lower distress and depression levels, and tended toward better social functioning.

Continuing Bonds

Researchers have established that individuals bereft of a loved one often derive much in the way of comfort and are better able to facilitate spiritual meaning making and reconnection with the loved one when they maintain a continuing bond (CB) with the deceased following death (Klass, Silverman, & Nickman, 1996). Field and Wogrin (2011) conceptualized the griever's use of CBs thusly:

> reorganizing or relocating the relationship [with the deceased loved one] such that it now exists at a purely mental representational level . . . [in order] to experience the deceased to some degree as continuing to serve a *safe haven* attachment function, to which the bereaved can turn as a comforting presence under times of stress. (p. 38)

Some studies suggest that in order for the bereaved to hold a consistent and comprehensible narrative of the loss that fits within the broader context of his or her life story, the bond with the deceased must not be severed but rather reestablished and maintained (Fraley & Shaver, 1999). However, an appreciation that CBs might be beneficial also must be coupled with an awareness that *bonding* is not synonymous with *binding* (Currier, Holland, & Neimeyer, 2006). A defining characteristic of CG is the maladaptive use of CBs, often representative of an individual with a highly dependent attachment style that is exhibited in intense separation distress when the primary attachment figure dies. Thus, a "clinician's toolbox" to facilitate reconstruction of the relationship with the deceased rather than relinquishment of it might well include such techniques as *imaginal dialogues, correspondence with the deceased*, and the *life imprint*, each of which we will briefly describe and illustrate.

Imaginal Dialogues

Imaginal dialogues commonly involve the therapist facilitating an enactment of a conversation between the mourner and the deceased, with the mourner playing both roles—his/her own and that of the deceased loved one. In this technique, the clinician guides the bereaved individual in a conversation that opens up important themes, often those related to unfinished business between the two people, or that invites forgiveness and/or mutual appreciation. Although such dialogues can be simply invited with the client imagining the deceased and then addressing him or her, the clinician also can make use of *empty chair* or *two-chair* work (Greenberg, Rice, & Elliott,

1993) to facilitate a shift in the griever's perspective, in the former case allowing the unoccupied seat to symbolically hold the loved one, and in the latter instance rotating the griever to the empty chair to respond as if in the voice of the deceased. A by-product of the clinician's choreographing of this type of oral interchange is that it can amplify the intensity of the contact. Perhaps the positive results achieved through use of imaginal conversations can be explained by the way in which they are spoken in the present tense, with the therapist prompting for depth and honesty from the sidelines of the conversation, in this way reanimating the relationship between the client and the deceased (Neimeyer, 2012a).

> *Sarah had lost her mother to cancer in her early teenage years, but now, in her mid-20s, found that she was beginning to lose even a sense of what her mother looked like, though she missed her still. Indeed, in a curious way, she found that her mother was "growing younger" as the years went on, as she replenished her visual memory with family photographs, many of them taken when her mother was a young woman in high school and college. Accepting the invitation of the therapist to "reopen the conversation with mom about the loss," Sarah spoke quietly and intensely of this irony to her mother, underscoring her continuing bond of love and expressing her wish for closer contact. Changing chairs at the therapist's suggestions, she then straightened and leaned forward, responding as her mother that she had great pride in the woman her daughter was becoming, tears coming to her eyes as she found the words and repeated them at the therapist's prompting. Returning to her seat, Sarah was moved by the encounter, and expressed how she was touched by the special symmetry of the evolving postmortem relationship with her mother: just as her mother was growing younger in her eyes, she was growing into maturity in her mom's. Something about this felt right, like a relationship coming full circle, and provided a different sort of comfort than she had previously known.*

Use of imaginal dialogues shows that, typically, these verbal exchanges are vividly emotional, highly clarifying, and nearly always affirming to the bereaved individual (Neimeyer, Burke, Mackay, & Stringer, 2010). With both the therapist and the client placing premium on the experience, this intensely experiential exchange is followed by client and therapist commentary to consolidate learning and growth. Benefits of using this technique are that it: a) serves to reaffirm the CB, providing a sense of attachment security; b) facilitates resolution of concerns about the death or the relationship, such as survivor guilt or self-blame; c) frees the bereaved to pursue personal goals of autonomy, effectiveness, and relatedness; and d) represents a key component in empirically supported Complicated Grief Therapy (CGT; Shear, Frank, Houch, & Reynolds, 2005).

Correspondence with the Deceased

Correspondence with the deceased, or "unsent letters" (Neimeyer, 2006; 2012b), is a straightforward attempt on the part of the survivor to reconnect with the deceased in narrative form, in an effort to say "hello again" (White, 1989), rather than a final good-bye. The most therapeutic letters appear to be those in which the griever speaks deeply from his/her heart about what is important as he or she attempts to reopen contact with the deceased rather than seek "closure" of the relationship. Some people find it beneficial to consider what the other has given them, intentionally or unintentionally, of enduring value. Additionally, letter writing offers an opportunity to use words that heretofore have remained unspoken, and to ask the questions that remain unasked. The following therapeutic prompts can help initiate this type of written dialogue, especially for those who may be stuck in their grief:

What I have always wanted to tell you is . . .
What you never understood was . . .
What I want you to know about me is . . .
What I now realize is . . .
The one question I have wanted to ask is . . .
I want to keep you in my life by . . .

Continuing bonds, by nature, are personal and individualized, and like imaginal dialogues of a spoken variety can invite a response from the other. Thus, many grievers use letter writing to initiate an ongoing correspondence "with" the deceased, letting the conversation evolve as their lives do. Others use such writing to begin a therapeutic journal, designed to branch out in a variety of literary directions. Still others take advantage of contemporary online media by opening an email account in the loved one's name to which personal messages can be sent, or by continuing to share postings about the deceased loved one via Facebook or other social networking sites.

When Fred lost his "sweetheart" Shirley after a 55-year marriage, he understandably grieved deeply. But he also felt relieved from the caregiving burden he had lovingly assumed during her long years of cancer and its treatment. Pursuing therapy to sort out these mixed feelings, he accepted the therapist's invitation to write about his conundrum to Shirley and seek her counsel, though the idea at first surprised him. In part, the first letters in the "exchange" read as follows:

Shirley, My Love,
      Well, today was the day to seek the shrink. . . . Dr. Neimeyer's waiting room invites calm as does his therapy suite. He

is thoroughly relaxing and non-threatening. Yet, as with any good therapist, you sense he's no push-over. He completely avoided the typical clinical protocol of intake forms, etc., and said simply, "How can we use this hour to help you?"

I jumped right in and told him about your death five months ago and my sojourn since. And that I was having some difficulty with doing as well as I was, with feelings of guilt [for feeling] release after the protracted and intense care-giving. . . . After asking a number of questions, he led me to the understanding that my recovery was not unusual [for someone in my position] following the release of the beloved from the great pain and suffering, [which] offers a new sense of freedom. He commented that my journaling was right on target with the most current grief therapies, and is what has put me in the relatively healthy place where I am. He read some of my writing and was obviously moved by it and said so. He said I dealt with you and your death in a moving and tender way. He did suggest that I stretch myself and conjure up what your thoughts and expressions would be to the things I am saying and writing now. So, that I will try. But it was so comforting to be really understood and affirmed. He said the next task I might consider would be to re-configure our relationship in light of your death. Not to say a final goodbye. But to find a way to continue the relationship on a different level and find your voice speaking to me and your presence still bearing upon me. Nothing spooky about that. Just simply to find your voice and your presence still with me. So, I shall try. Bear with me, my love.

Fred

He then continued with a new letter, only written with "Shirley's" words this time:

Freddie. It's about time you listened to me! How long have we known and loved each other. And me not to talk to you? That's unthinkable! Now, what Dr. Neimeyer says is exactly right. You just sit still and listen. That meditation you do each morning will probably help if you focus on it.

First of all, let's deal with the more mundane stuff—what you are doing with your time and energy. Now, that is fine with me as long as you don't do anything foolish. You don't have me to worry about. But that doesn't mean you can be reckless. There are still our children who would be heartbroken if anything happened to you. But go ahead and try some new ministry in the inner city if that's what God is calling you to do. Just don't be disappointed if no one stands and cheers! You have much to give and contribute. You have a loving heart and a good mind. Don't waste them on trivial things. . . . Rekindle the dream you had for the "beloved community" back in seminary days and earlier. I am with you on this one. Just be sure to include the little children as you go along in some way.

Well, tomorrow we will get into other stuff. But, sit on that tonight. And we will chat some more tomorrow.

Love always, Shirley

Narrative therapy techniques, such as letter writing that occurs between the bereaved and deceased, are used in various approaches to grief therapy, even those that otherwise differ in terms of their conceptualization of grief distress and how it should be treated (e.g., Boelen, de Keijser, van den Hout, & van den Bout, 2007; Neimeyer et al., 2010).

Life Imprints

Life imprints represent unique tools available to the clinician, ones that can be used to enable the griever to seek strands of continuity in the relationship to the deceased, as well as denoting potential points of transition (Neimeyer & Burke, 2012). The life imprint helps the griever see that his or her life is a reflection of bits and pieces of the many people whose characteristics and values he or she has unconsciously assimilated into a felt sense of identity. This "inheritance" transcends genetics, as we can powerfully or subtly be shaped not only by parents, but also by mentors, friends, siblings, or even children whom we have loved and lost. If life imprints are made up of parts of all of those with whom we have deep attachments, then it stands to reason that life imprints are not always positive. At times we can trace our self-criticism, distrust, fears, and emotional distance to once-influential relationships that are now with us only internally.

As a means of facilitating the process, grievers are asked to take a few moments privately to trace the imprint of an important figure in their lives, and then to discuss their observations with the therapist or another person, using the following fill-in-the-blank sequence of questions:

The person whose imprint I want to trace is: _____
This person has had the following impact on:
My mannerisms or gestures:
My ways of speaking and communicating:
My work and pastime activities:
My feelings about myself and others:

My basic personality:
My values and beliefs:
The imprints I would most like to affirm and develop are:
The imprints I would most like to relinquish or change are:

As with other techniques in the clinician's toolbox that are designed to foster CBs, variations and extensions of the life imprint can make the process more personalized. The clinician might suggest homework assignments that include:

Documentation—the client is asked to write a paragraph as between-session homework about each of the questions to reaffirm the lost connection.

Letters of gratitude—the survivor writes a "thank you" letter to the deceased for the "gifts" he/she has given.

Survey—the bereaved person interviews several other people about the imprint of the deceased on them to deepen appreciation of his or her life.

Directed telling—using an empty chair, the griever directly expresses the impact of the deceased loved one's life on his or her own.

Cara was a devoted African American mother of three living children whose fourth child, whom she named Spirit—"because that is how she came to me"—was stillborn at seven months of gestation. Although she had never known Spirit as a living being outside her womb, Cara decided to trace Spirit's imprint on herself, in part to recognize that her child had not lived for more than half a year inside her in vain. Chief among the imprints that Cara traced were Spirit's impact on her ways of communicating: after sharing the tragedy of her baby's living and dying with others in and beyond the family, including the therapist, she found that she was more emotionally expressive than before, letting people know she loved them, and initiating contact and attempting to resolve festering bad feelings in a way she never had previously. She also felt that Spirit had left a mark on her spirituality, as she was more convinced than ever that there were "other beings" that operated in our lives, including the guardian figure she believed she saw in shadowy outline in Spirit's earlier ultrasound, which she came to view as an ancestor figure who had come to usher her child into a different form of existence.[1]

ASSISTING SUFFERERS OF COMPLICATED SPIRITUAL GRIEF

As the field of bereavement studies is only now beginning to research spiritual crisis following loss, and has just recently developed and validated a means of assessing this construct (Burke, Neimeyer, Holland et al., in press), ideas for treating such distress are clearly germinal. However, in targeting issues related to a compromised relationship between the bereaved individual and God and/or the spiritual community, we might begin by creatively extending components of interventions that have been used with traumatized grievers. For instance, using modified procedures similar to those described above, the griever who struggles to make spiritual sense of the loss or who harbors negative emotions toward God might benefit from *an imaginal exploration of the death event from God's perspective.* For example, using a two-chair-type approach, the clinician could help the griever initiate a two-way conversation with God. With the therapist's guidance, the bereaved individual might gain greater understanding about God's perceived purposes or plan, or an increased acceptance about both the loved one's death and his or her future existence. Likewise, in the same vein as maintaining a CB with the deceased loved one, *letters to heaven* could offer the survivor an opportunity to use another medium to express both negative and positive emotions, ask questions, or expound on applicable Bible verses or other writings.

Devotional Writing

Elacqua and Hetzel (2010) propose a devotional writing approach, similar to that of *letters to heaven*, that allows the grievers to process their post-traumatic symptoms and feelings through God's perspective. The griever is encouraged to identify a specific area that he or she desires to explore (e.g., sleep problems, intrusive thoughts, the sovereignty of God, unanswered questions such as *Why, Lord?* or *What if?*) and then write his or her story to God. In this approach, God would respond, not the deceased, using Scripture to substantiate the responses. As the griever asks God a question or takes a concern to God, the griever finds Scripture to answer the question or address the concern. An example of devotional writing is found in the following excerpt from Elacqua and Hetzel's book of devotionals (originally designed for survivors of homicide loss) and Elacqua's (2013) book (applicable to many types of losses, including those arising from illness):

Believe in God

Let not your heart be troubled: ye believe in God, believe also in me.

John 14:1 (King James Version)

My parents were murdered on October 26, 2005. Even to this day, I still grieve their loss. Thoughts of returning to the hometown I grew up in bring a sense of loss, regret, and grief. I do feel that I have come far in the years of mourning. I have done many things to help me process my grief such as crying, joining support groups, participating in one-on-one counseling, attending homicide walks and retreats, speaking to many groups about my loss, writing, praying, and reading and meditating on God's Word. What I believe has helped me the most is my belief in God. Regardless of how much my heart is troubled, I choose to believe in God, and I pray Scripture to reinforce my faith.

I told God that "Scripture says, 'Do not let your hearts be troubled' (John 14:1a), but my heart is troubled, Lord!" I pled with God to give me the faith that will move mountains (Matthew 17:20). When I have struggled with painful feelings, I asked God to replace my anger, anxiety, and fear with the peace of God that surpasses all understanding (Philippians 4:7). I asked God to remove my sleepless nights and enable me to sleep in peace and safety (Psalm 4:8). I asked God to replace my weakness with His strength (Psalm 28:7). I asked God to take away the loneliness of life without Mom and Pop, and to give me the abundant life (John 10:10).

I desire justice, and God tells me in His Word that He is the Righteous Judge (Psalm 7:11; 9:8; 98:9). His Word reminds me that I do not need to worry about justice on earth because the final judgment happens in heaven (Revelation 20:11–15).

It is a long road to transformation, but I choose to believe that because my Heavenly Father gave me Jesus, His only Son, who died for my sins (John 3:16), and who I confess as my Savior (Romans 10:9), I have full confidence of victory over death. I will see my parents again in heaven with eternal life. God is all-powerful, and as the book of Revelation details, the victory has already been won.

Oh, Lord, thank You for Jesus. Thank You that in You there is peace, safety, strength, abundance, faith, and justice according to Your will. Lord, take my troubled heart and give me continual faith to believe in You. Amen.[2]

In addition to the client writing a spiritual devotional, Burke and Elacqua (2012) describe how this devotional set (found in *Hope Beyond Homicide: Remembrance Devotionals*) can be used as an in-session exercise, with the clinician (or the client) reading aloud the current week's devotional regarding an aspect of loss, followed by answering the prompts for discussion. The devotional readings could also be assigned for homework. Both methods help the client give voice to the emotions that arise during the process of meditating on loss and grief and the comfort that comes through God's Word, bringing to bear profound sources of spiritual wisdom.

Elacqua (2013) developed a 10-session intervention for counseling the bereaved using a biblical worldview. The sessions provide a means to explore the type of loss, various sources of support (e.g., effective and ineffective), and feelings and symptoms experienced pre- and post-loss, with practices to assist in coping. Spiritual interventions derived from Scripture are used to address topics that can often hinder the bereaved's relationship with the deceased, their family members, and the Lord (e.g., forgiveness, renewed mind, rebuilding a new life). The context is biblically based, with a foundation for exploring the client's relationship with God, promoting authenticity and transparency with him/herself, the counselor, others, and the Lord to encourage the client to find or develop a deeper intimate relationship with the Lord. One client expressed that *Hope beyond Loss* has encouraged her in her faith journey to "see that even in great loss or tragedy, God really can use horrible things for good, bring good out of it. He uses bad even to draw us near and bring intimacy with Him."

An accumulation of these types of letters or stories, written over time, could form the basis of a journal that could foster reflexive and ongoing engagement with the deeper meaning of love, loss, and faith for spiritually inclined mourners. Finally, because study results indicate that CSG involves complications not only in terms of the griever's relationship with God, but also with members of his/her spiritual community (Burke & Neimeyer, in press, Burke, Neimeyer, Young et al., in press; Burke et al., 2011), methods to address those relational deficits should also be employed. One such technique is for the clinician to facilitate *imaginal role-play* interactions between the bereaved individual and his or her spiritually inclined friends and family. Doing so can offer the survivor a chance to express concerns, hurts, and disappointments, while also providing a means for improving social and spiritual interactions in the future. Another such method is *directed journaling* (Lichtenthal & Neimeyer, 2012), in which religiously inclined individuals are prompted to write about the spiritual sense and "silver lining" they have found in the dark cloud of their bereavement, in a way that clarifies and promotes healing in their relationship to the divine and to their community of faith.

SUMMARY

As the second leading cause of death in women, cancer loss necessarily commands considerable attention in bereavement research. Living life without grieving the loss of a woman to cancer is an experience few Americans will have. And, although most caregivers and other bereaved survivors will eventually find their own way through grief following the death, others will require professional assistance to cope with the serious and debilitating nature of CG (Currier et al., 2008). Fortunately for these individuals, effective grief therapies do exist (Boelen et al., 2007; Field & Wogrin, 2011; Neimeyer, 2006; 2012a; 2012b; Neimeyer et al., 2010). In fact, empirically validated interventions designed specifically to meet the pre- and post-bereavement needs of families of patients with a terminal illness, such as cancer, are already available (Kissane et al., 2008).

Although more research is needed, recent studies have expanded the examination of problematic grief reactions and their relation to subsequent spiritual struggle both in detail (Burke & Neimeyer, in press; Burke, Neimeyer, Young et al., in press; Burke et al., 2011) and in comparison with other disorders (Neimeyer & Burke, 2011). Such research establishes a link between psychologically and spiritually oriented bereavement distress, suggesting that, on some level, they may share the common denominator of a stressed attachment. Thus, what begins as a loss of secure attachment to the loved one can eventuate in an insecure attachment to God (Kirkpatrick, 1995).

As an emergent construct, CSG has not been explored beyond the confines of the Christian faith tradition. However, an expanded program of research likely will reveal in greater depth the struggle experienced by some spiritually inclined grievers while also incorporating ever more accurate scales for measuring CSG, ones that go beyond Christianity to explore other belief systems.

An inability to make sense of the loss in either spiritual (Lichtenthal et al., 2010; Lichtenthal, Burke, & Neimeyer, 2011) or secular terms (Currier et al., 2006) can exacerbate grief. Conversely, meaning made, in terms of both the life and death of the loved one and God's role and intentions surrounding the death (for spiritually inclined grievers), appears to facilitate positive bereavement outcome (Lichtenthal et al., 2010; Lichtenthal et al., 2011).

Suffering the loss of a love relationship is surely one of the most painful human experiences to endure. Couple that with a severely compromised relationship with God and/or with one's faith community, and the picture is all the more challenging. We know that a subset of mourners will suffer substantially more than others at the hand of such affliction. It is for these individuals that more compassion, greater understanding, better assessment tools, and specialized treatment are specifically needed.

NOTES

1 A systematic empirical analysis of meaning reconstruction in Cara's six-therapy grief session can be found in the work of Alves, Mendes, Gonçalves, and Neimeyer (2012).

2 The 52-devotional book *Hope Beyond Homicide: Remembrance Devotionals* is available from the third author at www.hopebeyondhomicide.com.

REFERENCES

Abrums, M. (2000). Death and meaning in a storefront church. *Public Health Nursing, 17*, 132–142.

Alves, D., Mendes, I., Gonçalves, M., & Neimeyer, R. A. (2012). Innovative moments in grief therapy: Reconstructing meaning following perinatal death. *Death Studies, 36*, 785–818.

Attig, T. (2001). Relearning the world: Making and finding meanings. In Neimeyer, R. A. (Ed.), *Meaning reconstruction and the experience of loss* (pp. 33–53). Washington, DC: American Psychological Association.

Baumeister, R. F. (1991). *Meanings of life.* New York: Guilford Press.

Boelen, P. A., de Keijser, J., van den Hout, M., & van den Bout, J. (2007). Treatment of complicated grief: A comparison between cognitive-behavioral therapy and supportive counseling. *Journal of Clinical and Consulting Psychology, 75,* 277–284.

Boelen, P. A., & Prigerson, H. G. (2007). The influence of symptoms of prolonged grief disorder, depression, and anxiety on quality of life among bereaved adults: A prospective study. *European Archives of Psychiatry and Clinical Neuroscience, 257,* 444–452.

Bonanno, G. A., & Kaltman, S. (2001). The varieties of grief experience. *Clinical Psychology Review, 21,* 705–734.

Bonanno, G. A., & Mancini, A. D. (2006). Bereavement-related depression and PTSD: Evaluating interventions. In Barbanel, L., & Sternberg, R. J. (Eds.), *Psychological interventions in times of crisis* (pp. 37–55). New York: Springer.

Bowlby, J. (1969). *Attachment and loss* (Vol. 1). London: Hogarth Press.

Burke, L. A., & Elacqua, T. C. (2012). Spiritual devotionals. In Neimeyer, R. A. (Ed.), *Techniques of grief therapy* (pp. 175–177). New York: Routledge.

Burke, L. A., & Neimeyer, R. A. (in press). Complicated spiritual grief I: Relation to complicated grief symptomatology following violent death bereavement. *Death Studies.*

Burke, L. A., & Neimeyer, R. A. (2012a). Spirituality and health: Meaning making in bereavement. In Cobb, M., Puchalski, C., & Rumbold, B. (Eds.), *The textbook on spirituality in healthcare* (pp. 127–133). Oxford, UK: Oxford University Press.

Burke, L. A., & Neimeyer, R. A. (2012b) Prospective risk factors for complicated grief: A review of the empirical literature. In Stroebe, M. S., Schut, H., van der Bout, J., & Boelen, P., (Eds.), *Complicated grief: Scientific foundations for healthcare professionals* (pp. 145–161). New York: Routledge.

Burke, L. A., Neimeyer, R. A., Holland, J. M., Dennard, S., Oliver, L., & Shear, K. M. (in press). Inventory of complicated spiritual grief scale: Development and initial validation of a new measure. *Death Studies.*

Burke, L. A., Neimeyer, R. A., McDevitt-Murphy, M. E., Ippolito, M. R., & Roberts, J. M. (2011). In the wake of homicide: Spiritual crisis and bereavement distress in an African American sample. *International Journal Psychology of Religion, 21,* 289–307.

Burke, L. A., Neimeyer, R. A., Young, M. J., Piazza Bonin, B., & Davis, N. L. (in press). Complicated spiritual grief II: A deductive inquiry following the loss of a loved one. *Death Studies.*

Casarett, D., Pickard, A., Bailey, A., Ritchie, C., Furman, C., Rosenfeld, K., . . . Shea, J. A. (2010). Do palliative consultations improve patient outcomes? In Meier, D. E., Isaacs, S. L., & Hughes,. R. G. (Eds.), *Palliative care: Transforming the care of serious illness* (pp. 369–381). San Francisco, CA: Jossey-Bass.

Centers for Disease Control & Prevention (CDC). (2011). *Top ten cancers among women*. Retrieved from: http://www.cdc.gov/uscs.

Coleman, R. A., & Neimeyer, R. A. (2010). Measuring meaning: Searching for and making sense of spousal loss in later life. *Death Studies, 34,* 804–834.

Currier, J. M., Holland, J., & Neimeyer, R. A. (2006). Sense making, grief, and the experience of violent loss: Toward a mediational model. *Death Studies, 30,* 403–428.

Currier, J. M., Neimeyer, R. A., & Berman, J. S. (2008). The effectiveness of psychotherapeutic interventions for the bereaved: A comprehensive quantitative review. *Psychological Bulletin, 134,* 648–661.

Davis, C. G., & Nolen-Hoeksema, S. (2001). Loss and meaning: How do people make sense of loss? *American Behavioral Scientist, 44,* 726–741.

Elacqua, T. C. (Ed.). (in press). *Hope beyond loss.* Jackson, TN: Fellowship Bible Church.

Elacqua, T. C. (2013). *Hope beyond loss: A 10-session model for counseling the bereaved through a biblical worldview.* Jackson, TN: Elacqua.

Elacqua, T. C., & Hetzel, J. (Eds.). (2010). *Hope beyond homicide: Remembrance devotionals* (2nd ed.). Jackson, TN: Elacqua & Hetzel.

Ellis, J., & Lloyd-Williams, M. (2012). Palliative care. In Cobb, M., Puchalski, C., & Rumbold, B. (Eds.), *The textbook on spirituality in healthcare* (pp. 257–263). Oxford, UK: Oxford University Press.

Field, N. P., & Wogrin, C. (2011). The changing bond in therapy for unresolved loss: An attachment theory perspective. In Neimeyer, R. A., Harris, D., Winokuer, H., & Thornton, G. (Eds.). *Grief and bereavement in contemporary society: Bridging research and practice* (pp. 37–46). New York: Routledge.

Fraley, R. C., & Shaver, P. R. (1999). Loss and bereavement: Bowlby's theory and recent controversies concerning grief work and the nature of detachment. In Cassidy, J., & Shaver, P. R. (Eds.), *Handbook of attachment theory and research* (pp. 735–759). New York: Guilford Press.

Golsworthy, R., & Coyle, A. (1999). Practitioner's accounts of religious and spiritual dimension in bereavement therapy. *Counseling Psychology Quarterly, 14,* 183–202.

Greenberg, L., Rice, L. N., & Elliott, R. (1993). *Facilitating emotional change.* New York: Guilford Press.

Gündel, H., O'Connor, M. F., Littrell, L., Fort, C., & Lane, R. (2003). Functional neuroanatomy of grief: An fMRI study. *American Journal of Psychiatry, 160,* 1946–1953.

Harding, R., & Higginson, I. (2003). What is the best way to help caregivers in cancer and palliative care? A systematic literary review of interventions and their effectiveness. *Palliative Medicine, 17,* 63–74.

Hardison, H. G., Neimeyer, R. A., & Lichstein, K. L. (2005). Insomnia and complicated grief symptoms in bereaved college students. *Behavioral Sleep Medicine, 3,* 99–111.

Hays, J. C., & Hendrix, C. C. (2008). The role of religion in bereavement. In Stroebe, M. S., Hansson, R. O., Schut, H., Stroebe, W. & Blink, E. V. D., (Eds.), *Handbook of bereavement research and practice: Advances in theory and intervention* (pp. 327–348). Washington, DC: American Psychological Association.

Hill, P. C., & Pargament, K. I. (2008). Advances in the conceptualization and measurement of religion and spirituality: Implications for physical and mental health research. *Psychology of Religion and Spirituality, 1,* 2–17.

Holland, J. M., Neimeyer, R. A., Boelen, P. A., & Prigerson, H. G. (2009). The underlying structure of grief: A taxometric investigation of prolonged and normal reactions to loss. *Journal of Psychopathology and Behavioral Assessment, 31,* 190–201.

Kernohan, W., Waldron, M., McAfee, C., Cochrane, B., & Hasson, F. (2007). An evidence base for a palliative care chaplaincy service in Northern Ireland. *Palliative Medicine, 21,* 519–525. doi:10.1177/0269216307081500.

Kirkpatrick, L. A. (1995). Attachment theory and religious experience. In Hood, J. R. W. (Ed.), *Handbook of religious experience* (pp. 446–475). Birmingham, AL: Religious Education Press.

Kissane, D. W., Lichtenthal, W. G., & Zaider, T. I. (2008). Family care before and after bereavement. *Omega: Journal of Death and Dying, 1,* 21-32.

Kissane, D. W., Zaider, T. I., Li, Y., & Del Guadio, F. (2012). Family therapy for complicated grief. In Stroebe, M. S., Schut, H., van der Bout, J., & Boelens P., (Eds.), *Complicated grief: Scientific foundations for healthcare professionals* (pp. 248–262). New York: Routledge.

Klass, D., Silverman, P. R., & Nickman, S. (1996). *Continuing bonds: New understandings of grief.* Washington, DC: Taylor & Francis.

Latham, A., & Prigerson, H. (2004). Suicidality and bereavement: Complicated grief as psychiatric disorder presenting greatest risk for suicidality. *Suicide Life Threat Behavior, 34,* 350–362.

Lewis, C. S. (1961). *A grief observed.* New York: Harper Collins.

Lichtenthal, W. G., Burke, L. A., & Neimeyer, R. A. (2011). Religious coping and meaning-making following the loss of a loved one. *Counseling and Spirituality, 30,* 113–136.

Lichtenthal, W. G., Currier, J. M., Neimeyer, R. A., & Keesee, N. J. (2010). Sense and significance: A mixed-methods examination of meaning making following the loss of one's child. *Journal of Clinical Psychology, 66,* 791–812.

Lichtenthal, W. G., & Neimeyer, R. A. (2012). Directed journaling to facilitate meaning making. In Neimeyer, R. A. (Ed.), *Techniques of grief therapy* (pp. 161–164). New York: Routledge.

Mackay, M., & Stringer, J. (2010). Grief therapy and the reconstruction of meaning: From principles to practice. *Journal of Contemporary Psychotherapy, 40,* 73–85.

McDaid, C., Trowman, R., Golder, S., Hawton, K., & Sowden, A. (2008). Interventions for people bereaved through suicide: Systematic review. *The British Journal of Psychiatry, 193,* 438–443.

McIntosh, D. N., Silver, R. C., & Wortman, C. B. (1993). Religion's role in adjustment to a negative life event. *Journal of Personality and Social Psychology, 65,* 812–821.

Neimeyer, R. A. (Ed.). (2001). *Meaning reconstruction and the experience of loss.* Washington, DC: American Psychological Association.

Neimeyer, R. A. (2006). *Lessons of loss* (2nd ed.). New York: Routledge.

Neimeyer, R. A. (2012a). Chair work. In Neimeyer, R. A. (Ed.), *Techniques of grief therapy* (pp. 266–273). New York: Routledge.

Neimeyer, R. A. (2012b). Correspondence with the deceased. In Neimeyer, R. A. (Ed.), *Techniques of grief therapy* (pp. 259–261). New York: Routledge.

Neimeyer, R. A., & Burke, L. A. (2011). Complicated grief in the aftermath of homicide: Spiritual crisis and distress in an African American sample. *Religions.* Manuscript in review. (Invited submission for special issue: Spirituality and Health).

Neimeyer, R. A., & Burke, L. A. (2012). The life imprint. In Neimeyer, R. A. (Ed.), *Techniques of grief therapy: Creative Practices for Counseling the Bereaved.* New York: Routledge.

Neimeyer, R. A., Burke, L., Mackay, M., & Stringer, J. (2010). Grief therapy and the reconstruction of meaning: From principles to practice. *Journal of Contemporary Psychotherapy, 40,* 73–83.

O'Connor, M. F., Wellisch, D. K., Stanton, A. L., Eisenberger, N. I., Irwin, M. R., & Lieberman, M. D. (2008). Craving love? Enduring grief activates brain's reward center. *NeuroImage, 42,* 969–972.

Pargament, K., Koenig, H., & Perez, L. (2000). The many methods of religious coping: Development and initial validation of the RCOPE. *Journal of Clinical Psychology, 56,* 519–543.

Pargament, K. I., & Park, C. L. (1997). In times of stress: The religion-coping connection. In Spilka, B., & McIntosh, D. M. (Eds.), *The psychology of religion: Theoretical approaches* (pp. 43–53). Boulder, CO: Westview Press.

Park, C. L. (2005). Religion and meaning. In Paloutzian, C. L. P. R. F. (Ed.), *Handbook of the psychology of religion and spirituality* (pp. 295–314). New York: Guilford Press.

Parkes, C. M. (2011). The historical landscape of loss: Development of bereavement studies. In Neimeyer, R. A., Harris, D., Winokeur, H., & Thornton, G. (Eds.), *Grief and bereavement in contemporary society: Bridging research and practice* (pp. 1–8). New York: Routledge.

Prigerson, H. G., Beirhals, A. J., Kasl, S. V., Reynolds, C. F., Shear, K., Day, N., et al. (1997). Traumatic grief as a risk factor for mental and physical morbidity. *American Journal of Psychiatry, 154,* 616–623.

Prigerson, H. G., Frank, E., Kasl, S., Reynolds, C., Anderson, B., Zubenko, G. S., et al. (1995). Complicated grief and bereavement related depression as distinct disorders: Preliminary empirical validation in elderly bereaved spouses. *American Journal of Psychiatry, 152,* 22–30.

Prigerson, H. G., Horowitz, M. J., Jacobs, S. C., Parkes, C. M., Aslan, M., Goodkin, K., et al. (2009). Prolonged grief disorder: Psychometric validation of criteria proposed for DSM-V and ICD-11. *PLoS Medicine, 6,* 1–12.

Prigerson, H. G., & Jacobs, S. C. (2001). Traumatic grief as a distinct disorder: A rationale, consensus criteria, and a preliminary empirical test. In Stroebe, M. S., Hansson, R. O., Stroebe, W., & Schut, H. (Eds.), *Handbook of bereavement research* (pp. 613–645). Washington, DC: American Psychological Association.

Shear, K., Frank, E., Houch, P. R., & Reynolds, C. F. (2005). Treatment of complicated grief: A randomized controlled trial. *Journal of the American Medical Association, 293,* 2601–2608.

Shear, M. K., Dennard, S., Crawford, M., Cruz, M., Gorscak, B., & Oliver, L. (2006, November). *Developing a two-session intervention for church-based bereavement support: A pilot project.* Paper presented at the meeting of International Society for Traumatic Stress Studies, Hollywood, CA.

Shear, M. K., Simon, N., Wall, M., Zisook, S., Neimeyer, R., et al. (2011). Complicated grief and related bereavement issues for DSM-5. *Depression and Anxiety, 28,* 103–117.

Smith, S. H. (2001). "Fret no more my child . . . for I'm all over heaven all day": Religious beliefs in the bereavement of African American, middle-aged daughters coping with the death of an elderly mother. *Death Studies, 26,* 309–323.

Stein, C. H., Abraham, K. M., Bonar, E. E., McAuliffe, C. E., Fogo, W. R., Faigin, D. A., et al. (2009). Making meaning from personal loss: Religious, benefit finding, and goal-oriented attributions. *Journal of Loss and Trauma, 14,* 83–100.

Stroebe, M., Schut, H., & Stroebe, W. (2007). Health outcomes in bereavement. *Lancet, 370,* 1960–1973.

Stroebe, W., Stroebe, M. S., Abakoumkin, G., & Schut, H. (1996). The role of loneliness and social support in adjustment to loss: A test of attachment versus stress theory. *Journal of Personality and Social Psychology, 70,* 1241–1249.

Thoits, P. A. (1995). Stress, coping, and social support processes: Where are we? What next? *Journal of Health and Social Behavior, Extra issue,* 53–79.

Thompson, M. P., & Vardaman, P. J. (1997). The role of religion in coping with the loss of a family member to homicide. *Journal for the Scientific Study of Religion, 36,* 44–51.

van der Houwen, K., Stroebe, M., Stroebe, W., Schut, H., van den Bout, J., & Wijngaards-de Meij, L. (2010). Risk factors for bereavement outcome: A multivariate approach. *Death Studies, 34,* 195–220.

White, M. (1989). Saying hello again. In White, M. (Ed.), *Selected papers* (pp. 29–36). Adelaide, Australia: Dulwich Centre Publications.

Wortmann, J. H., & Park, C. L. (2008). Religion and spirituality in adjustment following bereavement: An integrative review. *Death Studies, 32,* 703–736.

Chapter 12

Women's Experiences of Treatment Decision Making for Breast Cancer

Katherine Swainston and Anna van Wersch

INTRODUCTION

Concerns throughout the 1970s that the standard use of radical mastectomy (removal of the breast) constituted overtreatment by breast surgeons sparked initial interest in treatment decision making for breast cancer (Lerner, 2001). Early results from randomized controlled trials motivated an increase in breast-conserving surgery, with such studies subsequently indicating comparable long-term outcomes for less invasive breast surgery (e.g., lumpectomy with radiotherapy) (e.g., Fisher et al., 2002) raising questions about women's involvement in surgical treatment decision making. Dissatisfaction with the existing decision-making model was further driven by the feminist movement as the roles of women in medical encounters were explored. Noting that radical mastectomy was predominantly performed by male surgeons, feminists began to critique the traditional patriarchal medical model (e.g., Kushner, 1975; Ruzek, 1978; Riessman, 1983).

Similarly, an increasingly consumerist view of health care led to a growing number of women challenging the authoritarian doctor-patient relationship and writing publicly about their experiences of breast cancer (Lerner, 2001). This added further impetus to the drive for women's involvement in treatment decision making and for full disclosure of surgical treatment options to women with breast cancer (Beisecker, Helmig, & Graham, 1994; Coulter, 1997). However, while such developments in thinking became integrated into health care policy and laws mandating informed consent, a lack of empirical research concerning the decision-making process remained (Katz & Hawley, 2007).

Research investigating breast cancer treatment decision making has increased exponentially in the last two decades and suggests that many women find this process to be difficult (e.g., Polacek, Ramos, & Ferrer, 2007). Women's role in making treatment decisions continues to be debated, yet the notion of shared decision making is currently advocated, and health care professionals are encouraged to facilitate this approach. Commonly considered to be positioned between paternalism and informed choice, shared decision making promotes women's involvement in their own care through women making decisions in partnership with physicians. However, confusion as to what constitutes shared decision making and variation in the roles and responsibilities ascribed to both parties (Charles, Whelan, Gafni, Willan, & Farrell, 2003) has resulted in inconsistent measurement of shared decision making and limits comparison across studies (Makoul & Clayman, 2006). Furthermore, numerous factors have been identified as potential contributors to women's decisional involvement and more generally to the complex and multifaceted nature of women's experiences of treatment decision making for breast cancer.

This chapter begins by reviewing the treatment decision-making pathway and subsequently explores the treatment decision-making time frame and women's role in the decision-making process. Patient-reported outcomes and the role of doctor-patient communication in the treatment decision-making process, as well as the impact of information and the use of decision aids in the context of breast cancer, are considered. The chapter subsequently explores how women maintain ownership of treatment decisions and how perceptions of the body may influence treatment preferences.

THE TREATMENT DECISION-MAKING PATHWAY

Firstly, the ways in which women experience treatment decision making for breast cancer may be influenced by the process of identification and diagnosis. The majority of breast cancers are believed to be detected by women themselves (e.g., Arndt et al., 2002) or as a result of screening in countries where mammography for women aged more than 50 years is part of a public health initiative (e.g., the OECD countries; Saika & Sobou, 2011). However, delays in seeking help following self-identification are commonly reported (e.g., O'Mahony & Hegarty, 2009) and have been associated with lower survival rates (Richards, Westcombe, Love, Littlejohns, & Ramirez, 1999). Furthermore, late presentation of symptoms may influence the treatment options available. This delay is less likely in the group of women who are referred for further diagnostic testing if a positive mammography result has been obtained via public health screening, as for them the entrance into the medical trajectory has already begun (Wang, Tan, & Chow, 2011).

In accordance with best practice, women attending a specialist breast unit should be seen by a multidisciplinary team (Association of Breast Surgery, 2009). Standard procedures indicate that a discussion with the woman about her breast symptoms should be followed by a triple examination involving breast palpation, mammography, or ultrasound scan (where appropriate) and either a fine needle aspiration (FNA) or core biopsy to assess breast tissue for cancerous cells. While the results of a core biopsy may not be known for several days, the diagnosis resulting from a fine needle aspiration may be given on the same day. Consequently, as surgery constitutes the primary method of treatment for breast cancer (NICE, 2009), surgical decisions are often made during women's initial consultation with the breast surgeon (Katz & Hawley, 2007), with surgery taking place shortly thereafter.

Despite breast conservation becoming the standard of care where possible (Fitzgal & Gnant, 2006), estimates indicate that up to one-third of women require mastectomy (Cordeiro, 2008). In such circumstances women may also be required to consider the possibility of reconstructing the breast during mastectomy surgery (immediate reconstruction). Women who are not suitable for immediate reconstruction (e.g., due to the need to complete other treatments) may still be required to contemplate their desire for delayed reconstructive surgery.

Recognition that women with breast cancer frequently benefit from multimodal treatment has led to an extension of the treatment decision-making process to encompass nonsurgical decisions, such as the use of chemotherapy, radiotherapy, hormonal therapy, and biological (targeted) therapy. Yet, even this decision-making process is undertaken within the first weeks following diagnosis (Katz & Hawley, 2007) as women are embarking upon postoperative recovery.

It is also noteworthy that treatment decisions vary in accordance with an individual woman's risk profile. The type and stage of breast cancer diagnosed, the size of a woman's breasts, a woman's age, and the health and psychological profiles of the woman, such as genetic vulnerability, are among the factors influencing the treatment options available. Specifically, histological results such as oestrogen receptor (ER) and human epidermal growth factor receptor 2 statuses (HER2) are particularly valuable in guiding decisions regarding adjuvant treatment (NICE, 2009).

THE DECISION-MAKING TIME FRAME

Advances in diagnostic processes and changes in health care policy (e.g., implementation of the two-week rule in the United Kingdom) have led to a shortening of the diagnostic and surgical decision-making time line. However, in accordance with the notion of shared decision making, women are expected to enact decisional involvement soon after receiving a breast cancer diagnosis, at a time when their information-processing abilities may be compromised. Qualitative studies exploring women's experiences highlight that the multitude of decisions women are required to make result in emotional challenges and that decisions made can have a lasting impact on women's lives (Halkett, Arbon, Scutter, & Borg, 2007).

The lack of time between diagnosis and initiation of the decision-making process may additionally influence women's preferred role in surgical treatment decision making. The restricted time frame and constraints of the health care system may inadvertently facilitate traditional doctor-patient relationships with an authoritarian doctor and passive patient (Street, 2003) limiting women's opportunities for decisional participation (Sharf & Vanderford, 2003). One qualitative study has shown that women felt a need to prepare for the decisions to be made (Halkett et al., 2007). However, for many women the shortened time frame from diagnosis to surgery may not allow this time for reflection, affecting their role in the treatment decision-making process. Similarly, as adjuvant and/or hormonal therapies are commenced shortly after surgery, women may have little time to engage in such decision making and may experience difficulties in doing so due to the physical and psychological impact of surgery.

WOMEN'S ROLE IN THE TREATMENT DECISION-MAKING PROCESS

The level of women's involvement in treatment decision making has received particular research attention with quantitative studies dominating this field; however, contradictory findings are commonplace. Rates of passivity vary, with some studies reporting this figure to be as low as 8 percent for surgical decisions (Lam, Fielding, Chan, Chow, & Ho, 2003), while others note that up to 52 percent of women in their sample delegated treatment decisions to health care professionals (Beaver et al., 1996). More recent studies have reported that 31 percent of women preferred to select their own treatment, 29 percent wanted collaboration with health care professionals, and 40 percent preferred a passive role (Vogel, Helmes, & Hasenburg, 2008). These findings suggest not only that may women's involvement differ given the treatment decision to be made but also that, despite health care policy currently promoting shared treatment decision making, this may not be in line with many women's desired level of involvement. Issues of generalizability, the use of forced-choice questionnaires to measure the multifactorial construct of decision making, and the lack of consideration that not all treatment options are available to all women with breast cancer constitute limitations of such quantitative findings.

Nonetheless, a recent qualitative exploration of women's experiences of breast cancer reported that the majority of women interviewed described passive levels of involvement for surgical treatment decisions (Swainston, Campbell, van Wersch, & Durning, 2012). Furthermore, none of the study participants described any involvement in nonsurgical treatment decision making and cited the multidisciplinary team as the decision makers in this context. This latter finding supports a previous qualitative exploration of decision making for chemotherapy, which found that women did not perceive an option in participating in such decisions yet experienced no desire to do so (Kreling, Fiqueiredo, Sheppard, & Mandelblatt, 2006). This may be partially explained by the fatigue, loss of confidence, and decreased capacity to engage in decision making that is reported to be characteristic of many women's experiences following breast cancer surgery, thereby influencing women's involvement in nonsurgical decision making (Mulcahy, Parry, & Glover, 2010).

PATIENT-REPORTED OUTCOMES IN TREATMENT DECISION MAKING

Health-related benefits have, nevertheless, been documented for women who actively engage in treatment decision making, with this level of involvement being linked to better long-term health outcomes (Andersen, Bowen, Morea, Stein, & Baker, 2009). Significantly higher quality of life has been reported by women who engaged actively in treatment decision making in comparison to those women who enacted a passive role (Hack, Degner, Watson, & Sinha, 2006).

Women who experience a lack of concordance between their actual and desired roles in the treatment decision-making process are more likely to report decisional regret (Lantz et al., 2005). However, the use of satisfaction surveys to assess women's desired and actual involvement has yielded contradictory findings. For example, while one study found that more than half of the women sampled did not attain their desired level of involvement (Degner et al., 1997), another has since reported that 60 percent of women surveyed achieved their desired role in the decision-making process (Temple et al., 2006). This discrepancy may be explained by methodological variation, changes to the health care system, and changes to women's perceptions of treatment decision making for breast cancer over time.

Where actual and desired levels of involvement are incompatible, women have been found to report decisional role regret, indicating that greater autonomy would have been preferred. From a qualitative perspective, contradictory findings are evident with one retrospective study noting that some women questioned the treatment decisions made for many years post-diagnosis (Thomas-McLean, 2004). However, this finding has not been supported in relation to women's experiences in the year post-diagnosis with no decisional regret being described (Swainston et al., 2012). In applying Festinger's (1957) theory of cognitive dissonance, it can be ascertained that these women either experienced no dissonance or that they evaded feelings of dissonance by avoiding reflection on, and engagement in, the treatment decision-making process, further corroborating the passive involvement identified.

Nonetheless, if achieving desired levels of involvement is linked to higher satisfaction levels with the decisions made, then this suggests that the decision-making process is as important as the decision itself (Sabo, St-Jacques, & Rayson, 2007). Doctors' consulting style as opposed to giving women a choice of surgical treatment options has been found to be particularly influential in women's long-term psychological adjustment (Sabo et al., 2007), highlighting the crucial role of communication.

THE ROLE OF DOCTOR-PATIENT COMMUNICATION

To uphold the principles of evidence-informed patient choice and informed consent, health care professionals are required to inform women of the benefits and risks of treatment options and offer opportunities for women to ask questions. Cancer patients, including women with breast cancer, have been found to rely predominantly on direct communication from health care professionals for information to aid decision making, particularly during the diagnostic and treatment stages of their experiences (e.g., O'Leary, Estabrooks, Olsen, & Cumming, 2007).

Research studies have indicated that doctors' advice is highly influential in treatment decision making for breast cancer (Temple et al., 2006). Women frequently cite acceptance of medical opinions and trust in the expertise of health care professionals as reasons for an unquestioning attitude and passive decisional involvement (e.g. Mendick, Young, Holcombe, & Salmon, 2010; Swainston et al., 2012). In referencing the expertise of health care professionals, women may be considered to have adopted an external locus of control in order to manage the uncertainty brought about by receiving a diagnosis of breast cancer (Shaha, Cox, Talman, & Kelly, 2008). Indeed, Moch (1995) asserts that the vulnerability women experience following a breast cancer diagnosis may lead some women to hand over responsibility for treatment decisions in the hope that they will receive the best possible care.

Women's initial attribution of breast cancer to death is also widely reported, and the resultant emotional state following diagnosis has been identified as important in health communication (e.g., Edwards & Hugman, 1997).

Emotional distress may either aid women's integration of information (Peters, Lipkus, & Diefenbach, 2006) or may hamper information processing and, in turn, treatment decision making (Ubel, 2002). In such highly emotional situations, women may use decisional heuristics (or shortcuts), which may lead to treatment decisions being based on fear rather than "evidence" (Slovic, Peters, Finucane, & MacGregor, 2005). Furthermore, in line with the emotional trade-off difficulty model (Luce, 2005) in delegating decisions to health care professionals, women may avoid weighing up difficult emotional trade-offs (e.g., long-term survival vs. mastectomy) and avoid the stress of autonomy when outcomes are uncertain. Accordingly, deferring to the expertise of health care professionals may be a rational decision in itself, if a woman assesses the relevant practitioners as being better placed to make a treatment decision (Kukla, 2005).

THE IMPACT OF INFORMATION

Research study findings suggest that medical information, including the information packs many women receive at the time of diagnosis, can confuse and overwhelm individuals, having a negative impact on treatment decision making (e.g., Hibbard & Peters, 2003; Payne, Large, Jarrett, & Turner, 2000). Yet, surveys have shown that despite such information frequently eliciting anxiety (e.g., Davey et al., 2002), many women hold a preference for more information (Degner et al., 1997). Women's satisfaction with the information received during the diagnosis and treatment process has been found to predict physical and social well-being and quality of life (Davies, Kinman, Thomas, & Bailey, 2008). On the one hand, unmet information needs have been linked to negative psychological outcomes, including anxiety and depression (Mesters, van den Borne, De Boer, & Pruyn, 2001), reduced well-being, and dissatisfaction with care (e.g., Beaver, Bogg, & Luker, 1999). On the other hand, positive outcomes of information provision include increases in knowledge, treatment compliance, satisfaction, and quality of life (e.g., Fallowfield, 1997).

Women who have unmet information needs following consultation with health care professionals have been found to be more likely to consult the Internet (Lee & Hawkins, 2010). The ever-increasing availability of informational resources, particularly electronic and media resources (e.g., Chen & Siu, 2001), is argued to have facilitated patient empowerment (Krupat et al., 1999) and led to greater patient involvement in health care decisions (Gatellari, Butow, & Tattersall, 2001). This may further symbolize a move away from traditional doctor-patient relations wherein the doctor acts as the information keeper (Mulcahy et al., 2010). Source choice has, however, been found to be influenced by age, education, and type of treatment chosen (O'Leary et al., 2007). For example, younger women are more likely to seek information from a variety of such sources, while older women have been found to be more satisfied with information from their health care providers (O'Leary et al., 2007). This may reflect a change in attitudes and that older women are perhaps more familiar with traditional doctor-patient interactions.

Actively seeking information is representative of Miller's (1995) monitor style, while the information and topic avoidance also reported in relation to women's experiences of breast cancer (e.g., Donovan-Kicken and Caughlin, 2011) and the tendency to be overwhelmed by threatening information are indicative of a blunter style of coping (Miller, 1995). Such avoidance of information may provide one explanation for the lack of knowledge reported following surgery about the rates of survival and recurrence associated with differing treatment options (Fagerlin et al., 2006), as well as women's acceptance of medical opinions.

Many women describe a step-by-step process of information acquisition and management throughout the health care trajectory (e.g., Swainston et al., 2012). This may constitute a positive coping strategy by which women enact control, lessen anxiety (Drageset, Lindstrom, & Underlid, 2009), and avoid feelings of cognitive dissonance (Festinger, 1957). The types of information women seek vary with the disease trajectory (Rees & Bath, 2000), though the highest rankings of information needs have been identified as those pertaining to chances for a cure, stage of the disease, and treatment options (O'Leary et al., 2007).

DECISION AIDS

Consumer decision aids are a means of engaging patients in considering treatment options by providing disease-specific knowledge and information on treatment regimens (e.g., Vodermaier et al., 2011). The results from a recent investigation of an interactive online decision aid suggest that the use of such tools may facilitate readiness to make a surgical treatment decision, helping to strengthen surgery intentions (Sivell et al., 2012). Computer programs designed to help inform discussions between patients and health care professionals as to the benefits of adjuvant therapy may also support the postsurgical decision-making process (Ravdin et al., 2001). Such tools take into account tumor size, histological grade, patient age, hormonal receptor status, and comorbidities to predict disease course and potentially effective treatment(s).

Reviews investigating women's use of consumer decision aids have reported higher knowledge levels, an increased likelihood of decisional involvement, less decisional conflict, and higher satisfaction with the treatment decision-making process (e.g. O'Leary et al., 2007; O'Brien et al., 2009; Vodermaier et al., 2011; Waljee, Rogers, & Alderman, 2007). Inconclusive findings have, however, been reported with regard to the impact of decision aids on psychological outcomes, including anxiety and depression symptoms, body image, and quality of life. Methodological issues (e.g., modest sample sizes and multiple treatment interference) may provide some insight into such findings; however, ultimately decision aids may not be available to all women, and some women may choose not to utilize such aids. Furthermore, current versions of decision aids do not include HER2 status, and variation in the use and interpretation of such Web-based tools may result in some women with early-stage breast cancer being under- or overtreated with chemotherapy (NICE, 2012).

MAINTAINING OWNERSHIP OF DECISIONS

In the traditional authoritarian health care system, where ultimate control and responsibility for treatment decisions and the availability of decision aids are with the health care provider, ownership of decisions is argued to be delegated rather than negotiated (Karnilowicz, 2011). Accordingly, women may find enacting a more autonomous role in treatment decision making difficult (Thomas-MacLean, 2004). However, rather than focusing on the responsibility for making treatment decisions, the concept of "conscientious autonomy" (Kukla, 2005) highlights the importance of ownership of, and commitment to, treatment decisions. In the context of breast cancer this may help to explain why some women opt to defer decisional responsibility to health care professionals without presenting as passively compliant and disengaged from the decision-making process. Indeed, in contrast to research studies indicating that passivity engendered a loss of control over the decision-making process (e.g. Halkett et al., 2007), other qualitative studies (e.g., Seale, 2005; Swainston et al., 2012) have found that some women consciously choose passivity but retain engagement with and a sense of ownership of treatment decisions. Women may maintain perceived control via having opportunities to ask questions, attending appointments, and being the one to act upon (or not) treatment decisions. Furthermore, as noted previously, as medical information increases in complexity, some women may delegate decisional responsibility to those who they perceive to have greater expertise, and accordingly may decide to follow the advice of health care professionals (Sinding et al., 2010). Consequently, women's distancing of themselves from decisional responsibility and handing over control to health care professionals may serve as a positive means of coping with the stress of diagnosis (Seale, 2005) and create a situation involving limited possibilities for self-directed action (Jadoulle et al., 2006).

THE BODY IN TREATMENT DECISIONS

Crouch and McKenzie (2000) purport that women's feelings and attitudes toward their bodies and their desire to preserve the integrity of their bodies is likely to influence treatment decision making. The focus of the medical model on the body as a physiological system, one with diseased body parts requiring treatment, indicates an objectification of the body and disease (Radley, 1996). Women's lexical choices in relation to breast cancer, such as "it" and "the cancer" (Cassell, 1976), provide support for this notion and suggest that treatment decisions are made about the body. Distancing the body from the self may constitute a coping mechanism employed to limit stress and anxiety and facilitate women handing over decisional responsibility, particularly regarding decisions that will alter the body (MacLachlan, 2004), as in the case of breast cancer.

Women have been found to speak of their breasts in differing ways, making reference to their functional nature as well as in gendered and medicalized terms (Langellier & Sullivan, 1998). Indeed, women's breasts are widely reported as being symbols of femininity and womanhood, as well as having importance in child-rearing and sexual relationships (Wilmoth, Coleman, Smith, & Davis, 2004). It has, however, been argued that the social construction of breasts as decorative rather than functional has led to women's breasts becoming objectified. Young (1992) further purports that this viewpoint is nurtured by health care professionals who portray breasts as objects that are replaceable either via reconstruction or external breast prostheses. While women's primary fear has been found to be cancer and not breast loss, the importance women ascribe to the opinions of health care professionals and women's perceptions of their bodies may affect decisions regarding surgical intervention.

WOMEN'S SURGICAL PREFERENCES

Research study findings indicate that some women fear breast loss prior to diagnosis, and numerous studies have identified breast surgery as disrupting women's identity (e.g., McCann, Illingworth, Wengström, Hubbard, & Kearney, 2010) and the connection between the body and the self. Commenting on one woman's desire to keep her breasts following a diagnosis of breast cancer, Moch (1995) notes that the importance ascribed to the woman's breasts resulted in a preference for her breasts not to be completely removed, with the resulting treatment decision being a lumpectomy. Accordingly, when making a choice about whether to undergo mastectomy or breast-conserving surgery, the meaning of women's breasts may influence the decision made.

However, rather than greater involvement in surgical treatment decision making resulting in less unnecessary surgery, an active role is associated with more invasive surgery (Katz et al., 2005). In choosing mastectomy, women may be seeking a form of ultimate predictability (Frank, 1995) over breast cancer and their bodies. Mastectomy has, nevertheless, been found to have a significant impact on women's body image when compared to breast-conserving surgery (e.g., Lindwall & Begbom, 2009). It is also un-common for a woman who has undergone a mastectomy to forgo the use of an external breast prosthesis or reconstructive surgery. It is argued that this represents a cultural expectation to disguise mastectomy and normal-ize appearance in order to regain womanhood and avoid stigmatization. Consequently, perceptions of the body, cultural influences, and reinforced objectification of the body by health care professionals (whether intentional or not) may be particularly influential in women's decisions to undergo breast reconstruction.

Further explorations of women's decisions to undergo mastectomy purport that women perceive this surgical intervention to enhance their chances of survival by providing the potential for a complete cure (Temple et al., 2006), lower their risk of local recurrence, and reduce the need for radiotherapy (Collins et al., 2009). Striving for survival has been linked to women's desire to fulfill child-rearing responsibilities (e.g., Fang, Shu, & Fetzer, 2011) and provides some support for the "tend-and-befriend" model (Taylor et al., 2000), as some women appear to make treatment de-cisions with the aim of protecting offspring and reducing distress.

CONCLUSION

Models of treatment decision making seemingly fail to take into account the multifaceted and complex nature of the ways in which women make treatment decisions for breast cancer. The suggestion that treatment decisions should be based solely on evidence neglects the role of context and women's material and social circumstances. Yet, recent research indi-cates that a woman's emotions, relationships, daily life (e.g. Sinding & Wiernikowski, 2009), perceptions of the body, and the meaning of her breasts may influence the treatment decision-making process. Similarly, family and significant others have been identified as influential in breast cancer treatment decision making, with some women's partners taking a dominant role in this process (Illingworth, Forbat, Hubbard, & Kearney, 2010). Such discussion raises questions around the concept of shared deci-sion making and its measurement, as such medical encounters suggest a triad as opposed to a dyad interaction (Charles, Gafni, & Freeman, 2010). Furthermore, it should not be forgotten that there are limits on patient choices, and policy decisions may render some treatment options available or unavailable to some women. The research presented in this chapter ad-ditionally leads to the question of whether autonomy is a realistic and re-quired goal for all women and the extent to which the existing medical model promotes autonomy in the treatment decision-making process. However, given the long-term implications of women's experiences of treatment decision making, it would seem that whichever role women take in this process, be it active, shared, or passive, the level of involvement needs to be of the women's choosing in order to facilitate coping and long-term satisfaction with treatment decisions.

REFERENCES

Andersen, M., Bowen, D., Morea, J., Stein, K., & Baker, F. (2009). Involvement in decision-making and breast cancer survivor quality of life. *Health Psychology, 28*, 29–37.

Arndt, V., Sturmer, T., Stegmaier, C., Ziegler, H., Dhom, G., & Brenner, H. (2002). Patient delay and stage of diagnosis among breast cancer patients in Germany—a population based study. *British Journal of Cancer, 86*, 1034–1040.

Association of Breast Surgery at BASO. (2009). Surgical guidelines for the management of breast cancer. *European Journal of Surgical Oncology, 35*, S1–22.

Beaver, K., Bogg, J., & Luker, K. A. (1999). Decision-making role preferences and information needs: A comparison of colorectal and breast cancer. *Health Expectations, 2*, 266–276.

Beaver, K., Luker, K. A., Owens, R. G., Leinster, S. J., Degner, L. F., & Sloan, J. A. (1996). Treatment decision making in women newly diagnosed with breast cancer. *Cancer Nursing, 19*, 8–19.

Beisecker, A. E., Helmig, L., & Graham, D. (1994). Attitudes of oncologists, oncology nurses, and patients from a women's clinic regarding medical decision-making for older and younger breast cancer patients. *Gerontologist, 34*, 505–512.

Cassell, E. J. (1976). Disease as an "it": Concepts of disease revealed by patients' representations of symptoms. *Social Science and Medicine, 10*, 143–146.

Charles, C., Gafni, A., & Freeman, E. (2010). Implementing shared treatment decision making and treatment decision aids: A cautionary tale. *Psicooncologia, 7*, 243–255.

Charles, C. A., Whelan, T., Gafni, A., Willan, A., & Farrell, S. (2003). Shared treatment decision-making: What does it mean to physicians? *Journal of Clinical Oncology, 21*, 932–936.

Chen, X., & Siu, L. L. (2001). Impact of the media and the internet on oncology: Survey of cancer patients and oncologists in Canada. *Journal of Clinical Oncology, 19*, 4291–4297.

Collins, E. D., Moore, C. P., Clay, K. F., Kearing, S. A., O'Connor, A. M., Llewellyn-Thomas, H. A., Barth, R. J., & Sepucha, K. R. (2009). Can women with early-stage breast cancer make an informed decision for mastectomy? *Journal of Clinical Oncology, 27*, 519–525.

Cordeiro, P. G. (2008). Breast reconstruction after surgery for breast cancer. *New England Journal of Medicine, 359*, 1590–1601.

Coulter, A. (1997). Partnerships with patients: The pros and cons of shared clinical decision-making. *Journal of Health Services Research and Policy, 2*, 112–121.

Crouch, M., & McKenzie, H. (2000). Social realities of loss and suffering following mastectomy. *Health, 4*, 196–215.

Davey, H. M., Barratt, A. L., Davey, E., Butow, P. N., Redman, S., Houssami, N., & Salkeld, G. (2002). Medical tests: Women's reported and preferred decision-making roles and preferences for information on benefits, side-effects, and false results. *Health Expectations, 5,* 330–340.

Davies, N. J., Kinman, G., Thomas, R. J., & Bailey, T. (2008). Information satisfaction in breast and prostate cancer patients: Implications for quality of life. *Psycho-Oncology, 17,* 1048–1052.

Degner, L. F., Kristjanson, L. J., Bowman, D., Sloan, J. A., Carriere, K. C., O'Neil, J., Bilodeau, B., Watson, P., & Mueller, B. (1997). Information needs and decisional preferences in women with breast cancer. *JAMA, 277,* 1485–1492.

Donovan-Kicken, E., & Caughlin, J. P. (2011). Breast cancer patients' topic avoidance and psychological distress: The mediating role of coping. *Journal of Health Psychology, 16,* 596–606.

Drageset, S., Lindstrom, T. C., & Underlid, K. (2009). Coping with breast cancer: Between diagnosis and surgery. *Journal of Advanced Nursing, 66,* 149–158.

Edwards, I. R., & Hugman, B. (1997). The challenge of communicating risk-benefit information. *Drug Safety, 17,* 216–227.

Fagerlin, A., Lakhani, I., Lantz, P. M., Janz, N. K., Morrow, M., Schwartz, K., Deapen, D., Salem, B., Liu, L., & Katz, S. J. (2006). An informed decision? Breast cancer patients and their knowledge about treatment. *Patient Education and Counselling, 64,* 303–312.

Fallowfield, L. (1997). Offering choices of surgical treatment to women with breast cancer. *Patient Education & Counseling, 30,* 209–214.

Fang, S-Y., Shu, B-C., & Fetzer, S. J. (2011). Deliberating over mastectomy: Survival and social roles. *Cancer Nursing, 34,* E21–E28.

Festinger, L. (1957). *A theory of cognitive dissonance.* Evanston, IL: Row Peterson.

Fisher, B., Anderson, S., Bryant, J., Margolese, R. G., Deutsch, M., Fisher, E. R., Jeong, J-H., & Wolmark, N. (2002). Twenty-year follow-up of a randomized trial comparing total mastectomy, lumpectomy, and lumpectomy plus irradiation for the treatment of invasive breast cancer. *The New England Journal of Medicine, 347,* 1233–1241.

Fitzgal, F., & Gnant, M. (2006). Breast conservation: Evolution of surgical strategies. *Breast Journal, 2,* 1S165–173.

Frank, A. W. (1995). *The wounded storyteller.* Chicago: University of Chicago Press.

Gatellari, M., Butow, P. N., & Tattersall, M. (2001). Sharing decisions in cancer. *Social Science & Medicine, 52,* 1865–1878.

Hack, T., Degner, L., Watson, P., & Sinha, L. (2006). Do patients benefit from participating in medical decision making? Longitudinal follow-up of women with breast cancer. *Psycho-Oncology, 15,* 9–19.

Halkett, G. K. B., Arbon, P., Scutter, S. D., & Borg, M. (2007). The phenomenon of making decisions during the experience of early breast cancer. *European Journal of Cancer Care, 16,* 322–330.

Hibbard, J. H., & Peters, E. (2003). Supporting consumer health care decisions: Data presentation approaches that facilitate the use of information in choice. *Annual Review of Public Health, 24,* 413–433.

Illingworth, N., Forbat, L., Hubbard, G., & Kearney, N. (2010). The importance of relationships in the experience of cancer: A re-working of the policy ideal of the whole-systems approach. *European Journal of Oncology Nursing, 14,* 23–28.

Jadoulle, V., Rokbani, L., Ogez, D., Maccioni, J., Lories, G., Bruchon-Schweitzer, M., & Constant, A. (2006). Coping and adapting to breast cancer: A six month prospective study. *Bulletin du Cancer, 93,* E67–E72.

Karnilowicz, W. (2011). Identity and psychological ownership in chronic illness and disease state. *European Journal of Cancer Care, 20,* 276–282.

Katz, S. J., & Hawley, S. T. (2007). From policy to patients and back: Surgical treatment decision making for patients with breast cancer. *Health Affairs, 26,* 761–769.

Katz, S. J., Lantz, P. M., Janz, N. K., Fagerlin, A., Schwartz, K., Liu, L., Deapen, D., Salem, B., Lakhani, I., & Morrow, M. (2005). Patient involvement in surgery treatment decisions for breast cancer. *Journal of Clinical Oncology, 23,* 5526–5533.

Kreling, B., Fiqueiredo, M. I., Sheppard, V. L., & Mandelblatt, J. S. (2006). A qualitative study of factors affecting chemotherapy use in older women with breast cancer: Barriers, promoters, and implications for intervention. *Psycho-Oncology, 15,* 1065–1076.

Krupat, E., Irish, J. T., Kasten, L. E., Freund, K. M., Burns, R. B., Moskowitz, M. A., & McKinlay, J. B. (1999). Patient assertiveness and physician decision-making among older breast cancer patients. *Social Science & Medicine, 49,* 449–457.

Kukla, R. (2005). Conscientious autonomy—displacing decisions in healthcare. *Hastings Center Report, 35,* 34–44.

Kushner, R. (1975). *Why me? What every woman should know about breast cancer to save her life.* New York: Henry Holt & Company.

Lam, W., Fielding, R., Chan, M., Chow, L., & Ho, E. (2003). Participation and satisfaction with surgical treatment decision-making in breast cancer among Chinese women. *Breast Cancer Research & Treatment, 80,* 171–180.

Langellier, K .M., & Sullivan, C. F. (1998). Breast talk in breast cancer narratives. *Qualitative Health Research, 8,* 76–94.

Lantz, P. M., Janz, M. K., Fagerlin, A., Schwartz, K., Liu, L., Lakhani, I., Salem, B., & Katz, S. J. (2005). Satisfaction with surgery outcomes and the decision process in a population based sample of women with breast cancer. *Health Service Research, 40,* 745–768.

Lee, S. Y., & Hawkins, R. (2010). Why do patients seek an alternative channel? The effects of unmet needs on patients' health-related internet use. *Journal of Health Communication, 15,* 152–166.

Lerner, B. H. (2001). *The breast cancer wars: Hope, fear, and the pursuit of a cure in twentieth-century America.* New York: Oxford University Press.

Lindwall, L., & Begbom, I. (2009). The altered body after breast cancer surgery. *International Journal of Qualitative Studies on Health and Well-Being, 4,* 1748–2631.

Luce, M. L. (2005). Decision making as coping. *Health Psychology, 24,* S23–S28.

MacLachlan, M. (2004). *Embodiment: Clinical, critical, and cultural perspectives on health and illness.* Maidenhead: Open University Press.

Makoul, G., & Clayman, M. L. (2006). An integrative model of shared decision-making in medical encounters. *Patient Education & Counselling, 60,* 301–312.

McCann, L., Illingworth, N., Wengström, Y., Hubbard, G., & Kearney, N. (2010). Transitional experiences of women with breast cancer within the first year following diagnosis. *Journal of Clinical Nursing, 19,* 1969–1976.

Mendick, N., Young, B., Holcombe, C., & Salmon, P. (2010). The ethics and responsibility of ownership in decision-making about treatment for breast cancer: Triangulation of consultation with patient and surgeon perspectives. *Social Science & Medicine, 70,* 1904–1911.

Mesters, I., van den Borne, B., De Boer, M., & Pruyn, J. (2001). Measuring information needs among cancer patients. *Patient Education & Counseling, 43,* 255–264.

Miller, S. M. (1995). Monitoring versus blunting styles of coping with cancer influence the information patients want and need about their disease. *Cancer, 76,* 167–177.

Moch, D. S. (1995). *Breast cancer: Twenty women's stories.* New York: NLN.

Mulcahy, C. M., Parry, D. C., & Glover, T. D. (2010). The "patient patient": The trauma of waiting and the power of resistance for people living with cancer. *Qualitative Health Research, 20,* 1062–1075.

National Institute for Health and Clinical Excellence (NICE). (2009). Early and locally advanced breast cancer: Diagnosis and treatment. *Clinical Guidelines, 80,* London: NICE.

National Institute for Health and Clinical Excellence (NICE). (2012). *Diagnostics consultation document. Gene expression profiling and expanded immunohisto-chemistry tests to guide the use of adjuvant chemotherapy in breast cancer management: MammaPrint, Oncotype DX, IHC4, and Mammostrat.* London: NICE.

O'Brien, M. A., Whelan, T. J., Villasis-Keever, M. A., Gafni, A., Charles, C., Roberts, R., Schiff, S., & Cai, W. (2009). Are cancer-related decision-aids effective? A systematic review and meta-analysis. *Journal of Clinical Oncology, 27,* 974–985.

O'Leary, K. A., Estabrooks, C. A., Olsen, K., & Cumming, C. (2007). Information acquisition for women facing surgical treatment for breast cancer: Influencing factors and selected outcomes. *Patient Education & Counselling, 69,* 5–19.

O'Mahony, M., & Hegarty, J. (2009). Factors influencing women in seeking help from a health care professional on self discovery of a breast symptom, in an Irish context. *Journal of Clinical Nursing, 18,* 2020–2029.

Payne, S., Large, S., Jarrett, N., & Turner, P. (2000). Written information given to patients and families by palliative care units: A national survey. *The Lancet, 355,* 1792.

Peters, E., Lipkus, I., & Diefenbach, M.A. (2006). The functions of affect in health communications and in the construction of health preferences. *Journal of Communication, 56,* S140–162.

Polacek, G. N. L., Ramos, M. C., & Ferrer, R. L. (2007). Breast cancer disparities and decision making among U.S. women. *Patient Education and Counselling, 65,* 158–165.

Radley, A. (1996). Displays and fragments: Embodiment and the configuration of social worlds. *Theory Psychology, 6,* 559–576.

Ravdin, P. M., Siminoff, L. A., Davis, G. J., Mercer, M. B., Hewlett, J., Gersen, N., & Parker, H. L. (2001). Computer program to assist in making decisions about adjuvant therapy for women with early breast cancer. *Journal of Clinical Oncology, 15,* 980–991.

Rees, C. E., & Bath, P. A. (2000). Information-seeking behaviours of women with breast cancer. *Oncologic Nursing Forum, 28,* 899–907.

Richards, M. A., Westcombe, A. M., Love, S. B., Littlejohns, P., & Ramirez, A. J. (1999). Influence of delay in survival of patients with breast cancer: A systematic review. *The Lancet, 353,* 1119–1126.

Riessman, C. (1983). Women and medicalisation: A new perspective. In Weitz, R. (Ed.), *The politics of women's bodies: Sexuality, appearance & behaviour* (pp. 46–63). Oxford: Oxford University Press.

Ruzek, S. B. (1978). *The women's health movement: Feminist alternatives to medical control.* New York: Praeger.

Sabo, B., St-Jacques, N., & Rayson, D. (2007). The decision-making experience among women diagnosed with stage I and II breast cancer. *Breast Cancer Research and Treatment, 102,* 51–59.

Saika, K., & Sobou, T. (2011). Time trends in breast cancer screening rates in the OECD countries. *Japanese Journal of Clinical Oncology, 41,* 591–592.

Seale, C. (2005). Portrayals of treatment decision-making on popular breast and prostate cancer web sites. *European Journal of Cancer Care, 14,* 171–174.

Shaha, M., Cox, C. L., Talman, K., & Kelly, D. (2008). Uncertainty in breast, prostate, and colorectal cancer: Implications for supportive care. *Journal of Nursing Scholarship, 40,* 60.

Sharf, B. F., & Vanderford, M. L. (2003). Illness narratives and the social construction of health. In Thompson, T. L., Dorsey, A., & Mill, K. (Eds.), *Handbook of health communication* (pp. 9–34). Mahwah, NJ: Lawrence Erlbaum.

Sinding, C., Hudak, P., Wiernikowski, J., Aronson, J., Miller, P., Gould, J., & Fitzpatrick-Lewis, D. (2010). "I like to be an informed person but . . .": Negotiating treatment decisions in cancer care. *Social Science & Medicine, 71,* 1094–1101.

Sinding, C., & Wiernikowski, J. (2009). Treatment decision-making and its discontents. *Social Work in Healthcare, 48,* 614–634.

Sivell, S., Edwards, A., Manstead, A. S. R., Reed, M. W. R., Caldon, L., Collins, K., Clements, A., & Elwyn, G. (2012). Increasing readiness to decide and strengthening behavioural intentions: Evaluating the impact of a web-based decision-aid for breast cancer treatment options. *Patient Education & Counselling, 88,* 209–217.

Slovic, P., Peters, E., Finucane, M. L., & MacGregor, D. G. (2005). Affect, risk, and decision-making. *Health Psychology, 24,* S35–40.

Street, R. L. (2003). Communication in medical encounters: An ecological perspective. In Thompson, T. L., Dorsey, A., & Mill, K. (Eds.), *Handbook of health communication* (pp. 63–89). Mahwah, NJ: Lawrence Erlbaum.

Swainston, K., Campbell, C., van Wersch, A., & Durning, P. (2012). Treatment decision-making in breast cancer: A longitudinal exploration of women's experiences. *British Journal of Health Psychology, 17,* 155–170.

Taylor, S. E., Klein, L. C., Lewis, B. P., Gruenewald, T. L., Gurung, R. A., & Updegraff, J. A. (2000). Biobehavioural responses to stress in females: Tend-and-befriend not fight-or-flight. *Psychological Review, 107,* 411–429.

Temple, W. J., Russell, M. L., Parsons, L. L., Huber, S. M., Jones, C. A., Bankes, J., & Eliasziw, M. (2006). Conservation surgery for breast cancer as the preferred choice: A prospective analysis. *Journal of Clinical Oncology, 24,* 3367–3373.

Thomas-MacLean, R. (2004). Memories of treatment: The immediacy of breast cancer. *Qualitative Health Research, 14,* 628–643.

Ubel, P. A. (2002). Is information always a good thing? Helping patients make "good" decisions. *Medical Care, 40,* V39–44.

Vodermaier, A., Caspari, C., Wang, L., Koehm, J., Ditsch, N., & Untch, M. (2011). How and for whom are decision-aids effective? Long-term psychological outcome of a randomised controlled trial in women with newly diagnosed breast cancer. *Health Psychology, 30,* 12–19.

Vogel, B. A., Helmes, A. W., & Hasenburg, A. (2008). Concordance between patients' desired and actual decision-making roles in breast cancer care. *Psycho-Oncology, 17,* 182–189.

Waljee, J. F., Rogers, M. A., & Alderman, A. K. (2007). Decision aids for breast cancer: Do they influence choice for surgery and knowledge of treatment options? *Journal of Clinical Oncology, 25,* 1067–1073.

Wang, W. V., Tan, S. M., Chow, W. L. (2011). The impact of mammographic breast cancer screening in Singapore: Comparison between screen-detected and symptomatic women. *Asian Pacific Journal of Cancer Prevention, 12,* 2735–2740.

Wilmoth, M. C., Coleman, E. A., Smith, S. C., & Davis, C. (2004). Fatigue, weight gain, and altered sexuality in patients with breast cancer: Exploration of a symptom cluster. *Oncology Nursing Forum, 31,* 1069–1075.

Young, I. M. (1992). Breasted experience: The look and the feeling. In Leder, D. (Ed.), *The body in medical thought and practice* (pp. 215–230). Dordrecht, Netherlands: Kluwer Academic Publishers.

Chapter 13

Distress and Suffering at the End of Life

Alicia Krikorian

INTRODUCTION

It is well known that at the end of life (EoL), in the context of a deterio-
rating illness, patients may encounter many stressors, uncontrolled
symptoms, and problems of diverse nature (Abraham, Kutner, & Beaty,
2006; Block, 2006; Delgado-Guay, Parsons, Li, Palmer, & Bruera, 2009;
Krikorian & Limonero, 2012; Oi-Ling, Man-Wah, & Kam-Hung, 2005;
Portenoy et al., 1994). Thus, it is not uncommon for them to frequently
feel uneasiness, distress, and even suffering (Block, 2006; Krikorian,
Limonero, & Maté, 2011; Wilson et al., 2007).

Distress has been defined as a "unique discomforting emotional response experienced by an individual in response to a specific stressor or
demand" (Rhodes & Watson, 1987). In the cancer context it is considered
a "multifactorial unpleasant emotional experience of a psychological
(cognitive, behavioral, emotional), social and/or spiritual nature that
may interfere with the ability to effectively cope with cancer, its physical
symptoms and its treatments" (Kelly, McClement & Chochinov, 2006;

NCCN, 2010). Rather than a single physical or emotional symptom, distress can be multifactorial in etiology and may represent physical, social, and emotional components (Vitek, Rosenzweig, & Stollings, 2007). It is a common experience in illness trajectories, particularly in cancer and palliative care (PC) contexts (Potash & Breitbart, 2002). Nearly all patients facing EoL may present feelings of grief, sadness, despair, fear, anxiety, loss, and loneliness (Block, 2006). In patients in a preterminal phase of a chronic illness, distress may become even more disabling than physical symptoms such as pain (Sirois, 2012). It may occur as a normal emotional response to stressors, lead to adjustment problems or to suffering, or constitute a mental health problem such as a depressive or anxiety disorder; therefore, it should be understood as a continuum ranging from normal negative feelings to incapacitating problems (Holland et al., 2013; Vitek et al., 2007).

Meanwhile, suffering is a multidimensional and dynamic experience of severe stress associated with significant threat and with insufficient regulatory processes that lead to exhaustion (Krikorian & Limonero, 2012). It is comprehensive and has physical, psychological, sociocultural, and spiritual/existential correlates (Cassell, 1991) that can manifest in a variety of behaviors or symptoms such as distress, uncontrolled physical symptoms, hopelessness, and a desire to hasten death, among many others (Chochinov, 2006; Krikorian et al., 2011). It can frequently occur at EoL (Abraham, Kutner, & Beaty, 2006; Baines & Norlander, 2000; Krikorian et al., 2011; Wilson et al., 2007).

ASSOCIATED FACTORS AND PREVALENCE

Distress is a prevalent problem during the illness trajectory. In cancer it can present from diagnosis to post-treatment phases in as much as one-third of the population, needing targeted psychosocial interventions when it becomes disabling (Holland et al., 2013; NCCN, 2010; Vachon, 2006).

Being a woman, of young age or older than 70 years old; being hospitalized; having some particular ethnic backgrounds or low income or education level; having a poor performance status or prognosis; and having practical, family, emotional, or physical problems have been found to constitute risk factors for cancer-related distress (Vachon, 2006).

Significant distress may impact quality of life (QoL) and is associated with adherence to treatment problems and low satisfaction with care. It may also reduce survival in cancer patients (Vachon, 2006). Therefore, its early detection and management become critical for the well-being and QoL of PC patients (Sloan et al., 2002).

Similarly, the experience of suffering and its severity fluctuate according to the individual's illness and individual characteristics (Wittmann et al., 2009). As stated, suffering is associated with problems in the physical, psychological, social, and spiritual dimensions (Cassell, 1991). Pain and uncontrolled physical symptoms may amplify or signal suffering, while preexisting and current psychiatric disorders, problems in the family dynamics, diminished social support, inadequate coping resources, personal vulnerabilities, and existential and spiritual concerns have been associated with greater suffering (Block, 2006; Krikorian et al., 2011; Wilson et al., 2007).

While normal responses of distress are practically universal at EoL both for the patient and the family (Block, 2006), suffering may present in as many as 90 percent of terminally ill patients (Baines & Norlander, 2000), and about half of them manifest moderate to severe levels of suffering (Benedict, 1989; Kuuppelomäki & Lauri, 1998). However, not all patients manifest suffering (Wilson et al., 2007).

Prevalence rates for adjustment and affective disorders in EoL are quite variable, depending on the population under study, assessment and methodological strategies, and treatment-related variables (such as availability of PC and mental health support) (Block, 2006; Wilson et al., 2007). Between 35 percent and 50 percent of patients in PC fulfill criteria for the diagnosis of a depressive or anxiety disorder, and about 25 percent for adjustment disorders (Kelly et al., 2006; Thekkumpurath, Venkateswaran, Kumar, & Bennett, 2008; Stefanek, Derogatis, & Shaw, 1987).

Depression is common in PC patients, and its diagnosis is a complex task, leading to frequent underrecognition in clinical practice. Prevalence estimates vary from 3 percent to 45 percent, indicating that it is not reliably detected, a problem that becomes critical given that diagnosis and treatment should be promptly made due to the short life expectancy of patients and their conditions of frailty (Rayner et al., 2009). Differential diagnosis is particularly difficult due to overlap with common physical symptoms, such as fatigue, insomnia, asthenia, and poor appetite, among others (Martínez, Barreto, & Toledo, 2001).

Establishing differences between normal sadness, grief reactions, and depression is of great importance. In Table 13.1, differences between normal sadness and depression are described. Depressive disorders are characterized by symptoms that are disproportionate to the context, and accepted diagnostic criteria should be followed. Diagnostic approaches such as the "inclusive" (using Research Diagnostic Criteria) and "substitutive" (using Endicott criteria) are useful, and evidence has shown that they are equally appropriate (Chochinov, Wilson, Enns, & Lander, 1994; Rayner et al., 2009). Table 13.2 shows the somatic criteria and the proposed substituting criteria (Endicott, 1983).

An increased risk of suicide can be found for some chronic life-threatening illnesses, such as AIDS, advanced cancer, and neurological progressive diseases (Kleespies, Hughes, & Gallacher, 2000). Depression

Table 13.1 Differences between normal sadness and depression

Sadness	Depression
Able to feel intimately connected with others	Feels isolated and alone
Feeling that someday this will end	Feeling of permanence
Able to enjoy happy memories and events	Regretful, rumination on "irredeemable" mistakes, feelings of guilt
Sense of self-worth is preserved	Extreme self-depreciation/ self-loathing
Variable over time (comes and goes)	Constant and unremitting
Maintains hope in the future	No hope/interest in the future
Able to enjoy and feel pleasure	Loss of interest and diminished capacity to enjoy
Maintains will to live	Suicidal thoughts/behavior, may have desire to hasten death

Source: Adapted from Rayner et al. (2011).

Table 13.2 Endicott criteria for diagnosis of depression in advanced cancer

Physical/somatic symptoms	Replaced by psychological symptoms
1. Change in appetite/weight	1. Tearfulness, depressed appearance
2. Sleep disturbance	2. Social withdrawal, decreased talkativeness
3. Fatigue, loss of energy	3. Brooding, self-pity, pessimism
4. Diminished ability to think or concentrate	4. Lack of reactivity, blunting

Source: Endicott, (1983).

and uncontrolled symptoms are associated with suicide and desire to die in the terminally ill (O'Mahony et al., 2005). The desire for hastened death may manifest as a patient's request for early cessation of active disease treatments, a transient or sustained expression of the desire for more rapid disease progression, or an active search for professional assistance in death-hastening activities (O'Mahony et al., 2005).

Anxiety and fear may also present as normal emotional reactions or constitute mental disorders. While low levels of anxiety can motivate the patient toward coping and adaptation, moderate and high levels can be problematic and disabling. Anxiety disorders may occur in between 15 percent and 28 percent of patients (Kerrihard, Breitbart, Dent, & Strout, 1999). Anxiety in PC may result from preexisting anxiety disorders, substance abuse, medications, delirium, or undertreated symptoms, especially pain (Block, 2006). Adequate and timely detection and management of anxiety responses are also relevant, given that they may intensify symptoms such as pain, vomiting, restlessness, sleep disturbances, disorganized activity, or death anxiety (Barreto & Bayés, 1990; Bayés & Limonero, 1999; Martínez et al., 2001) and contribute to overall suffering (Krikorian et al., 2011). Mild to moderate anxiety can be treated effectively with supportive psychotherapeutic interventions, while severe symptoms usually require medication (Breitbart & Jacobsen, 1996).

Anxious patients may present challenges to the patient-team relationship and communication. They often have difficulty taking in information about the illness and treatment; tend to ask the same questions repeatedly; overreact to information given, treatments, and symptoms; behave impulsively or inconsistently; and either ask for detailed information or avoid it for fear of their own emotions (Block, 2006). Consequently, an optimal and early recognition and management of anxiety may prevent relationship- and treatment-related difficulties and help the patient better cope with his/her circumstances.

About half of advanced cancer patients experiencing suffering also meet criteria for an anxiety or depressive disorder, while patients with mental disorders experience more severe suffering, according to the results of a study conducted by Wilson et al. (2007). Consequently, adequate detection and treatment of pathologic emotional responses is central to prevention and relief of suffering.

Another syndrome that may account for distress and suffering in PC is the rather recently described Demoralization Syndrome. It was proposed by Kissane and colleages (2004) and describes a disorder of meaning and hope. The proposed diagnostic criteria for the Demoralization Syndrome can be found in Table 13.3. Studies have evidenced how it differentiates from related problems such as depression and grief (Clarke & Kissane, 2002; Kissane et al., 2004; Lloyd-Williams, Reeve, & Kissane, 2008).

Table 13.3 Proposed diagnostic criteria for Demoralization Syndrome

Complaints of life's meaninglessness, pointlessness, or loss of purpose

Sense of pessimism, helplessness, and entrapment in the predicament

Loss of hope for improvement or recovery

Associated isolation, alienation, or lack of support

Potential to develop suicidal thoughts and plans

Phenomena persisting over more than two weeks

DISTRESS, THE SIXTH VITAL SIGN

Given the frequency and consequences of distress and suffering on the global well-being and health of patients, their screening and management have become of great importance. A growing awareness about the contribution of psychosocial and spiritual factors to illness, particularly in chronic life-threatening illnesses, has emerged. The focus on a biomedical approach has been shifting to a biopsychosocial and spiritual one (Sulmasy, 2002). Empirical evidence has demonstrated how psychosocial and spiritual variables contribute to illness, as well as the benefits of psychosocial interventions to patients, families, and caregivers (Bultz & Carlson, 2006; Howell & Olsen, 2011).

However, early detection and treatment are still lacking, and distress continues to be underrecognized (Howell & Olsen, 2011; Fallowfield, Ratcliffe, Jenkins, & Saul, 2001; Adler & Page, 2008). Consequently, an ongoing screening process of distress is needed throughout the illness trajectory, in particular one that is time effective and easy to perform for health practitioners in regular consultations with patients.

In 2001 the Canadian Strategy for Cancer Control (CSCC) decided to recognize emotional distress as a core indicator of a patient's health and well-being. Later, the Canadian Partnership Against Cancer (2009) and the NCCN (2010) endorsed distress as the "sixth vital sign," both nationally and internationally. It is intended to more closely monitor emotional distress in cancer care in order to ensure early identification of patients in need of a more detailed assessment process and targeted psychosocial interventions.

Some studies have been conducted in order to identify characteristics of patients with distress and associated problems in the context of "distress, the sixth vital sign" initiative. According to the results obtained by Giese-Davis et al. (2012), psychosocial problems were reported more often than practical ones, and younger single patients showed more risk for practical problems, while young women indicated more psychosocial problems; being married was found to be a buffering factor for distress. Meanwhile, Carlson, Waller, Groff, Zhong, & Bultz (2012) found that, after initial screening in 3,133 patients, distress, anxiety, depression, pain, and fatigue tended to decrease over time. Also, triage (personalized or computerized) and high symptom burden predicted more access to services and greater decrease of distress and other emotional responses. Similarly, Waller, Groff, Hagen, Bultz, & Carlson (2012) found that multiple and concurrent symptoms and psychosocial problems were more common in cancer patients attending a pain clinic than were controls. Altogether, these results point out the relevance of regular distress screening.

Assessment

Many distress screening instruments are currently available in cancer and PC contexts (Kelly et al., 2006; Mitchell, 2010; Thekkumpurath et al., 2008). In time, they have become more sophisticated, faster, and easier to use.

One-single-item measures are of special interest in the PC context, due to the patient's fragility. Chochinov, Wilson, Enns, & Lander (1997) adapted a single question from structured interviews: "Are you depressed?" It has been found to have a sensitivity ranging from 100 percent to 54 percent, and a specificity ranging from 100 percent to 67 percent to detect depressive mood (Thekkumpurath et al., 2008).

Also, the Visual Analog Scale (VAS) for mood screening (0= "worst possible mood" to 10= "best possible mood") has been examined. It was concluded that its performance was lower than other instruments, showing a sensitivity of 72 percent and a specificity of 50 percent (Chochinov et al., 1997).

The distress thermometer is one of the more widely accepted tools, valid and used in multiple populations (Snowden et al., 2011). It was developed by a panel of experts in collaboration with the NCCN. It is a simple pencil and paper measure, consisting of a 0-to-10 scale ("No Distress" to "Extreme Distress"). It allows for the identification of related problems, including practical, familial, emotional, and physical. The specificity and sensitivity of the single-item distress thermometer has been largely demonstrated (Kelly et al., 2006). Guidelines to manage each aspect of distress, according to its severity, are also provided by the NCCN (2010).

In order to screen for spiritual distress at EoL, a single-item measure consisting of a five-point Likert scale, using the question "Are you at peace?," was developed. It provides a nonthreatening gateway to elicit patient and family concerns in PC and EoL and was found to strongly correlate with emotional and spiritual well-being (Steinhauser et al., 2006).

Also, multidimensional screening instruments are available. One of the most widely used is the Hospital Anxiety and Depression Scale (HADS). It is a 14-item scale, with subscales for depression and anxiety, developed with focus on core depressive symptoms such as anhedonia (Zigmond & Snaith, 1983). Its performance has been found to be superior to other general psychological symptom measures in PC, although some concerns regarding its sensitivity and specificity in the PC context exist (Kelly et al., 2006; Lloyd-Williams & Riddleston, 2002; Thekkumpurath et al., 2008).

Recently, a group of experts collaborating with the Spanish Palliative Care Society (SECPAL) developed an instrument to screen for emotional distress in palliative and EoL care. The Detection of Emotional Distress scale (DED) is a theory-driven instrument that includes three questions directed to the patient that assess mood state and perceived coping of the situation and concerns, and record external signs of emotional distress identified by the clinician (Maté et al., 2009). DED was developed for use in Spanish and has demonstrated adequate reliability and convergent validity, as well as sensitivity and specificity (Limonero et al., 2012). An English version is now under development.

Other screening instruments for depression and anxiety commonly used are the Centre for Epidemiologic Studies Depression Scale (CES-D), the Beck Depression Inventory-II (BDI-II), and the Profile of Mood States (POMS). Some other more general instruments including items on distress, depression, and/or anxiety are the Palliative Care Outcome Scale (POS), the Edmonton Symptom Assessment Schedule (ESAS), the Structured Interview Assessment of Symptoms and Concerns in Palliative Care (SISC), and such QoL instruments as the FACIT, EORTC, and FACT questionnaires, along with many others (Kelly et al., 2006; Mitchell, 2010; Thekkumpurath et al., 2008).

Suffering assessment is less common and seems more complex. However, efforts to develop instruments adapted for the needs of PC and EoL patients have been made. A recent review of available instruments for suffering assessment was performed by Krikorian and Limonero (2012). Instruments such as the Pictorial Representation of Illness and Self Measure (PRISM) and SISC showed the strongest psychometric qualities and are coherent with current definitions of suffering.

The PRISM task consists of an A4-size whiteboard with a fixed yellow disk in the bottom right-hand corner (representing the self) and a mobile red disk (representing the illness). Patients are asked to imagine that the board represents their current life and are asked to place the red disk on the board to represent the place of the illness in their current life (Büchi, Sensky, Sharpe, & Timberlake, 1998). The distance between the disks' centers, referred to as Self–Illness Separation (SIS), is a valid and reliable quantitative measure of suffering (Krikorian & Limonero, 2012). It is a practical tool, easy to use and understand, that allows for a nondirective screening of suffering, even in patients with communication difficulties.

The SISC is a structured interview designed to assess common problems and concerns in PC. It is a 13-item instrument used to assess the presence and severity of different symptoms, including anxiety, depression, and suffering. It is reliable, and concurrent validity and sensitivity to individual differences were found to be adequate (Wilson et al., 2007). It allows for a comprehensive assessment in the context of an interview.

Screening for distress in the terminally ill should aim at identifying patients at risk for suffering and for mental health problems; it is intended for conducting more detailed assessment processes in at-risk patients that, in turn, will allow designing appropriate interventions. Some aspects that should be taken into account in the assessment process include:

The illness and its consequences—level of information and awareness; level of functioning and impact on important roles or the patient's personal identity; uncontrolled symptoms; difficulty with adherence to treatment recommendations.

Frequency and severity of negative emotions, as well as their impact on the patient's and caregiver's well-being; uncertainty and worries about the future.

Coping style and strategies used to manage issues in problematic areas; feelings of helplessness or inability to cope; exhaustion of coping resources.

Behaviors that signal difficulty processing emotions or current circumstances; behaviors not coherent with verbal communication; hostility and aggressive reactions toward family or health caregivers; tendency to continually ask the same questions or recall past stressful events; excessive or reduced emotional reactivity.

Spiritual issues—purpose and meaning in life; significance given to the illness process as a whole; unsolved issues; problems related to connection to significant ones and to higher powers that patients believe in; religious issues and related needs.

Persistence of practical problems that affect the patient or the family; lack of social or financial resources to effectively cope with practical problems.

Problems related to the family or the proximate social context.

Assessment should include examination of symptoms or signs that could lead to a diagnosis according to validated diagnostic criteria of disorders, such as adjustment, depression, and anxiety disorders (e.g., APA, 1994; or WHO, 1992); attention should be paid to comorbidities with personality disorders, which may be indicative of more pronounced emotional reactions or behavioral disorganization. Also, differential diagnosis with delirium, dementia, or other neuropsychiatric conditions; uncontrolled pain; cerebral metastases; and adverse drug reactions should be made (Rayner, Price, Hotopf, & Higginson, 2011).

Some somatic symptoms, such as pain and fatigue, are commonly associated with depression and anxiety. They may be due to physical disease or treatment, which should be taken into account when making a diagnosis of psychiatric disorders in PC. Finally, cultural variations (ethnic, regional, age-related) may occur in the presentation of emotional reactions, which should be also taken into consideration in the assessment process (Rayner et al., 2009; Rayner et al., 2011).

Management

Interventions should be tailored according to the severity and problems associated with distress and suffering. The NCCN distress guidelines (2010) offer a series of standards of care that include:

A regular screening process at different stages of the illness process to monitor levels of severity and identification of the nature of distress.

Recommendations oriented to educational programs for professionals in the health team, suggested levels of certification, and continued quality improvement processes.

Communication strategies within the health team for adequate referral to psychosocial centers within the institution or community.

An overview of evaluation and treatment is also suggested, according to the detected needs in the patient and family.

When mild distress is identified, referral to the oncology team is advised in order to perform a general psychosocial support, which may include counseling and problem-solving strategies.

If moderate to severe distress is observed, problem areas should be identified. If distress is directly related to unrelieved physical symptoms, then the use of specific guidelines for symptom control and supportive care is advised. If the primary health care team detects problems of a practical, psychological, social, or spiritual nature, then referral to corresponding specialized services is recommended (e.g., mental health team, social work, chaplaincy services). Specific guidelines for each problem area are also available, as well as for specific psychological and psychiatric syndromes and disorders like dementia, adjustment disorders, depression, and anxiety.

In every case, follow-up and communication with the primary health team and family/caregivers is suggested.

Other guidelines for distress management and psychosocial care in the PC context are available. The National Institute for Health and Clinical Excellence (NICE) was commissioned by the Department of Health of the United Kingdom to develop a guide for improving palliative and supportive care in adult cancer patients (2004). This manual was created as guidance for cancer services and includes, among other things, recommendations for quality support services in psychology, social work, and spiritual support. A four-level model for psychological assessment and intervention is described.

Levels I and II include interventions for mild distress that can be performed by health and social care professionals. Specific interventions include compassionate communication and general psychosocial support, as well as basic psychological techniques such as problem solving.

Level III (for moderate distress) includes interventions by accredited and trained professionals, such as counseling and more complex psychological interventions (e.g., anxiety management).

Table 13.4 Psychotherapeutic interventions for the PC context

Intervention	Reference
Dignity therapy	Chochinov et al., 2005
Narrative therapy	Viederman, 1983; Noble & Jones, 2005
Meaning-centered group psychotherapy	Breitbart et al., 2010
Meaning-centered individual psychotherapy	Breitbart et al., 2012
Counseling strategies	Undurraga, González, & Calderón, 2006
Interpersonal psychotherapy	Weissman, Markowitz, & Klerman, 2000
Meaning Making Intervention (MMI)	Lee, Cohen, Edgar, Laizner, & Gagnon, 2006
Managing Cancer and Living Meaningfully (CALM)	Nissim et al., 2012

Level IV should be performed by mental health practitioners in order to manage severe distress and mental disorders, using specialized psychological and psychiatric interventions such as psychotherapy.

Other intervention programs and psychotherapeutic models that can be useful in the PC and EoL context are mentioned in Table 13.4.

In the case of suffering, no standardized guidelines exist to date. However, some recommendations for suffering relief are available (Krikorian & Limonero, 2012). Patients in suffering and their families require a comprehensive and personalized approach to care, and assessment should include:

Biographical aspects
Physical and biomedical factors
Cultural, social, and familial environment factors
wPsychological factors
Spiritual factors
Time and illness-progression factors

Threats perceived by a patient and his or her family members in any dimension—physical, psychological, social, or spiritual—should be considered equally important. The particular needs manifested both by the patient and his/her family should be continually reassessed and taken into account. Threats should be rapidly identified and responded to, allowing patients and families to take a more active role in the care process, which in turn will provide them with a greater sense of control. Interdisciplinary care, rather than multidisciplinary care, may be more appropriate to suffering relief, given its complexity and the need to simultaneously manage matters in multiple dimensions (Krikorian & Limonero, 2012).

CONCLUSION

Distress and suffering at EoL are common experiences that should receive the proper attention given their pervasive consequences on well-being and QoL. Screening processes should be included in every service or institution dealing with life-threatening and life-limiting conditions. Also, standards of care and assessment and management guidelines should be implemented in order to accomplish early and effective treatments.

REFERENCES

Abraham, A., Kutner, J. S., & Beaty, B. (2006). Suffering at the end of life in the setting of low physical symptom distress. *Journal of Palliative Medicine, 9,* 658–665.

Adler, N. E., & Page, A. E. K. (Eds.). (2008). *Cancer care for the whole patient: Meeting psychosocial health needs.* Washington, DC: National Academies Press.

APA. (1994). Diagnostic and statistical manual of mental disorders (DSM-IV). 4th ed. Washington, DC: American Psychiatric Association.

Baines, B. K., & Norlander, L. (2000). The relationship of pain and suffering in a hospice population. *American Journal of Hospice and Palliative Care, 17,* 319–326.

Barreto, M. P., & Bayés, R. (1990). El psicólogo ante el enfermo en situación terminal. *Anales de psicología, 6,* 169–180.

Bayés, R., & Limonero, J. T. (1999). Aspectos emocionales del proceso de morir. In Fernández, E.G., & Palmero, F. (Eds.), *Emociones y salud* (pp. 265–278). Barcelona: Ariel.

Benedict, S. (1989). The suffering associated with lung cancer. *Cancer Nursing, 12,* 34–40.

Block, S. D. (2006). Psychological issues in end-of-life care. *Journal of Palliative Medicine, 9,* 751–772.

Breitbart, W., & Jacobsen, P. B. (1996). Psychiatric symptom management in terminal care. *Clinical Geriatric Medicine, 12,* 329–347.

Breitbart, W., Poppito, S., Rosenfeld, B., Vickers, A. J., Li, Y., Abbey, J., et al. (2012). Pilot randomized controlled trial of individual meaning-centered psychotherapy for patients with advanced cancer. *Journal of Clinical Oncology, 30,* 1304–1309. doi: 10.1200/JCO.2011.36.2517.

Breitbart, W., Rosenfeld, B., Gibson, C., Pessin, H., Poppito, S., Nelson, C., et al. (2010). Meaning-centered group psychotherapy for patients with advanced cancer: A pilot randomized controlled trial. *Psycho-Oncology, 19,* 21–28. doi: 10.1002/pon.1556.

Büchi, S., Sensky, T., Sharpe, L., & Timberlake, N. (1998). Graphic representation of illness: A novel method of measuring patients' perceptions of the impact of illness. *Psychotherapy and Psychosomatics, 67,* 222–225.

Bultz, B. D., & Carlson, L. E. (2006). Emotional distress: The sixth vital sign: Future directions in cancer care. *Psycho-Oncology, 15,* 93–95.

Canadian Partnership Against Cancer (CPAC), Cancer Action Journey Group. (2009). *Guide to implementing screening for distress, the 6th vital sign: Moving towards person-centered care. Part A. Background, recommendations and implementation.* Toronto, ON: CPAC.

Canadian Strategy for Cancer Control. (2001). *Canadian strategy for cancer control. Draft synthesis report.* Ottawa, ON.

Carlson, L. E., Waller, A., Groff, S. L., Zhong, L., & Bultz, B. D. (2012). Online screening for distress, the 6th vital sign, in newly diagnosed oncology outpatients: Randomised controlled trial of computerised vs personalised triage. *British Journal of Cancer, 107,* 617–625. doi: 10.1038/bjc.2012.309.

Cassell, E. J. (1991). Recognizing suffering. *Hastings Center Reports, 21,* 24–31.

Chochinov, H. M. (2006). Dying, dignity, and new horizons in palliative end-of-life care. *CA: A Cancer Journal for Clinicians, 56,* 84–103.

Chochinov, H. M., Hack, T., Hassard, T., Kristjanson, L. J., McClement, S., & Harlos, M. (2005). Dignity therapy: A novel psychotherapeutic intervention for patients near the end of life. *Journal of Clinical Oncology, 23,* 5520–5525.

Chochinov, H. M., Wilson, K. G., Enns, M., & Lander, S. (1994). Prevalence of depression in the terminally ill: Effects of diagnostic criteria and symptom threshold judgments. *American Journal of Psychiatry, 151,* 537–540.

Chochinov, H. M., Wilson, K. G., Enns, M., & Lander, S. (1997). "Are you depressed?" Screening for depression in the terminally ill. *American Journal of Psychiatry, 154,* 674–676.

Clarke, D. M., & Kissane, D. W. (2002). Demoralization: Its phenomenology and importance. *Australian and New Zealand Journal of Psychiatry, 36,* 733–742.

Delgado-Guay, M., Parsons, H. A., Li, Z., Palmer, J. L., & Bruera, E. (2009). Symptom distress in advanced cancer patients with anxiety and depression in the palliative care setting. *Support Care Cancer, 17,* 573–579.

Endicott, J. (1983). Measurement of depression patients with cancer. *Cancer, 53,* 2243–2248.

Fallowfield, L., Ratcliffe, D., Jenkins, V., & Saul, J. (2001). Psychiatric morbidity and its recognition by doctors in patients with cancer. *British Journal of Cancer, 84,* 1011–1015.

Giese-Davis, J., Waller, A., Carlson, L. E., Groff, S., Zhong, L., Neri, E., et al. (2012). Screening for distress, the 6th vital sign: Common problems in cancer outpatients over one year in usual care: Associations with marital status, sex, and age. *BMC Cancer, 12,* 441. doi: 10.1186/1471-2407-12-441.

Holland, J. C., Andersen, B., Breitbart, W. S., Buchmann, L. O., Compas, B., Deshields, T. L., et al. (2013). Distress management. *Journal of the National Comprehensive Cancer Network, 11,* 190–209.

Howell, D., & Olsen, K. (2011). Distress the 6th vital sign. *Current Oncology, 18,* 208–210.

Kelly, B., McClement, S., & Chochinov, H. M. L. (2006). Measurement of psychological distress in palliative care. *Palliative Medicine, 20,* 779–789.

Kerrihard, T., Breitbart, W., Dent, R., & Strout, D. (1999). Anxiety in patients with cancer and human immunodeficiency virus. *Seminars in Clinical Neuropsychiatry, 4,* 114–132.

Kissane, D. W., Wein, S., Love, A., Lee, X. Q., Kee, P. L., & Clarke, D. M. (2004). The Demoralization Scale: A report of its development and preliminary validation. *Journal of Palliative Care, 20,* 269–276.

Kleespies, P. M., Hughes, D. H., & Gallacher, F. P. (2000). Suicide in the medically and terminally ill: Psychological and ethical considerations. *Journal of Clinical Psychology, 56,* 1153–1171.

Krikorian, A., & Limonero, J. T. (2012). An integrated view of suffering in palliative care. *Journal of Palliative Care, 28,* 41–49.

Krikorian, A., Limonero, J. T., & Corey, M. (2013). Suffering assessment: A review of available instruments for use in palliative care. *Journal of Palliative Medicine, 16,* 130–142. doi: 10.1089/jpm.2012.0370.

Krikorian, A., Limonero, J. T., & Maté, J. (2011). Suffering and distress at the end-of-life. *Psycho-Oncology, 21,* 799–808.

Kuuppelomäki, M., & Lauri, S. (1998). Cancer patients' reported experiences of suffering. *Cancer Nursing, 21,* 364–369.

Lee, V., Cohen, S. R., Edgar, L., Laizner, A. M., & Gagnon, A. J. (2006). Meaning-making and psychological adjustment to cancer: Development of an intervention and pilot results. *Oncology Nursing Forum, 33,* 291–302.

Limonero, J. T., Mateo, D., Maté-Méndez, J., González-Barboteo, J., Bayés, R., Bernaus, M., et al. (2012). Assessment of the psychometric properties of the Detection of Emotional Distress Scale in cancer patients. *Gaceta Sanitaria, 26,* 145–152.

Lloyd-Williams, M., Reeve, J., & Kissane, D. (2008). Distress in palliative care patients: Developing patient-centred approaches to clinical management. *European Journal of Cancer, 44,* 1133–1138. doi: 10.1016/j.ejca.2008.02.032.

Lloyd-Williams, M., & Riddleston, H. (2002). The stability of depression scores in patients who are receiving palliative care. *Journal of Pain & Symptom Management, 24,* 593–597.

Martínez, E., Barreto, M. P., & Toledo, M. (2001). Intervención psicológica con el paciente en situación terminal. *Revista de Psicología y Salud, 13,* 117–131.

Maté, J., Mateo, D., Bayés, R., Bernaus, M., Casas, C., Gonzalez-Barboteo, J., et al. (2009). Elaboración y propuesta de un instrumento para la detección de malestar emocional en enfermos al final de la vida. *Psicooncología, 6,* 507–518.

Mitchell, A. J. (2010). Short screening tools for cancer-related distress: A review and diagnostic validity meta-analysis. *Journal of the National Comprehensive Cancer Network, 8,* 487–494.

National Comprehensive Cancer Network (NCCN). (2010). *NCCN clinical practice guidelines in oncology: Distress management. Version 1.2011*. Fort Washington, PA: NCCN. Retrieved from: http://www.nccn.org/professionals/physician_gls/pdf/distress.pdf.

National Institute for Health and Clinical Excellence. (2004). *Improving supportive and palliative care for adults with cancer. The manual*. London: NICE. Retrieved from www.nice.org.uk/nicemedia/pdf/csgspmanual.pdf.

NCCN—The National Comprehensive Cancer Network. (2010). *Distress management guidelines*. Retrieved from www.nccn.org.

Nissim, R., Freeman, E., Lo, C., Zimmermann, C., Gagliese, L., Rydall, A., et al. (2012). Managing Cancer and Living Meaningfully (CALM): A qualitative study of a brief individual psychotherapy for individuals with advanced cancer. *Palliative Medicine, 26,* 713–721. doi: 10.1177/0269216311425096.

Noble, A., & Jones, C. (2005). Benefits of narrative therapy: Holistic interventions at the end of life. *British Journal of Nursing, 14,* 330–333.

Oi-Ling, K., Man-Wah, D., & Kam-Hung, D. (2005). Symptom distress as rated by advanced cancer patients, caregivers, and physicians in the last week of life. *Palliative Medicine, 19,* 228–233.

O'Mahony, S., Goulet, J., Kornblith, A., Abbatiello, G., Clarke, B., Kless-Siegel, S., et al. (2005). Desire for hastened death, cancer pain, and depression: Report of a longitudinal observational study. *Journal of Pain & Symptom Management, 29,* 446–457.

Portenoy, R. K., Thaler, H. T., Kornblith, A. B., Lepore, J. M., Friedlander-Klar, H., Coyle, N., et al. (1994). Symptom prevalence, characteristics, and distress in a cancer population. *Quality of Life Research, 3,* 183–189.

Potash, M., & Breitbart, W. (2002). Affective disorders in advanced cancer. *Hematology and Oncology Clinics of North America, 16,* 671–700.

Rayner, L., Loge, J. H., Wasteson, E., Higginson, I. J., & EPCRC (European Palliative Care Research Collaborative). (2009). The detection of depression in palliative care. *Current Opinions in Supportive and Palliative Care, 3,* 55-60. doi: 10.1097/SPC.0b013e328326b59b.

Rayner, L., Price, A., Hotopf, M., & Higginson, I. J. (2011). The development of evidence-based European guidelines on the management of depression in palliative cancer care. *European Journal of Cancer, 47,* 702–712.

Rhodes, V. A., & Watson, P. M. (1987). Symptom distress—the concept: Past and present. *Seminars in Oncology Nursing, 3,* 242–247.

Sirois, F. (2012). Psychiatric aspects of chronic palliative care: Waiting for death. *Palliative and Supportive Care, 10,* 205–211. doi: 10.1017/S1478951511000885.

Sloan, J. A., Cella, D., Frost, M., Guyatt, G. H., Sprangers, M., & Symonds, T. (2002). Assessing clinical significance in measuring oncology patient quality of life: Introduction to the symposium, content overview, and definition of terms. *Mayo Clinic Proceedings, 77,* 367–370.

Snowden, A., White, C. A., Christie, Z., Murray, E., McGowan, C., & Scott, R. (2011). The clinical utility of the distress thermometer: A review. *British Journal of Nursing, 20,* 220–227.

Stefanek, M. E., Derogatis, L. P., & Shaw, A. (1987). Psychological distress among oncology outpatients. Prevalence and severity as measured with the Brief Symptom Inventory. *Psychosomatics, 28,* 530–532.

Steinhauser, K. E., Voils, C. I., Clipp, E. C., Bosworth, H. B., Christakis, N. A., & Tulsky, J. A. (2006). "Are you at peace?": One item to probe spiritual concerns at the end of life. *Archives of Internal Medicine, 166,* 101–105.

Sulmasy, D. (2002). A biopsychosocial-spiritual model for the care of patients at the end of life. *The Gerontologist, 42,* 24–33.

Thekkumpurath, P., Venkateswaran, C., Kumar, M., & Bennett, M. I. (2008). Screening for psychological distress in palliative care: A systematic review. *Journal of Pain & Symptom Management, 36,* 520–528.

Undurraga, F. J. P, González, M., & Calderón, J. (2006). Counseling: A comprehensive method to support the terminally ill. *Revista de Medicina Chilena, 134,* 1448–1454.

Vachon, M. (2006). Psychosocial distress and coping after cancer treatment. How clinicians can assess distress and which interventions are appropriate—what we know and what we don't. *American Journal of Nursing, 106*(3 Suppl.), 26–31.

Viederman, M. (1983). The psychodynamic life narrative: A psychotherapeutic intervention useful in crisis situations. *Psychiatry, 46,* 236–246.

Vitek, L., Rosenzweig, M. Q., & Stollings, S. (2007). Distress in patients with cancer: Definition, assessment, and suggested interventions. *Clinical Journal of Oncology Nursing, 11,* 413–418.

Waller, A., Groff, S. L., Hagen, N., Bultz, B. D., & Carlson, L. E. (2012). Characterizing distress, the 6th vital sign, in an oncology pain clinic. *Current Oncology, 19,* e53-9. doi: 10.3747/co.19.882.

Weissman, M. M., Markowitz, J. C., & Klerman, G. L. (2000). *Comprehensive guide to interpersonal psychotherapy.* New York: Basic Books.

WHO. (1992). The ICD-10 classification of mental and behavioral disorders: Clinical descriptions and diagnostic guidelines. Geneva: World Health Organisation.

Wilson, K. G., Chochinov, H. M., McPherson, C. J., LeMay, K., Allard, P., Chary, S., et al. (2007). Suffering with advanced cancer. *Journal of Clinical Oncology, 25,* 1691–1697.

Wilson, K. G., Graham, I. D., Viola, R. A., Chater, S., de Faye, B. J., Weaver, L. A., et al. (2004). Structured interview assessment of symptoms and concerns in palliative care. *Canadian Journal of Psychiatry, 49,* 350–358.

Wittmann, L., Sensky T., Meder L., Michel, B., Stoll, T., & Büchi, S. (2009). Suffering and posttraumatic growth in women with systemic lupus erythematosus (SLE): A qualitative/quantitative case study. *Psychosomatics, 50,* 362–374.

Zigmond, A. S., & Snaith, R. P. (1983). The hospital anxiety and depression scale. *Acta Psychiatrica Scandinava, 67,* 361–370.

Part IV

Women and Cancer: Relationships and Sexuality Issues

Chapter 14

Sex after Cancer: Women Renegotiating Sex outside the Coital Imperative

Jane M. Ussher, Emilee Gilbert, and Janette Perz

INTRODUCTION

Cancer is the leading cause of burden of disease in Australia, with more than 100,000 new cases diagnosed each year (Australian Institute of Health and Welfare [AIHW], 2010). However, five-year survival currently stands at more than 60 percent (AIHW, 2010), which has led to an increasing body of survivorship research examining the profound and enduring impact that cancer can have upon quality of life (QoL) and embodied subjectivity, leaving "no aspect of identity untouched" (Little, Jordens, & Sayers, 2003, p. 76; Little & Sayers, 2004). Indeed, it has been suggested that following cancer, an individual's experience of embodied subjectivity as functional, intact, and "normal" can move to a state of "dys-embodiment" (Williams, 1996, p. 23), in which the body and self are experienced as dysfunctional, ill, and at odds with the desired presentation of the self (Kelly & Field, 1996). Sexual well-being is a central component of QoL and embodied subjectivity, and it is now recognized that changes to sexuality can be the most problematic aspect of women's life post-cancer (Burwell, Case, Kaelin, & Avis, 2006), with the impact lasting for many years after successful treatment (Andersen, 2009; Bertero & Wilmoth, 2007) and often associated with serious physical and emotional side effects (Gilbert, Ussher, & Perz, 2010b; Gilbert, Ussher, & Perz, 2011). The purpose of this chapter is to draw on the findings of a recent research study to examine women's experience and construction of sexual well-being and intimacy after cancer, the impact of such changes on embodied subjectivity, and women's strategies of sexual renegotiation.

THE EXPERIENCE AND CONSTRUCTION OF CHANGES TO SEXUALITY AFTER CANCER

There is now substantial documentation of changes to women's sexuality following cancer. This can result from anatomical changes, such as vaginal shortening or reduced vaginal elasticity (Basson, 2010), pelvic nerve damage, clitoris removal, vaginal stenosis, and fistula formation (Holmes, 2005); and from physical changes, such as deceased bodily function (Holmes, 2005), fatigue (Lamb & Sheldon, 1994), dyspareunia (Bergmark, Avall-Lundqvist, Dickman, Henningsohn, & Steineck, 1999), infertility (Stead, Fallowfield, Selby, & Brown, 2007), and postcoital vaginal bleeding (Lamb & Sheldon, 1994). Negative body image or feelings of sexual unattractiveness (Bertero & Wilmoth, 2007), concern about weight gain or loss (Fobair et al., 2006) and loss of femininity (Archibald, Lemieux, Byers, Tamlyn, & Worth, 2006), and depression and anxiety (Garrusi & Faezee, 2008), as well as alterations to the sexual self (Wilmoth, 2001), can exacerbate the impact of these physical changes. In combination, this can result in changes to women's response (Stead, et al., 2007), including changes to desire (Sekse, Raaheim, Blaaka, & Gjengedal, 2010; Stead, et al., 2007), orgasm (Fobair et al., 2006), arousal (Weijmar Schultz, Van De Wiel, & Bouma, 1991), vaginal lubrication (Grumann, Robertson, Hacker, & Sommer, 2001; Ussher, Perz, & Gilbert, 2012a), genital swelling (Bergmark, et al., 1999), and genital sensitivity (Andersen & Hacker, 1983), leading to decreased frequency of sex (Green et al., 2000) and lack of sexual pleasure (Meyerowitz, Desmond, Rowland, Wyatt, & Ganz, 1999).

There are, however, a number of limitations of previous research on women's sexual well-being after cancer. The focus has been on physical changes, where functional sexuality is narrowly conceptualized as sexual intercourse (Fobair et al., 2006). This reflects the dominance of the "coital imperative" (McPhillips, Braun, & Gavey, 2001, p. 229), where "real sex" is defined as penis/vagina penetration (Hyde, 2007; Ussher, Perz, Gilbert, Wong, & Hobbs, 2012). Recent research has shown, however, that engaging in coital sex may not be women's primary focus of sexual concern after a cancer diagnosis, and that engagement in sexual intercourse does not necessary equate to sexual satisfaction (Wilmoth, 2001). At the same time, research has focused on sexual difficulties and dysfunction, negating the ways in which the meaning of sex is negotiated, or renegotiated, in the context of cancer (Gilbert, Ussher, & Perz, 2010a), which has led to a plea for research examining "successful strategies used by couples to maintain sexual intimacy" in the context of cancer (Beck, Robinson, & Carlson, 2009, p. 142).

There is some evidence that women can renegotiate sexual practices following cancer, based on accounts of a small number of participants taking part in studies focusing on sexual difficulties. For example, research with women partners of men with cancer has reported renegotiation of sex to include practices previously positioned as secondary to "real sex" (Gilbert et al., 2010a; Hawkins et al., 2009). It has also been reported that many women with breast cancer want information about how to use lubricants to combat vaginal dryness (Archibald et al., 2006; Ussher et al., 2012b), as well as where to purchase and how to use vibrators, dildos, or other sexual enhancement products as part of their post-cancer sexual repertoire (Herbenick, Reece, Hollub, Satinsky, & Dodge, 2008). However, there is a need for further research on women's sexual renegotiation after cancer, across a range of cancer types, as previous research has focused on cancers that directly affect the sexual or reproductive organs, such as breast and gynecological cancer. For while there are a few studies examining changes to sexuality in nonreproductive cancers, such as lung and colorectal cancer (e.g., Carolan, Meneses, Shell, & Zhang, 2008; Ramirez et al., 2010; Traa, De Vries, Roukema, & Den Oudsten, 2012), these studies are in the minority. Equally, while attention has been paid to "dys-embodiment" after illness (Leder, 1990; Williams, 1996, 1998), the impact of sexual changes after cancer on embodied subjectivity has been under-researched.

Previous research on women's sexuality after cancer has also primarily used quantitative methods of data collection. While quantitative methods can provide information on changes in large samples of individuals, they negate the lived experience and negotiation of sexual well-being after cancer (Gilbert et al., 2010b), leading to a call for qualitative research in this field (Traa et al., 2012). There has been some qualitative research that has examined women's lived experiences of changes to sexuality after cancer (see Archibald et al., 2006; Ussher et al., 2012a), and the ways in which sociocultural discourses shape the experience and interpretation of sexuality (Young, 1992). However, this research has focused on women with breast cancer, which limits generalizations that can be made across a range of cancer types. Equally, while sexual changes have been reported by the intimate partners of people with both reproductive and nonreproductive cancers (Gilbert, Ussher, & Hawkins, 2009; Hawkins et al., 2009), women partners are rarely included in research on cancer and sexuality. The focus of research has also primarily been on heterosexual women with cancer, with the experiences and concerns of lesbian and bisexual women marginalized or ignored (Brown & Tracy, 2008). Finally, sex is usually assumed to be of greater concern to younger women (Loe, 2004), leaving older women with cancer feeling as if their sexual needs are invisible or inappropriate, and rarely addressed by health professionals (Ussher et al., 2012a).

Mindful of the shortcomings of previous research, in this chapter we examine the lived experience and negotiation of sexual well-being and intimacy after cancer in heterosexual and nonheterosexual women with cancer, as well as women who are the partner of a person with cancer, across a range of cancer types and age groups, using qualitative research methods. We are adopting a material-discursive-intrapsychic (MDI) perspective (Gilbert et al., 2010b; Ussher, 2000), which acknowledges the materiality of physical changes in sexual well-being, as well as the tangible impact of cancer and cancer treatment; women's psychological and emotional experience; and the negotiation of such changes within relational context, where meaning is constructed in relation to cultural constructions of femininity, sexuality, and illness.

DESCRIPTION OF THE RESEARCH STUDY

Forty-one women took part in semi-structured interviews; 23 women with cancer and 18 women in an intimate relationship with a person with cancer. The participants were drawn from a larger mixed-method study examining changes to sexuality and intimacy in the context of cancer. The average age of participants was 51.5 years (49.5 for women with cancer; 53.9 for partners), and cancer was diagnosed on average five years prior to participation in the study. The majority (92.7%) identified as from an Anglo-European-Australian background, with one participant identifying as from an Asian background (2.4%), and two participants did not indicate their cultural background (4.9%). The following cancer types were reported by women with cancer and women partners—prostate (24.5%), breast (19.6%), leukemia (9.8%), bowel (2.4%), ovarian (9.8%), melanoma (7.3%), multiple myeloma (4.9%), non-Hodgkin lymphoma (2.4%), anal (4.9%), colon (2.4%), colorectal (2.4%), kidney (2.4%), lymphoma (2.4%), sarcoma (2.4%), and unknown primary (2.4%). Eighty-five percent of participants were currently in a relationship, with 37 participants identifying as heterosexual (90.2%), and four participants identifying as nonheterosexual, three as lesbians and one as polysexual.

We conducted a semi-structured in-depth interview on a face-to-face or telephone basis, to examine the experience and construction of changes to sexuality after cancer, and strategies of renegotiation. The interview questions included changes to sexuality and intimacy; emotional reactions to such changes; partner responses; support received from family, friends, or health professionals; and renegotiation of sex and intimacy. The analysis was conducted using theoretical thematic analysis (Braun & Clarke, 2006), using an inductive approach, with the development of themes being data driven, rather than based on preexisting research on sexuality and cancer. Two core themes of "changes to sexuality after cancer" and "renegotiating sex and intimacy" were developed, which are outlined below. In order to illustrate the extent and nature of sexual changes in women with cancer and women partners across age, cancer type, and sexual orientation, we are providing participant pseudonyms, as well as information on age, status as person with cancer (pwc) or partner (pt), cancer type, and identification as heterosexual (hetero), lesbian, or polysexual (poly) after substantive extracts.

STUDY FINDINGS

Changes to Sexuality after Cancer

In the interviews, a number of changes to sexual well-being were reported after the diagnosis or treatment for cancer. Women with cancer most commonly reported experiencing decreased sexual desire. As Mindy told us, "I'd rather do the washing but when it does happen, it's pleasurable and no pain" (49, pwc, breast, hetero). A small number of women with cancer attributed diminished desire to the early onset of menopause, with Ursula reporting that "the biggest effect is the instant menopause" (47, pwc, ovarian, hetero), which can lead to a "loss of passion." For the majority of women with cancer, as well as women partners, cancer diagnosis and treatment also meant that sex was positioned as secondary to survival; as Nelly reported, "My focus was very strongly on survival. I didn't want to die . . . sex really didn't matter" (57, pwc, lymphoma, hetero). Equally, Lara told us, "I think other things sort of took over a bit more" (26, pt, leukemia, hetero), and Ruby said, "sex is probably the last thing on your mind" (49, pwc, ovarian, hetero). This could result in a woman's sexuality being "shelved" for a time, as Vicky describes her experience after initial diagnosis:

> I even shelved my own sexual needs so I've, I was fully and utterly 100% celibate. It just didn't, it just got stopped, my sexuality just stopped . . . my sexuality was shelved, shelved but it was still there. (36, pwc, melanoma, lesbian)

Sexual pain was also reported by a number of women with cancer. For example, Frances told us, "we both feel that if we engage in sexual activity, am I going to be bedridden for a week as a result of one episode of sexual intercourse" (63, pwc, myeloma, hetero). Helen described sexual pain resulting from scarring following surgery:

> But when they did the surgery, they cut me straight down the front, so I have a zip. Um, and that zip has been extremely painful on and off over the years and if I get stressed, I still can't take any pressure, actually on the scar. It's the scar rather than the internal organs I'd say. So sex became very difficult and often it would hurt. (64, pwc, kidney, hetero)

Pain during coital sex resulting from vaginal dryness, a by-product of cancer treatment, was also reported by a number of women with cancer, particularly those with breast cancer. As Henna said, "I experienced a lot of dryness in the vagina, which causes me to be a little bit worried about the pain side of it" (59, pwc, ovarian, hetero). In a similar vein, Irene said, "It was unbelievably painful, I cannot tell you, it was unbelievably, it was excruciatingly painful to have intercourse. . . . I literally couldn't bear to be touched" (61, pwc, anal, hetero).

Concerns about body image were reported by many women with cancer, including scarring, weight gain, hair loss, and breast loss for women with breast cancer. For example, Kirsten said, "I have a scar that's on the very top of my inner thigh, and I hate the thing and I don't like looking at it" (24, pwc, lymphoma, hetero), and Cassie told us, "I've put on so much weight. I'm the heaviest I have ever been since I had children" (51, pwc, breast, hetero). Women partners were more likely to report tiredness as a source of sexual changes: "partners who care for people with cancer are too tired for sex" (Cynthia, 46, pt, myeloma, hetero), or to report changes in the sexual functioning of their male partners who had cancer: "he can get a soft erection but it's not strong enough for penetration" (Monica, 51, pt, prostate, hetero).

Coital Failure Equals Loss of Sex and Intimacy

If coital sex is not possible, or is painful, and sexual intimacy is not renegotiated, then the outcome can be a complete cessation of sexual and intimate contact after cancer (Gilbert et al., 2010a; Hawkins et al., 2009). One woman described cessation of sex because her partner would not countenance noncoital sexual exploration, because of his "terror of playing" (Helen, 64, pwc, kidney, hetero). Coital sex was also avoided because of pain experienced by women with cancer, as illustrated by Della (65, pwc, anal, hetero), who said she was "scared to be too intimate" with her husband because "I was very damaged in that area." Some partners also gave accounts of not wanting to ask their partners for coital sex because it would be inappropriate to put their own needs first, or because they did not want to make their partner feel guilty for saying "no": "I felt bad, I suppose. Why should I be just annoyed with not being able to have sex, or wanting him to touch me when he's got cancer? I don't have cancer" (Melanie, 37, pt, colon, hetero). In a small number of cases, women who had cancer described their partner as the one who did not want to engage in sex because they were afraid of being "poisoned" by chemotherapy drugs or because they were scared or disinterested. In all of these cases, couples had not renegotiated noncoital sexual practices, and all forms of intimacy had ceased.

Dys-embodied Sexual Subjectivity

As a result of these sexual changes following cancer, a number of participants reported that they had "lost" their former sexual selves and now felt that they were a "worse" version of their precancer sexual selves. For these participants, the post-cancer experience of sexual subjectivity was positioned as problematic because their sexual bodies had come to betray them: they failed to sexually function in their precancer forms, and they were no longer experienced as sexually attractive and confident—issues that were reported to have had a "devastating" impact on the sexual relationship. For these participants, the post-cancer sexual body and subjectivity "dys-appeared" (Leder, 1990, p. 84) and was largely characterized by "dys-order" and "dys-embodiment" (Williams 1996; 1998). In other words, the onset of cancer-related changes to the body and sexuality disrupted the once taken-for-granted "dis-appearance" of the body; as Williams (1996, p. 24) argues, it is "only when things 'go wrong' with our bodies, whether through illness or various other forms of bodily 'betrayal' and 'resistance,' do they become 'problematised' as the thematic *object* of attention" (emphasis in original). Thus, for some women, the post-cancer sexual body was experienced as being in a "dys-functional state" (Williams, 1998, p. 61), with the disruptions to sexuality reported to make them feel asexual, depressed, anxious, and stressed. For these women, post-cancer sexual subjectivity was also characterized by feelings of sexual loss—including loss of sexual confidence and loss of body image. For example, as Mindy said, "I felt that I'd lost, I'd lost me. . . . I got the breast cancer and then kind of then didn't know who I was. I just lost all my confidence" (49, pwc, breast, hetero). Similarly, Helen described her loss of sexual subjectivity below:

> Cancer changes lives. It's funny because I've got someone that I saw this morning, and she said to me, "You know, I don't know who I am any more. I'm not the person I was six years ago when this journey started, and I'm not even the person I was a month ago 'cause everything changes so rapidly." So there's this sense of fluidity, and people start to lose their sense of identity and who they are, and expressing it sexually can be very hard after treatment. (64, pwc, kidney, hetero)

At the center of women's accounts of post-cancer sexual dys-embodiment was a reported difficulty in accepting the changes that cancer brought about, and accepting the "new you." As Nelly said, "I feel completely different, and I don't like the way I'm totally different" (57, pwc, lymphoma, hetero). Cassie describes this lack of acceptance below, with her account highlighting the way in which health professionals can play a role in reinforcing the sense of changed sexual subjectivity post-cancer:

> It's not the same person that you were . . . you lose your identity, I think. Even the psychologist says, "Oh well, that was the old you and this is the new you. You just have to learn to accept it. This *is* the new you." And you think, "Well, I don't want to. I don't like this person." (51, pwc, breast, hetero)

The experience of dys-embodied sexual subjectivity also impacted upon the emotional well-being of women with cancer and their partners, with Deanna mentioning, "because of the depression, his moods are swinging . . . which flows through to how you're responding sexually" (56, pt, prostate, hetero). Similarly, for Hayley, "depression played a big part in a low point for our sexual relationship . . . he just really lost interest in all things that he used to be very interested in, and was negative all of the time and everything was a great effort to do anything, and so we weren't having a lot of regular sex at that period of time" (31, pt, leukemia, hetero).

The accounts above, underscored by reports of depression, anxiety, stress, and difficulty accepting changes to sexuality, point to the circular effect that changes to sexuality following cancer can have upon the experience of subjectivity more broadly—with changes to subjectivity in turn often compounding and reinforcing the experience of sexual dys-embodiment. Such accounts highlight the need for survivorship research on embodied subjectivity post-cancer to recognize the centrality of sexuality to subjectivity.

COUNTERNARRATIVE: SEXUALITY IS THE SAME AFTER CANCER

Negative changes to sexual well-being after cancer were not universal across the participants. A number of women reported that intimacy and sexuality had not changed, as illustrated by the accounts of Tracy and Charlotte, respectively: "I didn't actually feel much different" (26, pwc, colorectal, hetero), and "I don't think anything has really changed" (66, pt, prostate, hetero). These accounts were more common in early-stage cancer, and proportionately more common in accounts from lesbian or polysexual women. Thus, Tammy said, "I think essentially there haven't been as many changes as I thought there might be" (49, pwc, breast, lesbian), and Bronwyn told us:

And it [sex] didn't really stop, it didn't reduce. I mean there were times, when I was having chemo and stuff I felt crap, so it wasn't a happening thing. But pretty well, yeah, the attraction and the sexual part of our relationship continued. (50, pwc, breast, lesbian)

One of the factors that may account for the absence of significant sexual disruption is greater acceptance of bodily changes in lesbian women. Vicky (36, pwc, melanoma, lesbian) described having her "full back tattooed" with "butterflies and roses," and said that "my partner sees my tattoo and she absolutely loves it, she doesn't see the scar." Nina (48, pwc, breast, poly), who described herself as polysexual in a BDSM relationship with both men and women partners, said that despite having a "big hole" and a "big scar" in one breast, "the intimacy is greater than it was before," as she still had an active sex life and felt "very sexy." Another factor that may account for sexuality remaining the same is the inclusion of nonpenetrative sexual practices in the repertoire of lesbian and poly women. As Bronwyn commented, "sex is penetrative sexual intercourse, well as a lesbian, it's not, not necessarily. It can be, but it's often not," and as Nina said:

One of the things about BDSM is that there's like 500 things on the list to do, one of which is sexual intercourse. So there's lots of other options. Even when we weren't sick, when I wasn't sick, and there were, maybe we'd have sexual intercourse once a fortnight possibly, at the most, just do lots of other stuff.

These accounts stand in contrast to previous research with heterosexual women who experience absence of sexual desire, sensation, or pleasure following cancer yet continue to engage in coital sex, regardless of pain or discomfort (Jensen et al., 2004). While there has been little discussion in the research literature about why this is so (Hyde, 2007), women's adherence to the coital imperative is one plausible explanation. Coital sex is also central to the gendered subjectivity of heterosexual women, and the effects of cancer have been found to induce "invisible assaults to femininity" (Butler et al., 1998, p. 685). In this vein, women who cannot engage in coital sex, because of illness or pain, have been reported to describe themselves as an "inadequate woman" or "inadequate partner" (Ayling & Ussher, 2008, p. 294), expressing concern that their ability to fulfill relationship roles is disrupted (Juraskova et al., 2003).

Re-embodied Sexual Subjectivity

Sexual disruption and dys-embodiment were not universal for heterosexual women, however. For a number of participants, the disruption of cancer prompted them to positively reinvent their precancer sexual subjectivity, with many reporting that the onset of cancer led them to feel greater sexual confidence, have a more positive self-image, and become "stronger" and more "evolved" emotionally. While for these participants the sexual body also "dys-appeared" (Leder, 1990) post-cancer, the result of this dys-appearance was not sexual dys-embodiment, but sexual re-embodiment. Against William's (1996, p. 37) notion of "negotiated settlement"—in which "attempts" at re-embodiment can be made by individuals post-illness but ultimately render them "never quite able to return" to "their former embodied state" (p. 31)—for many of these women, cancer was the catalyst for the re-embodiment of a "better" sexual subjectivity. Indeed, these participants described cancer as "life-changing" and a "positive experience" that led them to feel "better for that," "changed quite a bit," and "empowered actually." As Tracy reported, "I feel like I know myself a lot better, and so that makes me more confident. . . . And for me I think it's ended in probably a much more positive self image actually" (26, pwc, colorectal, hetero). Central to participants' positive reconstruction of sexual subjectivity was an acceptance of the changes to sexuality and the body that cancer brought about, with accounts including, "I thought I just have to accept that I've got no sex drive"; "cancer is just a part of life, it's something you have to deal with"; "I do not dwell on the changes"; "think positively"; and "you just have to get through it" because "no use losing sleep about it, no use getting anxious or upset." For example, Sandra talked about how cancer enabled her to see herself "in a way I've never seen myself before" because she "left so much of my own garbage (behind)." Leaving this garbage meant that Sandra "saw how unimportant" her precancer sexual and bodily insecurities were, saying that, "I think I had so many insecurities that were superficial insecurities, like I don't look right, I don't speak right, I don't whatever it is, I don't, I use my hands when I talk, and I saw how unimportant they were" (55, pwc, sarcoma, hetero). Similarly, Kristen talked about having to accept that her post-surgical scars "are part of me":

> That scar I can't get rid of. I can't cover it up. It doesn't matter who sees me or what happens that's always going to be there, and it was hard to realize that, well, I have to accept that as part of me and not worry on it and not dwell about it and not dwell about what others are thinking and putting clothes on and thinking, "Can they see that through this or if I wear this can I . . . is someone going to know that the scar is there?" (24, pwc, non-Hodgkin's lymphoma, hetero)

This demonstrates that women are active agents in making sense of the changes to the body post-cancer, and that sexual subjectivity is not fixed or static but multiple and changing, as is also evident in accounts of oscillating sexual subjectivity.

Oscillating Sexual Subjectivity

While the majority of women reported that their post-cancer sexual subjectivity had changed either for the better or the worse, a minority were unsure about whether cancer-induced changes had led to a state of re-embodied or dys-embodied sexual subjectivity. At the center of these women's accounts was the experience of being in the process of coming to terms with the impact of cancer on sexual subjectivity, with accounts oscillating between positioning cancer-induced disruptions as a "gain" and as a "loss." Many of these participants were in the early stages of cancer and reported still "dealing with the aftermath" of cancer, and simply "persevering." As Emma described, "I'm still trying to work out who I am now, and kind of move on and, you know, who is this new person, and how do I deal with things?" (52, pwc, breast, cured, hetero). These women also positioned the cancer experience as both "so positive and so negative at the same time," with Monica reporting that "I have suffered a loss. . . . I just think it's something we've lost, but I feel that we've gained a lot of other things and I just . . . I don't know, I don't" (51, pt, prostate, hetero). Similarly, in her account below, Frances described the "real tussle" involved in coming to terms with her "new body" and changed sexual relationship—a tussle around "looking better than I ever looked before" but being restricted in her sexual expression:

It's interesting because I've always been grossly overweight and that, of course, obviously had an effect on my own personal perception of myself as a sexual being, but with this cancer I lost 50 kilograms and so suddenly I had a shape which I never had before and I could go into a store and buy clothing off the rack, which I couldn't do before, and so, here I was, looking better than I [chuckles], from my perspective, than I'd ever looked before and yet I couldn't [chuckles] express it in a sexual way, because I couldn't have physical sex in the normal way that we always had, and we've always had a very active sex life. So it was a, a real tussle, if you like, trying to come to grips with this new body, this new perception of myself but being made out of glass. (63, pwc, multiple myeloma, hetero)

These accounts point to the importance of positioning sexual subjectivity as a process that can unfold over the cancer trajectory, and one in which individuals move "from an initially embodied state" to a state that is now "a subtle, complex and sophisticated oscillation between states of dys-embodiment and attempts at re-embodiment" (Williams, 1996, p. 37).

These attempts at re-embodiment were also evident in accounts of sexual renegotiation.

RENEGOTIATING SEX: RESISTING THE COITAL IMPERATIVE AND EMBRACING INTIMACY

Renegotiation of sex or intimacy was reported by a significant proportion of women. A phallocentric model of sex, which places primacy on the erect penis, was explicitly abandoned within these accounts. For example, Nina (48, pwc, breast, poly) told us that she "deeply rejects" the notion that sex is "all defined in terms of the cock and what it does," wherein "sex starts when the guy gets an erection and ends when he's had an orgasm and that's it." In this vein, for many women, sexual renegotiation after cancer involved the exploration of noncoital or nonpenetrative sexual practices, suggesting resistance of the coital imperative. For example, Nelly (59, pwc, lymphoma, hetero) described herself and her partner in the following way:

> We were like, oh, two puppies playing together, even though I'm 59 and he's 74. Um, and even sort of simulated sex we'd get on top of each other and not actually have sex, but you know, sort of loving each other in a sex position.

Ruby (49, pwc, ovarian, hetero) told us that "if you borrow the Karma Sutra and someone thinks, 'Oh yeah, okay, let's see how that goes [laughs],'" which she described as "fun," concluding that her sex life was "very good" post-cancer. Many of the women partners gave similar accounts. For example, Dianne, age 65, whose husband was in active treatment for bowel cancer, told us that "he can always do that orally and if he likes to, also use his hand on me, and basically he doesn't need me to do a lot to him." Grace, age 65, whose partner has prostate cancer and had completed treatment, described engaging in mutually orgasmic masturbation:

> once or twice a week I'd say, "Do you want to rub yourself?" and Robert does the rubbing and uses a lubricant until he has an orgasm and I'll be involved with the rubbing . . . he enjoys all parts of my body and he'll rub my clitoris, and we've been more communicative about that in terms of the amount of pressure that I like.

While such practices are often labelled "foreplay" or "heavy petting," the majority of participants in the present study positioned noncoital genital intimacy as "sex," suggesting that renegotiated sexual practices are not seen as secondary to the "real thing"—in contrast to previous research with male prostate cancer survivors, who described noncoital practices as "proxy sex" (Oliffe, 2005, p. 2256).

A number of women described using sex toys, such as vibrators, to experience orgasm or sexual pleasure—something that they had not done before cancer. For example, Mindy (49, pwc, breast, hetero) told us that she had initially bought a vibrator to "keep all the (vaginal) muscles working," but that she and her husband also "had a bit of fun with it and now and again I'd think through the day, 'Oh, I should go and do that.'" Edith, age 69, whose husband had advanced melanoma and had completed treatment, said that "sexual aids are one way of both of us being able to participate," which was positioned as "important" when "the partner's unable to have an erection." Similarly, Hayley, age 31, whose partner had completed treatment for leukemia, told us that "he's had difficulties with erections after his chemo . . . so eventually talked me into [laughs] getting a vibrator and things like that and, but we now use together."

Other women described developing a focus on nongenital intimacy as a means of renegotiating sexuality after cancer, including accounts of cuddling, kissing, massage, and touching. Thus Henna (59, pwc, ovarian, hetero) said, "Well, I guess we sleep together, so that's a good thing [chuckles], and cuddle up, and touch, and that sort of thing is always good." Kirsten described "the little things" such as hugging as being important: "It's the little things, like he knows if something is not quite right and he'll just come and stand next to me and give me a hug . . . that makes a difference" (24, pwc, lymphoma, hetero). These accounts were common in interviews with heterosexual women whose male partner with cancer could no longer attain an erection. For example, Charlotte said, "You sort of lie together, you cuddle, you kiss, you fondle, and you know, being really very close together" (66, pt, prostate, hetero). In a similar way, Dianne (62, pt, bowel, hetero) said that:

> We spend time every day just kissing, cuddling, loving, and if there's no sex, there's no sex. If there's no heavy petting or anything, it doesn't matter. We're happy with whatever comes along that day.

Previous research with heterosexual couples has reported that noncoital sexual acts are conceptualized as less intimate than coital sex, whereas intercourse is associated with closeness and connectedness (Gavey, McPhillips, & Braun, 1999). However, in the present study many of our participants positioned genital and nongenital intimacy as a manifestation of closeness in the relationship. This was described in terms of "being really very close together" (Charlotte, 66, pt, prostate, hetero), or being "part of one another" (Pearl, 64, pt, prostate, hetero). Relationship closeness resulting from sex and intimacy was also positioned as central to coping with the impact of cancer. For example, Darcy (43, pt, breast, hetero) said that "the sexual relationship is part of that recovery and survival." Kristen (24, pwc, lymphoma, hetero) described sex as a "fantastic distraction," and Hayley (31, pt, leukemia, hetero) said engagement in sex was a "way of coping," which helps to "deal with lots of emotions, fear, and things like that." Renegotiated sex and intimacy could also serve to maintain normality in the face of cancer, providing reassurance that life was not "always about the cancer. It can be about desire and each other and those sorts of things" (Lara, 26, pt, leukemia, hetero). These accounts challenge the positioning of sex and intimacy as a trivial activity in the context of cancer, which can leave couples reluctant to raise sexual concerns with health professionals for fear of being rebuffed (Hordern & Street, 2007).

Communication was a key factor in sexual renegotiation after cancer, as Vicky illustrated:

> We tend to be very open communicators in the bedroom. We're also probably on the fringe of on the top echelon of wanting to explore and to try different things. So we'll see, we tend to see if a) does it work, b) does it feel good, c) if both a and b work well that's great. If a and b don't work, well then we don't do that one again. We stop. (36, pwc, melanoma, lesbian)

Conversely, participants who described an absence of sexual renegotiation were more likely to describe a lack of communication about sex, saying that they never discussed sex before cancer and did not discuss it now. Thus Helen (64, pwc, kidney, hetero) said that her husband "doesn't hear very well" and that the "whole issue of asking for what you want or giving someone what they want, be it sexually or anything else, he finds extraordinarily difficult." Those who had a preexisting close relationship, in particular, a good sexual relationship, were also more likely to describe successful renegotiation. For example, Emma (52, pwc, breast, hetero) said that she and her partner had "always been very close," and "always hugged a lot," which meant that it was not very different after cancer, other than "maybe you appreciate it even more." Partner support in relation to embodied changes experienced after cancer was positioned as an important aspect of renegotiating sex, as is evident in accounts of women who experienced absence of desire or vaginal dryness that led to pain during coital sex, with Della (65, pwc, anal, hetero) saying, "he's been fantastic, never put any pressure on me," and Mindy (49, pwc, breast, hetero) telling us, "he just says, 'look don't worry about it, it's okay.'" Women who had experienced hysterectomy, scarring, or mastectomy, also talked about the importance of partner acceptance.

> At the time I went through huge emotional ups and downs, and spoke to my husband about, "Oh this is terrible, I've lost all the bits

that I should have had." Yeah, so he was quite, very supportive about all that. He said, "It's alright, it's okay, you're still there." (Henna, 59, pwc, ovarian, hetero)

These findings confirm previous research that found that partner support is central to coping with changes to sexuality after cancer (Ussher, Perz, & Gilbert, 2012a) and reinforce the importance of conceptualizing cancer as a "we disease" (Kayser, Watson, & Andrade, 2007), wherein coping is examined from a relational perspective, and sexuality is acknowledged to be central to the couple relationship.

DISCUSSION

These findings support and extend previous research reporting significant changes in sexual well-being after diagnosis and treatment for cancer, for both women with cancer and women partners of a person with cancer. Decreases in frequency of sex, sexual arousal, interest, desire, pleasure, satisfaction, and intimacy were reported by the majority of women, confirming previous research (Gilbert et al., 2011; Ussher et al., 2012a). This suggests that acknowledgment of sexual changes, and the potential impact of such changes on subjectivity and relationships, should be a central part of health care provision for women with cancer and for women who are partners of a person with cancer (Hordern & Street, 2007), as these sexual changes can significantly impact psychological well-being, quality of life, and couple closeness.

A chronic illness such as cancer can potentially result in the construction of a number of new selves—selves that although altered by the cancer are experienced as more fully realized than the precancer self (Frank, 1993). Central to this research is the notion that individuals are not simply passive victims of cancer but take practical and symbolic actions to minimize the effects of illness on the body and subjectivity (Bury, 1991; Williams, 1996). Indeed, for Williams (1996), it is precisely because chronic illness shifts our "normal" taken-for-granted state of embodiment into a state of "dys-embodiment" that we can engage in the biographical work of not only preserving embodied subjectivity, but also of positively transforming it so that the precancer self is reconstructed and experienced as expanded and more functional. The self is "re-embodied" (Williams, 1996, p. 24), as was evident in accounts of many of the women in the present study. Here, there is a recognition of "vicissitudes" across the illness trajectory, involving a shift from the precancer state of embodiment, to an oscillation between dys-embodiment and attempts at re-embodiment (Williams, 1996, p. 23). Such vicissitudes underscore the mutability and fluctuations in embodied subjectivity, and recognize the importance of positioning subjectivity as a dynamic processes of becoming that can change over time and that is multiple and contradictory (Deleuze & Guattari, 1988; Fox, 1993, 2002).

While previous research has focused on embodied changes associated with sexuality after cancer, as well as their psychological consequences, the present study also focused on sexual renegotiation, suggesting that cultural constructions of "sex," in particular the coital imperative, are central to the experience of sex and intimacy after cancer. This is because embodied sexual changes cannot be conceptualized as separate from cultural discourse, or from the intrapsychic negotiation in which people with cancer and their partners engage, in order to make sense of sexual changes following cancer.

A significant proportion of women in the present study reported renegotiating sexual activity through exploring noncoital sexual practices and through focusing on intimacy. This suggests that, rather than the cancer-affected body being positioned as the site of failure or abjection (Manderson, 2005), it can be conceptualized as a "key site of transgression" (Williams, 1998, p. 63), serving to challenge the narrow definition of "sex" as penis-vaginal penetration, in order to return to prior modes of sexual enjoyment, or expand current practices in positive ways. This "progress narrative" of sex (Potts, Grace, Vares, & Gavey, 2006, p. 234), which acknowledges that sexuality can change and develop, as well as take on new meanings and different modes, has been reported in a minority of accounts in previous research outside of the context of cancer, where hetero-sex is positioned as "more than intercourse" or "beyond intercourse" (McPhillips et al., 2001, p. 234).

At the same time, while cultural representations of sexually active people invariably focus on young people (Sawin, 2012), the findings of the present study demonstrate that older women can continue to enjoy sex and want to explore different ways of achieving sexual pleasure, in the context of cancer, confirming previous reports that sexual desire and activity can continue into older age (Loe, 2004; Rheaume & Mitty, 2008; Watters & Boyd, 2009). Our finding that a number of women were satisfied with nonpenetrative sex also supports previous research, which reported that sex that is less focused on penetration, and more focused on genital touching and other forms of intimacy, may be preferred by many midlife and older women (Potts, Gavey, Grace, & Vares, 2003; Winterich, 2003). Cancer may serve to legitimate such women resisting the coital imperative.

However, it is also the case that penetrative sex is important for many women (Potts, Gavey, Grace, & Vares, 2004), reflected in accounts in the present study of some women wanting to continue to engage in sexual intercourse even if it caused pain, as has been reported in previous cancer research (Jensen et al., 2004). For other women, the inability to engage in coital sex was experienced as a significant loss. Health professionals therefore need to be aware that there are many ways of experiencing and negotiating changes to sexuality after cancer, and that it is important not to make assumptions about the sexual practices of individual women with cancer, based on factors such as age, relationship status, or sexual orientation.

Penetrative sex is also a common part of the sexual repertoire of many lesbians (Roberts, Sorensen, Patsdaughter, & Grindel, 2000); however, it is less likely to be the focus of sexual interaction (Rothblum, 1994), which may explain why bodily changes, such as vaginal dryness, have previously been reported to have less impact on lesbian sexual well-being or relationships (Boehmer, Potter, & Bowen, 2009; Winterich, 2003). In the present study, there was less evidence of changes to sexual practices post-cancer in nonheterosexual relationships, as nonpenetrative practices and nongenital intimacy were already a central part of the lesbian and polysexual repertoire. There was also less evidence of body image concerns. This confirms previous findings that lesbians with cancer report lower levels of sexual concern and less disruption in sexual activity (Arena et al., 2007), as well as less concern about their appearance, than heterosexual women with cancer (Arena et al., 2007; Fobair et al., 2001). Further research is needed to examine sexual changes and renegotiation after cancer in a broader population of lesbian, bisexual, polysexual, and transgender women, who have been described as an "overlooked health disparity" (Brown & Tracy, 2008, p. 1009) in the context of cancer.

In conclusion, the findings outlined in this study are of significance to clinicians, as sexual well-being is central to psychological well-being and quality of life, and sexual intimacy has been found to make the experience of cancer more manageable and assist in the recovery process (Schultz & Van de Wiel, 2003). Therapists and other health professionals can play an important role in ameliorating concerns surrounding sexual well-being after cancer, offering specific suggestions related to sexual enhancement products, emotional adjustment to sexual changes, and information for partners (Herbenick et al., 2008; Ussher et al., 2012b). In this vein, the present study was part of a broader research program within which a self-help intervention to address sexual concerns following cancer was developed and administered, either on its own or as part of a minimal intervention—a one-hour session with a trained health professional. The self-help booklet Sexuality, Intimacy, and Cancer (2010) contains information about the changes to the sexual body and sexual feelings following cancer; the impact of treatment; strategies of maintaining or renegotiating sexuality; strategies for communicating with partners and health professionals; information for partners; information for single people; and information for those in heterosexual and same-sex relationships. This resource was reported to be very beneficial by participants who took part in the research, both on its own and as part of the session with the therapist, who was able to discuss specific sexual concerns. In particular, participants reported that the intervention normalized sexual changes after cancer, facilitated communication about sex, increased understanding, and assisted with renegotiation, as is evidenced by the following accounts: "It reaffirmed for me that how I am is 'all right'—that there is nothing wrong with me. Great opportunity to open up conversation about it" (Zoe, 48, pwc, breast, hetero); "we now have more open communication about how we see each other and what we both need and want sexually" (Kristen, 24, pwc, non-Hodgkin's lymphoma, hetero); "I guess I'm pretty old fashioned and . . . probably very naive as well, but I just found it really opened my eyes to a lot that I didn't know. So that was very helpful" (Imogen, 64, pt, lung, hetero).

This type of intervention could be provided to women with cancer and their partners by health professionals who are engaged in generic cancer care, following the PLISSIT model of providing permission, limited information, specific suggestions, and intensive therapy (Annon, 1981). It legitimates the discussion of sex and intimacy within couple relationships, and discussion with health professionals ("permission"), as well as providing "limited information" and "specific suggestions" about changes to sexuality following cancer. It could be utilized in a similar manner by therapists who are providing care outside of a cancer context, but whose clients, or the client's partner, may have a diagnosis of cancer, and as a result have experienced sexual changes and concerns. Finally, this type of resource may be useful as part of a sexually focused therapy with women who have cancer, providing written information that can supplement therapist suggestions and interventions, and normalize the experience of sexual changes in the context of cancer. Sexual changes after cancer may be one of the most devastating long-term consequences of survivorship, but there are many ways in which intimacy and sexual relationships can be maintained or renegotiated, with or without therapeutic intervention.

ACKNOWLEDGMENTS

This research was funded by an Australian Research Council Linkage Grant, LP0883344, in conjunction with the Cancer Council New South Wales and the National Breast Cancer Foundation. We received in-kind support from Westmead Hospital and Nepean Hospital.

The chief investigators on the project were Jane Ussher, Janette Perz, and Emilee Gilbert, and the partner investigators were Gerard Wain, Gill Batt, Kendra Sundquist, Kim Hobbs, Catherine Mason, Laura Kirsten, and Sue Carrick. We thank Tim Wong, Caroline Joyce, and Emma Hurst for research support and assistance.

Portions of this chapter were adapted, with permission from Wolters Kluwer, from:

Ussher, J. M., Perz, J., Gilbert, E. (2012). Changes to sexual well-being and intimacy after breast cancer. *Cancer Nursing, 35*(6), 456–465.

Ussher, J. M., Perz, J., Gilbert, E., Wong, W. K. T., & Hobbs, K. (2003). Renegotiating sex and intimacy after cancer: Resisting the coital imperative. *Cancer Nursing, 36*(6), 454–462.

REFERENCES

Andersen, B. L. (2009). In sickness and in health: Maintaining intimacy after breast cancer recurrence. *The Cancer Journal, 15,* 70–73.

Andersen, B. L., & Hacker, N. F. (1983). Psychosexual adjustment after vulvar surgery. *Obsetrics and Gynaecology, 62,* 457–462.

Annon, J. S. (1981). PLISSIT therapy. In Corsine, R. J. (Ed.), *Handbook of Innovative Psychotherapies* (pp. 629–639). New York: Wiley and Sons.

Archibald, S., Lemieux, S., Byers, E. S., Tamlyn, K., & Worth, J. (2006). Chemically-induced menopause and the sexual functioning of breast cancer survivors. *Women & Therapy, 29,* 83–106.

Arena, P. L., Carver, C. S., Antoni, M. H., Weiss, S., Ironson, G., & Durán, R. E. (2007). Psychosocial responses to treatment for breast cancer among lesbian and heterosexual women. *Women & Health, 44,* 81–102. doi: 10.1300/J013v44n02_05.

Australian Institute of Health and Welfare (AIHW). (2010). Cancer in Australia 2010: An overview (Vol. Cancer series no. 60. Cat. no. CAN 56). Canberra: AIHW.

Ayling, K., & Ussher, J. M. (2008). "If sex hurts, am I still a woman?" The subjective experience of vulvodynia in hetero-sexual women. *Archives of Sexual Behavior, 37,* 294–304. doi: 10.1007/s10508-007-9204-1.

Basson, R. (2010). Sexual function of women with chronic illness and cancer. *Women's Health, 6,* 407–429. doi: 10.2217/whe.10.23

Beck, A. M., Robinson, J. W., & Carlson, L. E. (2009). Sexual intimacy in heterosexual couples after prostate cancer treatment: What we know and what we still need to learn. *Urologic Oncology: Seminars and Original Investigations, 27,* 137–143. doi: 10.1016/j.urolonc.2007.11.032.

Bergmark, K., Avall-Lundqvist, E., Dickman, P. W., Henningsohn, L., & Steineck, G. (1999). Vaginal changes and sexuality in women with a history of cervical cancer. *The New England Journal of Medicine, 340,* 1383–1389.

Bertero, C., & Wilmoth, M. C. (2007). Breast cancer diagnosis and its treatment affecting the self. *Cancer Nursing, 30,* 194–202.

Boehmer, U., Potter, J., & Bowen, D. J. (2009). Sexual functioning after cancer in sexual minority women. *The Cancer Journal, 15,* 65–69.

Braun, V., & Clarke, V. (2006). Using thematic analysis in psychology. *Qualitative Research in Psychology, 3,* 77–101.

Brown, J. P., & Tracy, J. K. (2008). Lesbians and cancer: An overlooked health disparity. *Cancer Causes & Control, 19,* 1009–1020.

Burwell, S. R., Case, D. L., Kaelin, C., & Avis, N. E. (2006). Sexual problems in younger women after breast cancer surgery. *Journal of Clinical Oncology, 24,* 2815–2821.

Bury, M. (1991). The sociology of chronic illness: A review of research and prospects. *Sociology of Health & Illness, 13,* 451–468.

Butler, L., Banfiled, V., Sveinson, T., Allen, K., Downe-Wanboldt, B., & Alteneder, R. R. (1998). Conceptualizing sexual health in cancer care. *Western Journal of Nursing Research, 20,* 683–705.

Carolan, M., Meneses, K. D., Shell, J. A., & Zhang, Y. (2008). The longitudinal effects of cancer treatment on sexuality in individuals with lung cancer [Clinical report]. *Oncology Nursing Forum, 35,* 73–79.

Deleuze, G., & Guattari, F. (1988). *A Thousand Plateaus: Capitalism and schizophrenia.* London: Athlone.

Fobair, P., O'Hanlan, K., Koopman, C., Classen, C., Dimiceli, S., Drooker, N., . . . Spiegel, D. (2001). Comparison of lesbian and heterosexual women's response to newly diagnosed breast cancer. *Psycho-Oncology, 10,* 40–51. doi: 10.1002/1099-1611(200101/02)10:1<40::aid-pon480>3.0.co;2-s.

Fobair, P., Stewart, S. L., Chang, S., D'Onofrio, C., Banks, P. J., & Bloom, J. R. (2006). Body image and sexual problems in young women with breast cancer. *Psycho-Oncology, 15,* 579–594.

Fox, N. (1993). *Postmodernism, sociology, and health.* Milton Keynes: Open University Press.

Fox, N. (2002). Refracting "health": Deleuze, Guatarri, and the body-self. *Health, 6,* 347–363.

Frank, A. W. (1993). The rhetoric of self-change: Illness experience as narrative. *The Sociological Quarterly, 34,* 39–52.

Garrusi, B., & Faezee, H. (2008). How do Iranian women with breast cancer conceptualise sex and body image? *Sex and Disability, 26,* 159–165.

Gavey, N., McPhillips, K., & Braun, V. (1999). Interruptus coitus: Heterosexuals accounting for intercourse. *Sexualities, 2,* 35–68. doi:10.1177/136346099002001003.

Gilbert, E., Ussher, J. M., & Hawkins, Y. (2009). Accounts of disruptions to sexuality following cancer: The perspective of informal carers who are partners of a person with cancer. *Health: An Interdisciplinary Journal, 13,* 523–541.

Gilbert, E., Ussher, J. M., & Perz, J. (2010a). Renegotiating sexuality and intimacy in the context of cancer: The experiences of carers. *Archives of Sexual Behavior, 39,* 998–1009. doi: 10.1007/s10508-008-9416-z.

Gilbert, E., Ussher, J. M., & Perz, J. (2010b). Sexuality after breast cancer: A review. *Mauritius, 66,* 397–407.

Gilbert, E., Ussher, J. M., & Perz, J. (2011). Sexuality after gynaecological cancer: A review of the material, intrapsychic, and discursive aspects of treatment on women's sexual-wellbeing. *Maturitas, 70,* 42–57. doi: 10.1016/j.maturitas.2011 .06.013.

Green, M. S., Naumann, R. W., Elliot, M., Hall, J. B., Higgins, R. V., & Grigsby, J. H. (2000). Sexual dysfunction following vulvectomy. *Gynecologic Oncology, 77,* 73–77. doi: 10.1006/gyno.2000.5745.

Grumann, M., Robertson, R., Hacker, N. F., & Sommer, G. (2001). Sexual functioning in patients following radical hysterectomy for stage IB cancer of the
cervix. *International Journal of Gynecological Cancer, 11*, 372–380.

Hawkins, Y., Ussher, J. M., Gilbert, E., Perz, J., Sandoval, M., & Sundquist, K.
(2009). Changes in sexuality and intimacy after the diagnosis of cancer. The
experience of partners in a sexual relationship with a person with cancer.
Cancer Nursing, 34, 271–280.

Herbenick, D., Reece, M., Hollub, A., Satinsky, S., & Dodge, B. (2008). Young
female breast cancer survivors. Their sexual function and interest in sexual
enhancement products and services. *Cancer Nursing, 31*, 417–425.

Holmes, L. (2005). Sexuality in gynaecological cancer patients. *Cancer Nursing
Practice, 4*, 35–39.

Hordern, A. J., & Street, A. F. (2007). Communicating about patient sexuality and
intimacy after cancer: Mismatched expectations and unmet needs. *Medical
Journal of Australia, 186*, 224–227.

Hyde, A. (2007). The politics of heterosexuality—a missing discourse in cancer
nursing literature on sexuality: A discussion paper. *International Journal of
Nursing Studies, 44*, 315–325. doi: 10.1016/j.ijnurstu.2006.03.020.

Jensen, P. T., Groenvold, M., Klee, M. C., Thranov, I., Petersen, M. A., & Machin, D.
(2004). Early-stage cervical carcinoma, radical hysterectomy, and sexual
function. *Cancer, 100*, 97–106. doi: 10.1002/cncr.11877.

Juraskova, I., Butow, P., Robertson, R., Sharpe, L., McLeod, C., & Hacker, N.
(2003). Post-treatment sexual adjustment following cervical and endometrial cancer: A qualitative insight. *Psycho-Oncology, 12*, 267–279. doi: 10
.1002/pon.639.

Kayser, K., Watson, L. E., & Andrade, J. T. (2007). Cancer as a "we-disease": Examining the process of coping from a relational perspective. *Families, Systems,
& Health, 25*, 404–418.

Kelly, M., & Field, D. (1996). Medical sociology, chronic illness and the body. *Sociology of Health & Illness, 18*, 241–257. doi: 10.1111/1467-9566.ep10934993.

Lamb, M. A., & Sheldon, T. A. (1994). The sexual adaptation of women treated for
endometrial cancer. *Cancer Practice, 2*, 103–113.

Leder, D. (1990). *The absent body.* Chicago: University of Chicago Press.

Little, M., Jordens, C. F. C., & Sayers, E. (2003). Discourse communities and the
discourse of experience. *Health, 7*, 78–86.

Little, M., & Sayers, E. (2004). While there's life . . . hope and the experience of
cancer. *Social Science and Medicine, 59*, 1329–1337.

Loe, M. (2004). Sex and the senior woman: Pleasure and danger in the Viagra era.
Sexualities, 7, 303–326. doi: 10.1177/1363460704044803.

Manderson, L. (2005). Boundary breaches: The body, sex and sexuality after stoma
surgery. *Social Science and Medicine, 61*, 405–415.

McPhillips, K., Braun, V., & Gavey, N. (2001). Defining (hetero)sex: How imperative is the coital imperative? *Women's Studies International Forum, 24*,
229–240.

Meyerowitz, B., Desmond, K., Rowland, J., Wyatt, G., & Ganz, P. (1999). Sexuality following breast cancer. *Journal of Sex and Marital Therapy, 25,* 237–250. doi: 10.1080/00926239908403998.

Oliffe, J. (2005). Constructions of masculinity following prostatectomy-induced impotence. *Social Science and Medicine, 60,* 2249–2259. doi: 10.1016/j .socscimed.2004.10.016.

Potts, A., Gavey, N., Grace, V., & Vares, T. (2004). The downside of Viagra: Women's experiences and concerns. *Sociology of Health and Illness, 25,* 697–719.

Potts, A., Gavey, N., Grace, V. M., & Vares, T. (2003). The downside of Viagra: Women's experiences and concerns. *Sociology of Health & Illness, 25,* 697–719. doi: 10.1046/j.1467-9566.2003.00366.x.

Potts, A., Grace, V. M., Vares, T., & Gavey, N. (2006). "Sex for life"? Men's counter-stories on "erectile dysfunction," male sexuality and ageing. *Sociology of Health & Illness, 28,* 306–329. doi: 10.1111/j.1467-9566.2006.00494.x.

Ramirez, M., McMullen, C., Grant, M., Altschuler, A., Hornbrook, M. C., & Krouse, R. S. (2010). Figuring out sex in a reconfigured body: Experiences of female colorectal cancer survivors with ostomies. *Women & Health, 49,* 608–624. doi: 10.1080/03630240903496093.

Rheaume, C., & Mitty, E. (2008). Sexuality and intimacy in older adults. *Geriatric Nursing, 29,* 342–349. doi: 10.1016/j.gerinurse.2008.08.004.

Roberts, S. J., Sorensen, L., Patsdaughter, C. A., & Grindel, C. (2000). Sexual behaviors and sexually transmitted diseases of lesbians. *Journal of Lesbian Studies, 4,* 49–70. doi: 10.1300/J155v04n03_03.

Rothblum, E. D. (1994). Transforming lesbian sexuality. *Psychology of Women Quarterly, 18,* 627–641. doi: 10.1111/j.1471-6402.1994.tb01051.x.

Sawin, E. M. (2012). The body gives way, things happen: Older women describe breast cancer with a non-supportive intimate partner. *European Journal of Oncology Nursing, 16,* 64–70. doi: 10.1016/j.ejon.2011.03.006.

Schultz, W. C. M., & Van de Wiel, H. B. M. (2003). Sexuality, intimacy and gynaecological cancer. *JSMT, 29,* 121–128.

Sekse, R. J. T., Raaheim, M., Blaaka, G., & Gjengedal, E. (2010). Life beyond cancer: Women's experiences 5 years after treatment for gynaecological cancer. *Scandinavian Journal of Caring Sciences, 24,* 799–807. doi: 10.1111/j.1471-6712 .2010.00778.x.

Sexuality intimacy and cancer self-help guide. (2010). Sexuality, intimacy and cancer: A self-help guide for people with cancer and their partner. Retrieved from http://www.uws.edu.au/chr/centre_for_health_research/research/ cancer_and_sexuality.

Stead, M. L., Fallowfield, L., Selby, P., & Brown, J. M. (2007). Psychosexual function and impact of gynaecological cancer. *Best Practice & Research Clinical Obstetrics & Gynaecology, 21,* 309–320. doi: 10.1016/j.bpobgyn.2006.11.008.

Traa, M. J., De Vries, J., Roukema, J. A., & Den Oudsten, B. L. (2012). Sexual (dys) function and the quality of sexual life in patients with colorectal cancer: A systematic review. *Annals of Oncology, 23,* 19–27. doi: 10.1093/annonc/mdr133.

Ussher, J. M. (2000). Women's madness: A material-discursive-intra psychic approach. In Fee, D. (Ed.), *Psychology and the postmodern: Mental illness as discourse and experience* (pp. 207–230). London: Sage.

Ussher, J. M., Perz, J., & Gilbert, E. (2012a). Changes to sexual well-being and intimacy after breast cancer. *Cancer Nursing*. doi:10.1097/NCC.0b013e3182395401.

Ussher, J. M., Perz, J., & Gilbert, E. (2012b). Information needs associated with changes to sexual well-being after breast cancer. *Journal of Advanced Nursing*. doi: 10.1111/j.1365-2648.2012.06010.x.

Ussher, J. M., Perz, J., Gilbert, E., Wong, W. K. T., & Hobbs, K. (2012). Renegotiating sex after cancer: Resisting the coital imperative. *Cancer Nursing, 35.*

Watters, Y., & Boyd, T. V. (2009). Sexuality in later life: Opportunity for reflections for healthcare providers. *Sexual and Relationship Therapy, 24,* 307–315. doi: 10.1080/14681990903398047.

Weijmar Schultz, W. C. M., Van De Wiel, H. B. M., & Bouma, J. (1991). Psychosexual functioning after treatment for cancer of the cervix: A comparative and longitudinal study. *International Journal of Gynecological Cancer, 1,* 37–46. doi: 10.1111/j.1525-1438.1991.tb00037.x.

Williams, S. J. (1996). The vicissitudes of embodiment across the chronic illness trajectory. *Body and Society, 2,* 23–47.

Williams, S. J. (1998). Bodily dys-order: Desire, excess and the transgression of corporeal boundaries. *Body & Society, 4,* 59–82. doi: 10.1177/1357034x98004002004.

Wilmoth, M. C. (2001). The aftermath of breast cancer: An altered sexual self. *Cancer Nursing, 24,* 278–286.

Winterich, J. A. (2003). Sex, menopause, and culture: Sexual orientation and the meaning of menopause for women's sex lives. *Gender & Society, 17,* 627–642. doi: 10.1177/0891243203253962.

Young, I. M. (1992). Breasted experience: The look and the feeling. In Leder, D. (Ed.), *The Body in Medical Thought and Practice* (pp. 215–232). Dordrecht, Netherlands: Kluwer Academic Publishers.

Chapter 15

Family Caregiver Support to Cancer Patients: The Relevance of Adult Children

Ricardo Joao Texeira and Maria Graca Pereira

INTRODUCTION

Cancer is a disease of global importance with 7.6 million deaths related to the disease occurring in 2008 (World Health Organization, 2012). More than 3 million new cases of cancer were diagnosed in Europe in 2006 (Ferlay et al., 2007), and around 1.6 million new cases were estimated in the United States in 2012. Although there are a high number of cancer deaths, survival has increased considerably, with estimated five-year survival rates ranging from 51 percent in the United Kingdom to 67 percent in the United States (American Cancer Society, 2012; Cancer Research UK, 2012). Consequently, an increasing number of patients and families have had to deal with the disease and respective consequences, as well as with the fear of recurrence for longer periods of time. The advances in medicine, in recent decades, have contributed to the changing of the myth of cancer as a terminal illness. This disease is increasingly considered a chronic condition, implying that the family will assume a key role in providing differentiated care (especially emotional support) to the oncological patient (Raveis, Karus, & Pretter,

1999). It is natural that, after a cancer diagnosis, fears and concerns arise leading patients' families to readjust themselves, in order to protect and satisfy their needs (Lewis, 2010). From this readaptation of the family, in functional and structural terms, it is a common stand that a primary caregiver assumes a part of the ongoing physical and/or psychosocial support and care to the patient. Thus, the experience of cancer generates suffering, worries, and losses, both in the patient and their family members, but particularly in the primary care provider.

During the 1990s, significant changes emerged in the demography of caregiving in the United States (Wolff & Kasper, 2006). By 1999, for example, the proportion of adult children as primary caregivers had increased to 41.3 percent. During the same decade, the proportion of patients receiving help in instrumental activities of daily living decreased, whereas the proportion receiving help for five or more personal activities of daily living increased. Consistent with the trend for more adult children to assume the caregiving role of their parents and for older adults to manifest poorer health, the proportion of caregivers providing help on a daily basis increased substantially between 1989 and 1999, with this change being most noticeable among adult children caregivers (Stephens & Franks, 2009). Although the share of men among adult children caregivers has increased slightly during the 1990s, the caregiver role remains highly gendered, with almost three quarters of all adult children caregivers being women in 1999 (Wolff & Kasper, 2006). Even though men also provide caregiving assistance, female caregivers spend as much as 50 percent more time providing care than do their male counterparts (Wolff & Kasper, 2006). Since the early 1980s, a great deal of attention has been paid to middle-aged women who provide parent care and simultaneously occupy other family and professional roles. These women have often been mentioned as "women in the middle" (Brody, 2004). This label can refer to the generational position of these women, between the older generation of their parents and the younger generation of their children, but it can also refer to their chronological age, since these women are in the middle years of the life span (Brody, 2004). Although awareness of "women in the middle" began more than 30 years ago, the issues and concerns raised at that time appear to be even more applicable to today's women and those who will enter midlife in the near future. According to census data, one-half of American middle-aged women are married and in the paid labor force, and more than one-third are married and have a child under the age of 18 (Stephens & Franks, 2009). Therefore, today's middle-aged women are more in the middle than ever before (Brody, 2004).

The importance of the support provided by the adult children of cancer patients, their perceptions, reactions, and experiences, was the keystone for this chapter. The present work constitutes an important contribution to the study of the biopsychosocial impact of parental cancer on the personal and familial life of adult children caregivers. The act of caring is an attitude that represents a moment of attention, zeal, concern, responsibility, and emotional involvement to the other. Although the caregiver is usually the family member who provides the majority of the care that the cancer patient requires, the primary caregiver is not always the only family member who provides care, since this attitude may be present, indeed very often, in children. The caregiving of family members has psychological, physical, social, and family implications (Deeken, Taylor, Mangan, Yabroff, & Ingham, 2003; Payne & Ellis-Hill, 2001). In the context of cancer, these effects can directly influence caregivers' quality of life (Clark et al., 2006), especially considering that 30 percent of family caregivers experience distress (Blanchard, Toseland, & McCallion, 1996). According to Clark et al. (2006), family caregivers tend to restrict their social activities, to neglect their own health, and to develop psychological morbidity. The stress and burden of adult children, greatly depending on the stage and disease progression of the parent, are aspects to consider, since this situation induces discomfort in the caregiver as well as in his/her own nuclear family (Goodman, 2005).

Most studies in psycho-oncology focus on the perspective of the cancer patient. Care providers (formal and informal) also received some attention in research, although studies centered in family caregiving are a trend, particularly in the case of spouses, parents (in the case of pediatric oncology), and children, usually young children and/or teenagers. Research has not been exploring the particular perspective of the adult children of cancer patients. Thus, this chapter seeks to explore this phenomenon, starting from the assumption that there are different interpretations and experiences during the life cycle. Research on parental cancer is underlined by the notion that this is a significant psychosocial stressor that can be a serious challenge in terms of coping and adjustment, at least in the short term. However, according to Leedham and Meyerowitz (1999), it is still unknown if parental cancer (when diagnosed in childhood or adolescence) has psychosocial effects that last into adulthood. Data, although limited, suggest a low probability of adverse effects on patients' offspring's psychological health. Still, for the authors, some continuing effects of this experience may be too subtle for evaluation by common measures of psychological adjustment. In addition, the data in this field of study have produced limited practical information to health care professionals who work with cancer patients. Thus, there are very limited theoretical and practical available resources to be offered to patients who ask how they can be sure that, over time, their children will be alright (Leedham & Meyerowitz, 1999).

According to Veach and Nicholas (1998), it is estimated that three out of four families face the problem of oncological disease throughout the life span. In addition, researchers note that many family members are deeply and painfully affected by the cancer of a loved one (Leedham & Meyerowitz, 1999). Only recently, clinicians and researchers began to conceptualize the family of the cancer patient as a treatment unit, instead of just the patient. However, the impact of cancer in the family remains a relatively under-studied phenomenon. After a few pioneering studies, we now know more about the impact of cancer in the offspring of patients with regard to how they interpret and adapt their family environment, as well as their own family coping styles, especially when they enter adulthood (Kahle & Jones, 2000; Mosher & Danoff-Burg, 2005).

A review of the literature suggests that children of cancer patients suffer a profound impact from the experience with an ill parent. For example, children and adolescents of cancer patients were indicated as a hidden risk group who may suffer from vegetative disorders, psychological symptoms, avoidance behavior, school problems, and probable long-term changes in levels of self-esteem and cognitive functioning (Leedham & Meyerowitz, 1999). However, little is known about how adolescents, in the transition to adulthood, and adult children perceive and adapt to parental cancer and whether they perceive it as a catalyst for change in their family context.

As mentioned, most of the studies on the impact of cancer in the family have focused on samples of patients and/or spouses, having explored insufficiently the adult children perspective (Faulkner & Davey, 2002). For Mosher and Danoff-Burg (2005), it is important to study separately these experiences of care between spouses and adult children, as research documents differentiated perceptions of burden and adaptive resources for these groups. In addition, most of the studies that focused on the family context of cancer patients have neglected the sample selection and merely compared between the two types of family systems in terms of oncological disease: those who appear to have reduced levels of distress and those with high levels of distress. For example, studies have shown that families characterized by high cohesion and low levels of conflict seem to show lower levels of distress and higher levels of adaptation to the crisis of cancer when compared to families with the opposite characteristics (Schulz, Schultz, Schultz, & Von Kerekjarto, 1996). Other variables, such as the level of flexibility among family systems, open communication among family members, and a strong sense of cohesion, were associated with high levels of adaptation in families with a history of cancer (Rustad, 1984; Schulz et al., 1996). Despite the relevance of this acquaintance in under-standing the relationships between context and family functioning, the literature lacks studies comparing families affected by cancer and adequate controls, or those families without disease (Kahle & Jones, 2000). In fact, only when the scope of the investigation is extended to include a greater number of chronic diseases will the results of comparative studies of affected and nonaffected families by chronic illnesses be more enlightening. Results from preliminary studies indicate that families, whose members suffer from a chronic illness, tend to experience higher levels of conflict and lower levels of cohesion when compared to control families (Dura & Beck, 1988; Peters & Esses, 1985). However, these studies normally involve small samples and address diseases such as chronic pain, diabetes, and arthritis. Therefore, more studies are needed to confirm the preliminary results and to ascertain generalizations for those who have a parent with cancer. In fact, one may conclude that how patients and their partners react and adapt when confronted with a diagnosis of cancer has been a much wider focus of investigation than the focus on patients' children. The few studies conducted with adult children, and a larger number with children in preschool and/or adolescents, allow us to draw conclusions that contribute to the growing field of research on the implications of parental cancer in adult children, while encouraging future investigations.

FAMILY CAREGIVERS OF ONCOLOGICAL PATIENTS

Psychological Distress

Cancer occurs in the context of a family system, producing negative effects on the functioning of the system and each of its members. As a system, the behavior of each of its members is inseparable from the behavior of others, and there is a circularity in the relationship between patient and family (Bloom, 1996). Therefore, the diagnosis of cancer in a person is able to affect the entire family system, and depending on how well the system adjusts and adapts, this diagnosis can have positive or negative effects on the patient. The negative impact on the family system is associated with the crisis that originated when the diagnosis was confirmed. This will correspond to a situation in which the adjustment and the internal or external balance of the system (or the individual) was disturbed, triggering a series of structural, psychological, economic, and social changes, at family and individual levels (Rolland, 2004).

According to Lewis (2010), the families of cancer patients experience the same demands and challenges as the patients themselves. The way families adapt and cope with the illness of one of the members has a major impact on the physical and psychosocial well-being of their members, as well as in the clinical course of the disease itself (Tansella, 1995). The 1980s contributed greatly to the study of the relationship between family and disease, both in terms of diversity of perspectives around the phenomenon, as well as in the development theoretical models. However, the research unit was much more focused on the patient than on the family system as a whole. For example, research with members of the family system emerged with samples of the parental subsystem, particularly in situations of pediatric cancer (Fuemmeler, Brown, Williams, & Barredo, 2003; Given et al., 1993), and of the marital subsystem, in which the spouse was the primary caregiver (Axelsson & Sjöden, 1998; Douglass, 1997). In addition, the knowledge of the genetic mechanisms of some forms of cancer has been alerting the community to various dangers, especially with regard to the possible effect of carcinogens (Singhal, Vachani, Antin-Ozerkis, Kaiser, & Abelda, 2005), and investigation in this field has led to the modification of policies to prevent disease and promote health in oncology (Patenaude, 2005). According to Baanders and Heijmans (2007), the diagnosis and treatment of cancer often involve needs and caregiving tasks that directly affect patients' family members. The consequences of the caregiver role are multiple, from the household economy to the physical and mental health (Nijboer et al., 1998). Studies indicate that the diagnosis of cancer causes, very often, distress in patients and informal caregivers, in the form of depression, severe levels of anxiety, and stress (Edwards & Clarke, 2004). However, Vanderwerker, Laff, Kadan-Lottick, McColl, and Prigerson (2005) report that there is little research effectively available on the prevalence of mental disorders among caregivers of cancer patients, since practically all studies used only symptoms inventories. The literature review carried out by Keller, Henrich, Sellschopp, and Beutel (1996) found psychological symptomatology in spouses of cancer patients, especially mood disorders and anxiety, as well as physical and psychosomatic symptoms. The authors estimate that between 20 percent and 30 percent of spouses have psychologically debilitating mood disorders. In turn, Kissane, Bloch, Burns, Mckenzie, and Posterino (1994) reported that 35 percent of spouses had depression and 28 percent of children have high levels of depression and hostility. Akechi et al. (2006) reported that, among relatives of cancer patients treated in mental health services, nearly 90 percent were spouses, presenting complaints compatible with adjustment disorders and major depression. Using recognized instruments for assessing psychological morbidity, the studies of Nijboer et al. (1998) and Chentsova-Dutton et al. (2002) found that six months after surgery, 20 percent of cancer patients' caregivers had depression, and 23 percent of caregivers of hospitalized patients showed scores above the cutoff for depression. In Vanderwerker's et al. (2005) study, the mental health of 200 caregivers of advanced cancer patients was assessed with a rigorous psychiatric interview, and results showed that 13 percent of caregivers suffered from a psychiatric disorder. In terms of diagnostic criteria, 8 percent had a panic disorder, 4.5 percent major depression, 4 percent post-traumatic stress disorder (PTSD), and 3.5 percent generalized anxiety. It is important to emphasize that only 46 percent of caregivers who had a psychiatric disorder sought help in mental health services. Caring for a loved one can be a highly stressful and even traumatic experience, but despite the most recent attention to the psychosocial consequences of informal caregiving, there is still a paucity of studies on the prevalence of mental disorders and the use of mental health services (Goodman, 2005). Spouses and other family members, including children, are key elements in the familial and social support to cancer patients, evidencing that most of them deal well with the caregiver role. However, as Pitceathly and Maguire (2003) note, an important minority has high levels of distress, developing affective disorders. Caregiver gender is also a particularly important variable in studies with care providers, since women seem to be the most vulnerable. In particular, women with a history of previous psychological morbidity tend to have a more negative perception of the impact of the disease (Loscalzo, Kim, & Clark, 2010). The distress in the caregiver also has an association with disease progression to palliative care (Payne & Ellis-Hill, 2001). The lack of a support network in caregivers (Nijboer et al., 1998) and the existence of relational difficulties with the patient (Kuscu et al., 2009) are considered risk factors.

Burden

Several studies have shown the important contribution that informal caregivers provide for patients with chronic diseases, particularly the elderly and cancer patients, taking into account the changes that have been occurring in the health care system of many countries (Ducharme et al., 2006). However, it is noteworthy that this obligation to care for a sick family member carries a set of changes in the family, for which some caregivers are not prepared. The diagnosis of cancer causes a cascade of changes in the routines, rituals, and rules of the family, as well as in the redistribution of roles and new responsibilities. These changes lead to a series of biopsychosocial disorders labeled in the literature as "burden." The concept of burden was first introduced in the literature by Grad and Sainsbury (1966), who defined it as any negative consequences to the family of the sick person. It arises as a result of mandatory care for a sick family member, particularly in contexts of prolonged illness (Chou, 2000). More currently, burden has been defined in a multidimensional perspective, as a physical, psychological, emotional, social, or financial problem sensed by the caregiver (Lidell, 2002).

The responses of caregivers, in the face of this need to provide care, may be influenced by two phenomena which consist in the existence of a prior relationship between the provider and the receiver of the care, and in the personal characteristics of both (Yeh, Johnson, & Wang, 2002). In this perspective, the concept of burden includes how caregiving activities affect the financial status and the social, emotional, and physical well-being of the family member who plays the role of caregiver. In turn, Chou (2000) defines burden as a mediating force between the physical commitment of the patient and the impact that caring has on the lives of caregivers and their families. This author divides burden in objective and subjective terms. Objective burden is related to events and activities associated with negative experiences of care, and subjective burden is related to the feelings aroused in caregivers during the performance of their caring responsibilities.

Stetz (2003) states that the role of family caregivers tends to grow as a result of the advances in technology and increased survival rates of cancer patients. This increased responsibility required of family members and significant others promotes significant distress on informal caregivers, given their insufficient psychological preparation in the face of the demands that the disease imposes. This mainly psychological burden is described by Tebb (1995) as the inability to be resilient, to the extent that each provider realizes that his/her physical, social, mental, and spiritual condition is suffering as a result of the dedication to the tasks of caregiving. Deeken et al. (2003) stress that this overload, caused by the experience of caring for a sick family member, is felt in an extremely subjective way. These differences emerge as a result of the influence of various factors, such as the personality of the caregiver, available social resources, functional status of the family, and the existence of other commitments that compete with the development of the caregiver activities. For the patient's family, the disease represents a high burden. As mentioned, this burden includes economic issues, since a large number of informal carers are forced to implement significant changes in their lives, such as leave or change jobs, in order to provide care to the sick family member. The increased responsibilities related to these sources of burden can easily cause an imbalance between demands and resources of caregivers, leading to serious consequences such as: emotional imbalance, physical illness, and drastic lifestyle changes (Lidell, 2002).

In the case of adult children, and in addition to the aspects mentioned above, these caregivers may be working outside their home and feel torn between the demands of the job and the needs of their ill parent, not to mention the needs of their own family. Therefore, care providers may report feeling more tired at work, compared to the period preceding the onset of parental illness, and show a decreased ability to concentrate as well as increased absenteeism, which may cause greater uncertainty about their professional future (Stetz, 2003). This overload of work and responsibilities, imposed on adult children, can make it impossible for them to provide adequate emotional support to the patient and may actually contribute to the adult children's distress. More specifically, when family caregivers experience higher burden, it is more likely that the patients do not feel their needs satisfied—in other words, there seems to be an inverse correlation between the activity level of the patient and the psychological needs of family caregivers (Deeken et al., 2003). Generally, the literature on family caregivers indicates that it is mainly adult daughters who are heavily involved in informal support and care for dependent parents (Mosher & Weiss, 2010). In fact, these adult children caregivers have been referred to in the literature as the "sandwich generation" or, as previously mentioned, "women in the middle," because of the burden involved in balancing the different demands of multiple roles (Brody, 2004). For example, the results of Kim, Baker, Spillers, and Wellisch (2006) with caregivers of cancer patients, reveal that employed caregivers who have children report higher levels of stress and burden when compared to employed or unemployed caregivers who are childless. In turn, the study of Raveis et al. (1999) reveals that daughters with caregiving responsibilities, employed and with multiple obligations, do not tend to reduce the time of care; instead, they tend to eliminate their leisure time, reduce working hours, or even stop working.

Social Support

In the last decades there has been a significant amount of research on the relationship between stressful life experiences and psychological well-being. In populations more exposed to stressors and adversity, one can better understand the etiology of distress. It is necessary to take into account the vulnerabilities vs. strengths of personality, the type of stressor, and the resources available to respond to stress, whether in the form of social resources or coping strategies (Lloyd, 1995). It is particularly well known the moderating role of social support in individuals with chronic illnesses and their families, since social contact is essential to organic balancing, and the adaptation to the social environment is a factor that can actually decrease disease vulnerability (Symister & Friend, 2003). At the family level, it is known that support strongly contributes to the adjustment and adaptation to stressful events (Moores & Meadow-Orlans, 2002).

The nature of social networks and family relationships of oncology patients represents an important resource for understanding the experience of having cancer (Bloom, 1996). The family, in the oncological setting, is fundamental. In this sense, the family can be equated as an entity that supports but that also needs to be supported. For example, Manne (1994), in a review about spouses' social support in oncology, highlights the importance of understanding the support given and received within a marital relationship. In oncology, the lack of a support network is considered a risk factor in family caregivers. Although in the majority of cases there is some kind of network support, this may not be sufficient or appropriate to the caregiver needs (Pitceathly & Maguire, 2003). According to Fadden, Bebbington, and Kuipers (1987), the burden of family caregivers can be high enough to absorb social activities and leisure time as a consequence.

The importance of social support is undeniable, and emotional support is its most important component. Emotional support to the cancer patient is a crucial active ingredient of the expression of feelings and sorrows and is, therefore, an important part of coping (Grulke et al., 2005). This consideration is imperative for family caregivers, since those who provide informal care to cancer patients are more likely to face greater emotional demands. According to Thomas and Morris (2002), although the diagnosis and treatment of cancer promotes burden, anxiety, and fear in patients and close relatives, it is important to stay positive and focused on hope, despite the fears. Therefore, these authors suggest that emotional support may be crucial for those who are closely involved in caring for a family member with cancer. Caring for a parent with cancer, being employed and married (or living with a partner) are social roles that involve constant interaction and social obligations that potentially can compete with time and attention of the caregiver. A wide circle of social relationships can provide important resources and social support, but holding several roles can hinder the performance of these different functions, creating, ultimately, tension and role confusion (Raveis et al., 1999).

Literature regarding the investigation of social support in adult children caregivers of cancer patients is scarce. However, some studies have given some attention to this topic. For example, Lewandowski (1992) considers the level of disease-related information provided to the adult children, family communication patterns, and the quantity and quality of available social support to be important mediators that influence the way in which these children are affected by having a parent with cancer. Shifren (2008) investigated the parent-child relationships at the time of care, and the children's current perception of social support. The results showed that children who began caregiving in adolescence portrayed their parents as more warm and caring than those who began at earlier ages. Less caregiving tasks were associated with a better perception of current affective support, as well as informational support available to caregivers in adulthood. Shorter durations of the experience of care were associated with stronger relationships in adulthood. Reports of a warm relationship with the patient were associated with higher levels of perceived support in adulthood. Another important result was that the warm relationship of the sick parent with the child caregiver in the first 16 years of life was associated with reports of an increased amount of family and friends available to provide support in adulthood. More recently, the qualitative study conducted by Wong, Ratner, Gladstone, Davtyan, and Koopman (2010) revealed five important themes featuring received and perceived social support during parental illness: listening and understanding, encouragement and security, tangible assistance, communication about cancer and treatment, and return to normal life experiences. The differences in the perception of respondents about the effects of specific forms of received social support underline the need for individualized support to cancer patients' offspring, based on the specific needs and circumstances of each individual.

Family Functioning

The family of the oncological patient faces many issues related to cancer and its treatments, including the caregiving tasks and associated burden (Nijboer et al., 1998), the effects on family interactions (Soothill et al., 2003), changes in family roles (Northouse, Schafer, Tipton, & Metivier, 1999), and communication difficulties (Porter, Keefe, Hurwitz, & Faber, 2005), as well as financial and psychological stresses (Lidell, 2002). At the same time, as with other families, family members need to deal with issues not related to cancer, such as their own health problems and caring for children or other family members (Soothill et al., 2003). Thus, cancer affects not only the cancer patient but also has a strong impact on the lives of family members. Family (dis)functioning represents one of the most important areas of stress for families dealing with the problem of oncological disease, only surpassed by the cancer itself. Unfortunately, almost half of the family members who deal with this disease experience distress in levels similar to the ones felt by the patient, creating a greater strain on the family system (Schulz et al., 1996).

As mentioned previously, almost 30 percent of cancer patients' families experience significant levels of distress, resulting in psychological symptoms requiring professional intervention (Blanchard et al., 1996). Literature indicates that one of the most difficult hurdles for many families to overcome is based on the (in)ability in adapting the system to the demands of the disease. Indeed, the degree of flexibility, or structural adaptation, is considered a basic component of how cancer will impact the family over time (Rait & Lederberg, 1989).

In the last two decades, the focus of family literature moved from a perspective centered on family functioning deficits to a perspective based on their resources and strengths (Walsh, 2003). The resilience of families, and their ability to thrive in the post-adversity, have been studied mainly from the perspective of family stress and coping (Patterson, 2002). Families facing adverse events, such as a cancer diagnosis, can respond with a strengthening of their relations. This finding is consistent with the concepts of positive feedback (Nichols & Schwartz, 2008), deviation amplification mechanisms (Maruyama, 1963), as well as with complexity theory (Warren, Franklin, & Streeter, 1998). These theories postulate that serious adverse events have the potential to trigger second-order change processes that produce fundamental changes in systems, leading to a higher level of functioning, and not necessarily to homeostasis. Family functioning seems to change throughout the course of the disease and treatments, depending on the demands associated with the stage of the disease/treatment (Barakat & Kazak, 1999). In fact, a strong association was found between family cohesion, flexibility, and adjustment in cancer survivors, whether they had recently completed treatment or if they were survivors for more than five years (Rait et al., 1992).

Literature showed that family members' coping is likely to be influenced by other family members. For example, a study with long-term survivors of leukemia, which included the mothers of patients, indicated that families could deal effectively with the disease 10 years after the end of treatment (Kupst et al., 1995). Furthermore, the coping and adjustment of mothers was the strongest predictor of the coping and adjustment of patients, showing the transactional nature of the family coping. Feelings of uncertainty and loneliness, as well as PTSD symptoms, were also reported by parents of childhood cancer survivors, showing the network effects of the disease on the family (Kazak et al., 2004).

According to Rolland (2004), acute and chronic illnesses have the power to affect family functioning. In an acute illness, the readjustments operated in the family occur in a very short time, requiring from the family a faster mobility in the ability to manage the crisis. When the disease is chronic, progressive, and incapacity increases gradually, like in the oncological disease, the adaptation and changing of roles within the family occur progressively. For Rolland (2004), the family is subjected to increasing tension, both because of the risk of burden and the continuous increase of tasks over time.

The family may present feelings of confusion and insecurity in their relationship with the patient, and difficulties may occur in responding to the patient's needs. The family reaction to cancer will be influenced by the role and function of the sick member, since it is different if a mother, a father, or a son/daughter falls ill. In the case of parental cancer, and considering the emotional bond between the patient and the rest of the family, Augusto and Carvalho (2002) find that in a patriarchal family structure, where incomes depend exclusively on the father, the cancer causes a decrease in income and a possible change in household expenditure. When the patient is the mother, the disease tends to produce an emotional and assistential void. As mentioned, a cancer in the family may be perceived as a life event that affects all family members, resulting in changes in the family system, and can manifest itself in various areas of family dynamics: level of interactions, goals, roles, rules, and borders. If the process of adjustment to illness does not occur, and the family is unable to establish and maintain balance, then it will have to resort to mediating factors that might facilitate this adaptation, like support from members of various communities and institutions (McCubbin, Thompson, Thompson, & Fromer, 1998).

Parental cancer has a profound impact, especially on children and adolescents (Huizinga, Visser, van der Graaf, Hoekstra, & Hoekstra-Weebers,

2005). Children often assume caregiver tasks, facing the hard and painful circumstances of the disease, many times motivated by the hope of healing, but also with disappointments, sorrows, and workloads (Johnson & Catalano, 1983). These experiences, according to several authors, tend to intensify disease progression and entry into adulthood (Thomas & Morris, 2002; Thomas, Morris, & Harman, 2002). In addition, patients with children living at home are concerned about the consequences of parental cancer on them and may experience feelings of dissatisfaction about their parenting tasks (Kelley, Sikka, & Venkatesan, 1997).

PTSD AND POST-TRAUMATIC GROWTH

Research shows that children of parents with a chronic disease are at increased risk of developing emotional and behavioral problems than are children with healthy parents. The risk for these problems, however, depends on individual and family variables related to the disease itself (Rolland, 2004). Although quantitative studies contribute to the understanding of the impact of oncological disease on children, they seem, however, biased to the extent that they resort essentially to psychopathological assessment tools, taking a perspective of vulnerability/disability (Mosher & Danoff-Burg, 2005; Power & Dell Orto, 2004). Thus, it is legitimate to ask how it is possible to find transformation and personal growth through the cancer experience, if participants are only assessed in order to "fit" into a pathological diagnosis.

As previously reported, most studies have been addressing the impact of cancer on spouses. The empirical results indicate that many spouses experience social (i.e., isolation) and psychological distress (i.e., anxiety, worry, stress, depression) equal or even higher than the patient (Wagner, Bigatti, & Storniolo, 2006). Furthermore, emotional distress can continue long after the cancer treatment has ended (Harden, 2005). The psychosocial suffering can be explained by the fact that the diagnosis of cancer often generates a crisis in spouse caregivers by increasing the need to deal with social isolation, expenditures, and new responsibilities brought by the cancer diagnosis, and to simultaneously provide emotional support to the family, without being able to express their own sufferings (Harden, 2005).

Cancer is currently seen as a possible trigger of post-traumatic stress disorder (PTSD) symptoms (American Psychiatric Association, 2000), both in patients and in first-degree relatives. For example, Boyer et al. (2002) found that 21 percent of patients with breast cancer and 13 percent of their daughters reported symptoms consistent with PTSD. The prevalence of PTSD symptoms in daughters was comparable to the results found in previous studies in women with breast cancer, reporting that mothers with PTSD symptoms increase the likelihood of their daughters manifesting these symptoms too. According to a review conducted by Mosher and Danoff-Burg (2005), research suggests that first-degree relatives of patients with breast cancer have significantly higher levels of cancer-related intrusive thoughts and avoidance, compared with women without a family history of oncological disease (Zakowski et al., 1997). In turn, the study by Lindberg and Wellisch (2004) found that 4 percent of first-degree relatives of patients with breast cancer showed levels of symptoms consistent with a diagnosis of PTSD, most likely cancer related. Furthermore, 7 percent of first-degree relatives showed symptoms consistent with subclinical levels of PTSD, potentially associated with cancer. Lerman et al. (1993) found that 53 percent of first-degree relatives of patients with breast cancer had intrusive thoughts, whose levels were comparable to those found in studies involving individuals exposed to other types of trauma.

Given the great variability in distress levels among first-degree relatives of patients with cancer (Lerman et al., 1993), it is important to assess the main predictors of their responses to stress. For example, one study showed that avoidance was a partial mediator in the relationship between social constraints and two types of distress (cancer-related intrusive thoughts and general distress) among first-degree relatives of patients with breast cancer (Schnur, Valdimarsdottir, Montgomery, Nevid, & Bovbjerg, 2004). In a social-cognitive perspective, studies suggest that the negative reactions of misunderstanding or lack of support from others during the expression of thoughts and feelings associated with stress may result in an attempt to avoid such thoughts and feelings (Mosher & Danoff-Burg, 2005). Thus, this inadequate exposure to the stressor may prevent its cognitive processing, thus prolonging the distress. The current age of a woman can also be associated with the severity of her distress, as pointed to by Lerman, Kash, and Stefanek (1994) in their study with first-degree relatives of patients with breast cancer. The authors found higher levels of intrusive thoughts among women who were 50 or more years old, compared with younger women. This finding is especially noteworthy in light of the evidence about an inverse association between psychological distress and adherence to mammography among first-degree relatives of patients with cancer (George, 2000). According to Baider, Ever-Hadani, and De-Nour (1999), when compared with women who had a mother or sister with breast cancer, women who had a history of breast cancer in both reported higher levels of intrusive thoughts.

The death of a parent with cancer may be another potential predictor of PTSD, especially when it was preceded by a long and painful decline in the health of the parent as well as by long-term caregiving. Zakowski et al.'s (1997) study reveals that the daughters of deceased patients with breast cancer were found to show more intrusion, avoidance, and cancer-related thoughts about perceived risk. The results suggest that the perceived risk of breast cancer mediated the effect of the parent's death in the intrusive thoughts and avoidance. In the cross-sectional study by Erblich, Bovbjerg, and Valdimarsdottir (2000), the healthy caregiving daughters with maternal history of breast cancer reported higher values on the concerns directly related to breast cancer, when compared to noncaregiver daughters. The unique aspects of the experience of cancer, and the overlap between normative reactions to cancer and PTSD responses, confounds the interpretation of these studies' findings. For example, the normal reactions of pain and suffering before a diagnosis of cancer can be confused with PTSD symptoms because both usually involve hyperarousal, avoidance, and intrusive thoughts (Kangas, Henry, & Bryant, 2002). Certainly that avoiding of the "reminders" of trauma may be impossible for family members of cancer patients, mainly due to external cues such as doctor visits, drug prescriptions, and treatment side effects. Still, it is important to note that in the context of cancer, the usual definition of reexperienced symptoms may not be the same as in other contexts because intrusive thoughts may consist of future concerns related to health issues, rather than ruminations on the past experiences. Although there are records of intrusive thoughts on adult children caregivers of cancer patients, its exact nature is still unknown (Kangas et al., 2002).

According to Joseph and Linley (2008), PTSD theories do not consider the positive consequences of trauma. For the authors, it is essential that any theory about positive changes does not contradict what is known about the development of PTSD, but should accommodate the knowledge about this disorder and growth. Therefore, in order to develop an understanding of growth through adversity, it is necessary to integrate in any growth theory the symptoms of PTSD and how these symptoms relate to positive psychological changes. Studies focused on the concept of distress show that, effectively, cancer can be seen as a psychosocial transition (Cordova, 2008), which potentially could result in adjustment difficulties, but also in personal growth and empowerment. According to Parkes (1971), the term "psychosocial transition" refers to basic life experiences that require individuals to restructure their ways of seeing the world and their plans in life. In fact, this notion is evident in several reports of cancer survivors, and in their elaborations about positive attributions around their efforts to fight the disease (Cordova, 2008). For example, a qualitative study shows that some breast cancer survivors experience spiritual growth as they build a sense of connection with others or a higher power, thus finding a renewed purpose for their lives (Gall & Cornblat, 2002).

The term "post-traumatic growth" was introduced by Calhoun and Tedeschi (2008) to describe positive changes after a disease or other stress enhancing experiences. The study of potential catalysts for a positive personal transformation had a strong focus on the experience of cancer, especially in patients (Cordova, 2008), but little is known about the potential psychosocial gains among relatives. However, to Mosher, Danoff-Burg, and Brunker (2006), evidences suggests that cancer-related experiences can precipitate personal growth, not only in patients but also in their spouses and children. For example, among women with breast cancer, a higher post-traumatic growth was associated with a younger age, higher income, and more contact with others, as well as better emotional expression and lower perceived cancer-related stress (Manne et al., 2004). Among spouses, post-traumatic growth was associated with a younger age, more intrusive thoughts, and perceptions of illness as a traumatic event, as well as a greater use of positive reappraisal and emotional processing as coping strategies (Manne et al., 2004). In this line, Weiss (2002) found that, after the diagnosis, most husbands of breast cancer patients tend to report positive changes with a small to medium intensity.

In the last decade, the studies by Leedham and Meyerowitz (1999) assumed special relevance in the context of the parent-child relationship in parental cancer settings. The authors assessed the benefits derived from the cancer experience, with 93 percent of the adult daughters of the sample indicating that parental cancer had caused at least one positive change in their lives—in other words, almost all seemed to derive benefits from the experience of parental cancer. This study suggests that research questions could include an analysis of both psychosocial consequences (positive and negative) and their respective predictors in this population.

One of the most relevant studies in this field was conducted by Mosher et al. (2006). The authors assessed the predictors of post-traumatic growth in adult daughters of patients with breast cancer, as well as their coping strategies and caregiving tasks. It is important to note that, according to the theoretical model of Calhoun and Tedeschi (2008), optimists (i.e., people who have higher positive expectations regarding the results) use coping strategies that promote post-traumatic growth. Furthermore, having enough time to process the implications of a diagnosis of cancer in a social context of good emotional support is seen as the main explanatory hypothesis for growth. However, it is noteworthy that neither optimism nor social support was associated with post-traumatic growth in studies with cancer patients (Cordova, 2008).

In comparison, the degrees of post-traumatic growth between an adult daughter whose mother was diagnosed with breast cancer and the cancer patient herself are very similar (Cordova, 2008). In the study by Mosher et al. (2006), personal characteristics (age, income, education, marital status, optimism) were not correlated with post-traumatic growth, although a better perception about cancer-related stress and greater social support have proven to be promoters of growth. These results enhance Calhoun and Tedeschi's model (2008), in which a strong commitment to a stressor, in a context of good social support, enables post-traumatic growth. Also consistent with this model was the fact that an active emotional management of parental stressors associated with cancer encourages greater post-traumatic growth. More specifically, higher post-traumatic growth led to a greater probability of developing planning strategies for a coping-oriented approach, active coping, social-support seeking, and emotional processing (Mosher et al., 2006). According to Calhoun and Tedeschi (2008), caregivers rely on several resources when faced with cancer-related stressors, and a tendency for action may contribute to post-traumatic growth (Shakespeare-Finch & Barrington, 2012).

CONCLUSIONS AND IMPLICATIONS

A diagnosis of cancer is a shattering event, not only for the patient but also for the family. The literature is extensive with respect to the psychological effects of diagnosis and treatment of cancer in patients and their partners. However, the study of the consequences for their children, regardless of age, when a parent (or both) is suffering from cancer, has received much less attention. Most research in this field has focused on studies with adult children whose mothers had breast cancer, in which the healthy parent was excluded. The literature sustains, however, that these adult children may develop psychological morbidity, as they are confronted with a very distressing event. The impact can be so intense that many children develop symptoms consistent with a diagnosis of PTSD (Lindberg & Wellisch, 2004). The prevalence of these symptoms was, in some research studies, particularly alarming (Mosher & Danoff-Burg, 2005). Our studies with adult children caregivers showed that, in a parental cancer setting, they suffer from significant psychological morbidity. Perhaps the most important contribution of our studies is the fact that they focused on the influence of different paths on how parental cancer can affect adult children. Although there is some research on coping, adjustment difficulties, and optimism in children dealing with parental cancer, the literature mainly includes theoretical studies that lack a comparison group. Some researchers have discussed the possible mechanisms of influence, but conceptually, without consistent empirical data.

Our line of research shows that psychological morbidity of adult children with parental cancer is more prevalent in women with lower monthly income. In clinical terms, we found that higher levels of PTSD symptoms and caregiver burden are associated with shorter durations of parental illness and caregiving responsibilities. We also found that children with more dependent parents showed more distress, PTSD symptoms, burden, and a worse perception of social support, especially on an intimate level. Regarding the predictors of burden, we found that being a woman, caregiving for shorter periods of time, and having a more dependent parent are related to less satisfaction than are factors that enhance burden. Finally, with these variables, we found that the dissatisfaction with social support, in adult children caregivers, has a mediating effect, helping to explain the relationship between distress/PTSD symptoms and burden (Teixeira & Pereira, 2012).

A second line of our research sought to examine the physiological effects of caregiving in adult children in oncology. Thus, we found that, compared with a group of adult children without chronically ill parents, the group of children caregivers of parents with cancer has a distinct psychophysiological outline. In fact, adult children caregivers appear to be at increased risk for stress-related disorders relative to the comparison group, mainly due to the results obtained in the cardiovascular response to idiographic unpleasant stimulus (Teixeira & Pereira, submitted a). These results contribute to the advancement of knowledge around the physiological mechanisms involved in psychological morbidity in caregivers of cancer patients, with the ultimate goal of improving the diagnosis and prognosis in this population. The results are also in line with research reporting that more than half of family caregivers in oncology suffer from chronic health problems, such as heart disease and hypertension (Mellon & Northouse, 2001; Thornton, Perez, & Meyerowitz, 2004), and that these health problems can be aggravated by caregivers' stress (Haley, LaMonde, Han, Burton, & Schonwetter, 2003).

At the family level, our results highlight that family functioning requires constant adjustments, and that these may influence the levels of distress of the patient as well as other family members (Teixeira & Pereira, submitted b). Considering the comparison group, adult children caregivers presented indicators of higher family imbalance, particularly in terms of cohesion and flexibility, as well as a greater tendency for enmeshment. Whereas cancer can be a traumatic experience for patients and families, our research examined the main family predictors of post-traumatic symptomatology in adult children caregivers. The results showed that being a woman and presenting a family functioning characterized by a higher enmeshment and chaos significantly potentiates PTSD symptoms. These results emphasize that a chaotic family functioning indirectly interferes (partial mediating effect) with the association between difficulties in family communication/satisfaction, promoting higher levels of PTSD symptoms in children dealing with parental cancer.

Literature supports that the experience of cancer, both for patients and their first-degree relatives, may be a trigger for substantial psychological distress. In addition, studies show that the same experience can also be seen as a psychosocial transition with perceived benefits in different dimensions (Janoff-Bulman, 2006). Our results with adult children caregivers revealed a significant positive association between post-traumatic growth (associated with the experience of parental cancer) and psychological morbidity. Being a woman, perceiving the parent as more dependent and with a longer disease duration, in addition to suffering from more intensive PTSD symptoms, were factors that highlighted the key predictors of post-traumatic growth in adult children caregivers (Teixeira & Pereira, in press). Taking into account a possible stress-buffering effect of post-traumatic growth (Silva, Moreira, & Canavarro, 2012), our results indicate that the relationship between distress and social support was moderated by post-traumatic growth (Teixeira & Pereira, 2013). These data contribute to the discussion over the nature of the experience of post-traumatic growth, and if this is best explained as a process or as an outcome (Tedeschi & Calhoun, 2004). Anyway, as part of our studies, it seems clear that post-traumatic growth reflects a cognitive adaptation as a response to the caregiving experience.

The purpose of our chapter was also to contribute to psychological intervention. More specifically, our results seem to highlight the crucial importance of social support in this population. This may help health professionals in the development of programs promoting social support, in order to mitigate the effects of psychological symptoms that can accompany the caregiver's burden in oncology. Psychosocial interventions for family caregivers of cancer patients seem to promote important clinical outcomes, particularly in specific components of quality of life, significantly reducing the burden (Northouse, Katapodi, Song, Zhang, & Mood, 2010). In adult children, this reduction may allow an improvement of coping, self-confidence, and marital and family relationships, as well as a decrease in psychological tension and distress. Psychosocial interventions with adult children caregivers should reduce their distress, which, in turn, will most likely result in more positive benefits to the patients themselves. In psychophysiological terms, our data indicate that the risk associated with increased heart rate in adult children caregivers of patients in oncology is not only statistically significant but also clinically relevant, and might be part of the medical evaluation. These results can drive health professionals to pay attention to caregivers' cardiac activity, and to recommend lifestyle changes or pharmacological treatment in order to reduce cardiovascular risk.

Considering family functioning as perceived by adult children caregivers, and taking into account the literature that supports a relationship between these variables and PTSD reactions (Uruk, Sayger, & Cogdal, 2007), family proximity should also be of particular importance for interventions with families suffering from traumatic symptoms associated with cancer. At this level, our data suggest that adult children dealing with parental cancer, and their families, may benefit from prevention and intervention programs focused on improving family functioning. Following that hypothesis, through healthy relationships within the family these adult children can learn more adaptive ways of coping with cancer-related distress by trying not to dwell in family functioning with extreme characteristics. Thus, psychological intervention for family caregivers of cancer patients, in addition to including information about how to care, how to maintain marital and family relationships, and how to take care of oneself, could benefit from the participation of the patients themselves, since both are affected by the disease (Northouse et al., 2010). Our results also suggest that adult children who are caregivers of parents with cancer may benefit from interventions improving their ability to accept and to find meaning and personal growth from the experience of care. Promoting positive changes may enhance the mental health of caregivers, while health care professionals can encourage personal growth, for example, by focusing on aspects of health promotion. These are well known to have an impact on the post-traumatic anxiety and depression effects, in the long term.

There seems to be a general consensus in the literature that when patients and caregivers are treated simultaneously, important synergies are achieved, contributing to the welfare of each one (Hagedoorn, Sanderman, Bolks, Tuinstra, & Coyne, 2008). Thus, it will be of interest to health professionals who deal with family members of cancer patients to address the needs of adult children caregivers. Meeting their physical and mental health needs may ensure that patients will receive the best possible care from a prepared, motivated, and balanced family caregiver.

One of the main proposals for progress in parental cancer research as a psychosocial phenomenon is through longitudinal studies. Such studies will certainly make the results easier to generalize by evaluating the stressors over time and by fostering an understanding of the dynamic nature of social support in early burden of adult children caregivers. Furthermore, longitudinal studies may also clarify the direction of effects between family functioning in the context of oncology and PTSD symptoms, as well as help to clarify the effects of current and progressive experiences of post-traumatic growth. Another direction for future research should focus on the effective evaluation of PTSD severity in samples of adult children caregivers. Additionally, research could provide evidence regarding the needs of adult children showing moderate to severe symptoms of PTSD, and the kind of interventions that could be more effective. Ideally, randomized controlled trials should be used in these types of studies. Additional research should also include the assessment of PTSD symptoms in patients themselves, as the literature claims that the symptoms of parents can mediate the response of children to adverse situations related to the development of cancer. In fact, empirical studies on the treatment of adult caregivers in oncology with a diagnosis of PTSD are extremely rare, despite the data of Vanderwerker et al. (2005) showing that 4 percent of caregivers suffer from the disorder. For example, in the United States, psychotherapy is recommended as primary treatment, combined with psychopharmacological treatment for caregivers with PTSD (Davidson, Stein, Shalev, & Yehuda, 2004).

Future studies may also focus on the experiences of post-traumatic growth, considered through some core clinical variables, such as the stage of disease, different types of treatment received, or even different types of pathology. Regarding the latter and according to Levesque and Maybery (2012), it is conceivable that a parent's brain cancer, with the cognitive changes that it imposes, is more traumatic for adult children than other types of cancer. This fact may raise different patterns of perceived benefits and post-traumatic growth. Studies with larger samples, by cancer type, may certainly lead to interesting paths for future research. Furthermore, these studies can focus on the subjective experience of the traumatic event, as it is the individual perception of it and the responses to it that determine the arising consequences. The relationship/balance between positive and negative outcomes in caregivers of parents with cancer is important, as it will clarify the most important aspects of post-traumatic growth. This will, in turn, maximize the clinical applications of this data. Further research with samples composed by family caregivers in oncology would certainly benefit from studies that address individual differences, previously associated in the literature with the experience of post-traumatic growth (e.g., coping strategies and optimism). Additionally, beyond studying post-traumatic growth in adult children caregivers, future research should also include other family members, as well as the cancer patient. Moreover, and considering the existing literature with qualitative data reported by individuals who experienced post-traumatic growth in caregiving contexts (Levesque & Maybery, 2012; Puterman & Cadell, 2008), future studies would certainly benefit from the inclusion of mixed methodologies of data collection.

At the research-action level, there is a need for further studies identifying caregivers and oncology patients who may be at increased risk for worse psychosocial outcomes. Generally, a large proportion of caregivers receive basic information about the provision of care in health institutions. However, efforts should be made to identify families at higher risk, as those may benefit the most from psychosocial interventions. For this to be a reality, it is necessary that researchers and clinicians work together to determine ways of implementing evidence-based interventions in oncology settings (i.e., where the caregivers can benefit from them). Finally, researchers, clinicians, and funding agencies must cooperate to put the knowledge obtained from efficacy studies into practice, so that evidence-based interventions can also become the focus of effectiveness studies (Northouse et al., 2010).

REFERENCES

Akechi, T., Akizuki, N., Okamura, M., Shimizu, K., Oba, A., Ito, T., . . . Uchitomi, Y. (2006). Psychological distress experienced by families of cancer Patients: Preliminary findings from psychiatric consultation of a Cancer Center Hospital. *Japanese Journal of Clinical Oncology, 36*(5), 329–332.

American Cancer Society. (2012). Cancer facts & figures 2012. Retrieved from http://www.cancer.org/acs/groups/content/@epidemiologysurveilance/documents/document/acspc-031941.pdf.

American Psychiatric Association. (2000). *Diagnostic and statistical manual of mental disorders* (4th rev ed.). Washington, DC: American Psychiatric Association.

Augusto, B., & Carvalho, R. (2002). Cuidados continuados—Família, centro de saúde e hospital como parceiros do cuidar [*Continued care—family, health center, and hospital as partners in care*]. Coimbra: Formasau.

Axelsson, B., & Sjöden, P.-O. (1998). Quality of life of cancer patients and their spouses in palliative home care. *Palliative Medicine, 12*(1), 29–39.

Baanders, A. N., & Heijmans, M. J. (2007). The impact of chronic diseases: The partner's perspective. *Family & Community Health, 30*(4), 305–317.

Baider, L., Ever-Hadani, P., & De-Nour, A. K. (1999). Psychological distress in healthy women with familial breast cancer: Like mother, like daughter? *International Journal of Psychiatry in Medicine, 29*(4), 411–420.

Barakat, L., & Kazak, A. (1999). Family issues. In Brown, R. T. (Ed.), *Cognitive aspects of chronic illness in children* (pp. 333–354). New York: Guilford Press.

Blanchard, C. G., Toseland, R. W., & McCallion, P. (1996). The effects of a problem-solving intervention with spouses of cancer patients. *Journal of Psychosocial Oncology, 14*(2), 1–21.

Bloom, J. R. (1996). Social support of the cancer patient and the role of the family. In Baider, L., Cooper, C. L., & De-Nour, A. K. (Eds.), *Cancer and the family* (2nd ed., pp. 53–70). Chichester: John Wiley & Sons.

Boyer, B. A., Bubel, D., Jacobs, S. R., Knolls, M. L., Harwell, V. D., Goscicka, M., & Keegan, A. (2002). Posttraumatic stress in women with breast cancer and their daughters. *American Journal of Family Therapy, 30*(4), 323–338.

Brody, E. M. (2004). *Women in the middle: Their parent care years* (2nd ed.). New York: Springer.

Calhoun, L., & Tedeschi, R. (2008). The paradox of struggling with trauma: Guidelines for practice and directions for research. In Joseph, S., & Linley, P. A. (Eds.), *Trauma, recovery, and growth: Positive psychological perspectives on posttraumatic stress* (pp. 325–337). Hoboken, NJ: John Wiley & Sons.

Cancer Research UK. (2012). CancerStats key facts. Retrieved from http://publictions.cancerresearchuk.org/downloads/Product/CS_KF_ALLCANCERS.pdf.

Chentsova-Dutton, Y., Shucter, S., Hutchin, S., Strause, L., Burns, K., Dunn, L., . . . Zisook, S. (2002). Depression and grief reactions in hospice caregivers: From pre-death to 1 year afterwards. *Journal of Affective Disorders, 69*(1-3), 53–60.

Chou, K.-R. (2000). Caregiver burden: A concept analysis. *Journal of Pediatric Nursing, 15*(6), 398–407.

Clark, M., Rummans, T. A., Sloan, J. A., Jensen, A., Atherton, P. J., Frost, M. H., . . . Brown, P. D. (2006). Quality of life of caregivers of patients with advanced-stage cancer. *American Journal of Hospice & Palliative Medicine, 23*(3), 185–191.

Cordova, M. J. (2008). Facilitating posttraumatic growth following cancer. In Joseph, S. & Linley, P. A. (Eds.), *Trauma, recovery, and growth: Positive psychological perspectives on posttraumatic stress* (pp. 185–205). Hoboken, NJ: John Wiley & Sons.

Davidson, J., Stein, D., Shalev, A., & Yehuda, R. (2004). Posttraumatic stress disorder: Acquisition, recognition, course, and treatment. *Journal of Neuropsychiatry and Clinical Neurosciences, 16*(2), 135–147.

Deeken, J. F., Taylor, K. L., Mangan, P., Yabroff, K. R., & Ingham, J. M. (2003). Care for the caregivers: A review of self-report instruments developed to measure the burden, needs, and quality of life of informal caregivers. *Journal of Pain and Symptom Management, 26*(4), 922–953.

Douglass, L. G. (1997). Reciprocal support in the context of cancer: Perspectives of the patient and spouse. *Oncology Nursing Forum, 24*(9), 1529–1536.

Ducharme, F., Levesque, L., Lachance, L., Zarit, S., Vezina, J., Gangde, M., & Caron, C. (2006). Older husbands as caregivers of their wives: A descriptive study of the context and relational aspects of care. *International Journal of Nursing Studies, 43*(5), 567–579.

Dura, J., & Beck, S. (1988). A comparison of family functioning when mothers have chronic pain. *Pain, 35*(1), 79–89.

Edwards, B., & Clarke, V. (2004). The psychological impact of a cancer diagnosis on families: The influence of family functioning and patients' illness characteristics on depression and anxiety. *Psycho-Oncology, 13*(8), 562–576.

Erblich, J., Bovbjerg, D. H., & Valdimarsdottir, H. B. (2000). Looking forward and back: Distress among women at familial risk for breast cancer. *Annals of Behavioral Medicine, 22*(1), 53–59.

Fadden, G., Bebbington, P., & Kuipers, L. (1987). Caring and its burdens. A study of the spouses of depressed patients. *British Journal of Psychiatry, 151*, 660–667.

Faulkner, R., & Davey, M. (2002). Children and adolescents of cancer patients: The impact of cancer on the family. *The American Journal of Family Therapy, 30*(1), 63–72.

Ferlay, J., Autier, P., Bonoil, M., Heanue, M., Colombet, M., & Boyle, P. (2007). Estimates of the cancer incidence and mortality in Europe in 2006. *Annals of Oncology, 18*(3), 581–592.

Fuemmeler, B. F., Brown, R. T., Williams, L., & Barredo, J. (2003). Adjustment of children with cancer and their caregivers: Moderating influences of family functioning. *Families, Systems & Health, 21*(3), 263–276.

Gall, T. L., & Cornblat, M. W. (2002). Breast cancer survivors give voice: A qualitative analysis of spiritual factors in long-term adjustment. *Psycho-Oncology, 11*(6), 524–535.

George, S. A. (2000). Barriers to breast cancer screening: An integrative review. *Health Care for Women International, 21*(1), 53–65.

Given, C. W., Stommel, M., Given, B., Osuch, J., Kurtz, M. E., & Kurtz, J. C. (1993). The influence of cancer patients' symptoms and functional states on patients' depression and family caregivers' reaction and depression. *Health Psychology, 12*(4), 277–285.

Goodman, A. (2005). Caregiver psychological burden: An opportunity for appropriate referral. *Oncology Times, 27*(24), 20–26.

Grad, J., & Sainsbury, P. (1966). Problems of caring for the mentally ill at home. *Proceedings of the Royal Society of Medicine, 59*(1), 20–23.

Grulke, N., Boiler, H., Hertenstein, B. H. K., Arnold, R., Tschuschke, V., & Heimpel, H. (2005). Coping and survival in patients with leukemia undergoing allogeneic bone marrow transplantation—long term follow-up of a prospective study. *Journal of Psychosomatic Research, 59*(5), 337–346.

Hagedoorn, M., Sanderman, R., Bolks, H. N., Tuinstra, J., & Coyne, J. C. (2008). Distress in couples coping with cancer: A meta-analysis and critical review of role and gender effects. *Psychological Bulletin, 134*(1), 1–30.

Haley, W. E., LaMonde, L. A., Han, B., Burton, A. M., & Schonwetter, R. (2003). Predictors of depression and life satisfaction among spouse caregivers in hospice: Application of a stress process model. *Journal of Palliative Medicine, 6*(2), 215–224.

Harden, J. (2005). Developmental life stage and couples' experiences with prostate cancer. *Cancer Nursing, 28*(2), 85–98.

Huizinga, G. A., Visser, A., van der Graaf, W. T. A., Hoekstra, H. J., & Hoekstra-Weebers, J. E. H. M. (2005). The quality of communication between parents and adolescent children in the case of parental cancer. *Annals of Oncology, 16*(12), 1956–1961.

Janoff-Bulman, R. (2006). Schema-change perspectives on posttraumatic growth. In Calhoun, L. G., & Tedeschi, R. G. (Eds.), *Handbook of posttraumatic growth* (pp. 81–99). Mahwah, NJ: Lawrence Erlbaum Associates.

Johnson, C. L., & Catalano, D. J. (1983). A longitudinal study of family supports to impaired elderly. *The Gerontologist, 23*(6), 612–618.

Joseph, S., & Linley, P. A. (2008). Reflections on theory and practice in trauma, recovery, and growth: A paradigm shift for the field of traumatic stress. In Joseph, S., & Linley, P. A. (Eds.), *Trauma, recovery, and growth: Positive psychological perspectives on posttraumatic stress* (pp. 339–356). Hoboken, NJ: John Wiley & Sons.

Kahle, A., & Jones, G. (2000). Adaptation to parental chronic illness. In Goreczny, A., & Hersen, M. (Eds.), *Handbook of pediatric and adolescent health psychology* (pp. 387–400). Boston: Allyn & Bacon.

Kangas, M., Henry, J. L., & Bryant, R. A. (2002). Posttraumatic stress disorder following cancer: A conceptual and empirical review. *Clinical Psychology Review, 22*(4), 499–524.

Kazak, A., Alderfer, M., Rourke, M., Simms, S., Streisand, R., & Grossman, J. (2004). Posttraumatic stress disorder (PTSD) and posttraumatic stress symptoms (PTSS) in families of adolescent childhood cancer survivors. *Journal of Pediatric Psychology, 29*(3), 211–219.

Keller, M., Henrich, G., Sellschopp, A., & Beutel, M. (1996). Between distress and support: Spouses of cancer patients. In Baider, L., Cooper, C. L., & De-Nour,

A. K. (Eds.), *Cancer and the family* (2nd ed., pp. 187–223). Chichester: John Wiley & Sons.

Kelley, S. D. M., Sikka, A., & Venkatesan, S. (1997). A review of research on parental disability: Implications for research and counseling practice. *Rehabilitation Counseling Bulletin, 41*(2), 105–121.

Kim, Y., Baker, F., Spillers, R. L., & Wellisch, D. K. (2006). Psychological adjustment of cancer caregivers with multiple roles. *Psycho-Oncology, 15*(9), 795–804.

Kissane, D. W., Bloch, S., Burns, W. I., Mckenzie, D., & Posterino, M. (1994). Psychological morbidity in the families of patients with cancer. *Psycho-Oncology, 3*(1), 47–56.

Kupst, M. J., Natta, M. B., Richardson, C. C., Schulman, J. L., Lavigne, J. V., & Das, L. (1995). Family coping with pediatric leukemia: Ten years after treatment. *Journal of Pediatric Psychology, 20*(5), 601–617.

Kuscu, M. K., Dural, U., Onen, P., Yaşa, Y., Yayla, M., Basaran, G., . . . Bekiroğlu, N. (2009). The association between individual attachment patterns, the perceived social support, and the psychological well-being of Turkish informal caregivers. *Psycho-Oncology, 18,* 927–935.

Leedham, B., & Meyerowitz, B. (1999). Responses to parental cancer: A clinical perspective. *Journal of Clinical Psychology in Medical Settings, 6*(4), 441–461.

Lerman, C., Daly, M., Sands, C., Balshem, A., Lustbader, E., Heggan, T., . . . Engstrom, P. (1993). Mammography adherence and psychological distress among women at risk for breast cancer. *Journal of the National Cancer Institute, 85*(13), 1074–1080.

Lerman, C., Kash, K., & Stefanek, M. (1994). Younger women at increased risk for breast cancer: Perceived risk, psychological well-being, and surveillance behavior. *Journal of the National Cancer Institute Monographs, 16,* 171–176.

Levesque, J. V., & Maybery, D. (2012). Parental cancer: Catalyst for positive growth and change. *Qualitative Health Research, 22*(3), 397–408.

Lewandowski, L. A. (1992). Needs of children during the critical illness of a parent or sibling. *Critical Care Nursing Clinics of North America, 4*(4), 573–585.

Lewis, F. M. (2010). The family's "stuck points" in adjusting to cancer. In Holland, J. C., Breitbart, W. S., Jacobsen, P. B., Lederberg, M. S., Loscalzo, M. J., & McCorkle, R. (Eds.), *Psycho-Oncology* (2nd ed., pp. 511–515). New York: Oxford University Press.

Lidell, E. (2002). Family support—a burden to patient and caregiver. *European Journal of Cardiovascular Nursing, 1*(2), 149–152.

Lindberg, N. M., & Wellisch, D. K. (2004). Identification of traumatic stress reactions in women at increased risk for breast cancer. *Psychosomatics, 45*(1), 7–16.

Lloyd, C. (1995). Understanding social support within the context of theory and research on the relationship of life stress and mental health. In Brugha, T. S. (Ed.), *Social support and psychiatric disorder: Research findings and guidelines for clinical practice* (pp. 41–60). New York: Cambridge University Press.

Loscalzo, M. J., Kim, Y., & Clark, K. L. (2010). Gender and caregiving. In Holland, J. C., Breitbart, W. S., Jacobsen, P. B., Lederberg, M. S., Loscalzo, M. J., & McCorkle, R. (Eds.), *Psycho-Oncology* (2nd ed., pp. 522–526). New York: Oxford University Press.

Manne, S. (1994). Couples coping with cancer: Research issues and recent findings. *Journal of Clinical Psychology in Medical Settings, 1*(4), 317–330.

Manne, S., Ostroff, J., Winkel, G., Goldstein, L., Fox, K., & Grana, G. (2004). Post-traumatic growth after breast cancer: Patient, partner, and couple perspectives. *Psychosomatic Medicine, 66*(3), 442–454.

Maruyama, M. (1963). The second cybernetics: Deviation-amplifying mutual causal processes. *American Scientist, 5*(2), 164–179.

McCubbin, H. I., Thompson, E. A., Thompson, A. I., & Fromer, J. E. (1998). *Stress, coping, and health in families: Sense of coherence and resiliency.* Thousand Oaks, CA: Sage.

Mellon, S., & Northouse, L. L. (2001). Family survivorship and quality of life following a cancer diagnosis. *Research in Nursing & Health, 24*(6), 446–459.

Moores, D. F., & Meadow-Orlans, K. P. (2002). *Educational and developmental aspects of deafness.* Washington: Gallaudet University Press.

Mosher, C. E., & Danoff-Burg, S. (2005). Psychosocial impact of parental cancer in adulthood: A conceptual and empirical review. *Clinical Psychology Review, 25*(3), 365–382.

Mosher, C. E., Danoff-Burg, S., & Brunker, B. (2006). Post-traumatic growth and psychosocial adjustment of daughters of breast cancer survivors. *Oncology Nursing Forum, 33*(3), 543–551.

Mosher, C. E., & Weiss, T. R. (2010). Psychosocial research and practice with adult children of cancer patients. In Holland, J. C., Breitbart, W. S., Jacobsen, P. B., Lederberg, M. S., Loscalzo, M. J., & McCorkle, R. (Eds.), *Psycho-Oncology* (2nd ed., pp. 532–536). New York: Oxford University Press.

Nichols, M. P., & Schwartz, R. C. (2008). *Family therapy: Concepts and methods* (8th ed.). Boston: Allyn & Bacon.

Nijboer, C., Tempelaar, R., Sanderman, R., Triemstra, M., Spruijt, R. J., & van den Bos, G. A. (1998). Cancer and caregiving: The impact on the caregiver's health. *Psycho-Oncology, 7*(1), 3–13.

Northouse, L. L., Katapodi, M. C., Song, L., Zhang, L., & Mood, D. W. (2010). Interventions with family caregivers of cancer patients: Meta-analysis of randomized trials. *CA: A Cancer Journal for Clinicians, 60*(5), 317–339.

Northouse, L. L., Schafer, J. A., Tipton, J., & Metivier, L. (1999). The concerns of patients and spouses after the diagnosis of colon cancer: A qualitative analysis. *Journal of Wound, Ostomy, and Continence Nursing, 26*(1), 8–17.

Parkes, C. M. (1971). Psycho-social transitions: A field for study. *Social Science & Medicine, 5*(2), 101–115.

Patenaude, A. F. (2005). *Genetic testing for cancer: Psychological approaches for helping patients and families.* Washington, DC: American Psychological Association.

Patterson, J. M. (2002). Integrating family resilience and family stress theory. *Journal of Marriage and the Family, 64*(2), 349–361.

Payne, S., & Ellis-Hill, C. (2001). Being a carer. In Payne, S., & Ellis-Hill, C. (Eds.), *Chronic and terminal illness: New perspectives on caring and carers* (pp. 1–21). New York: Oxford University Press.

Peters, L., & Esses, L. (1985). Family environment as perceived by children with a chronically ill parent. *Journal of Chronic Diseases, 38*(4), 301–308.

Pitceathly, C., & Maguire, P. (2003). The psychological impact of cancer on patients' partners and other key relatives: A review. *European Journal of Cancer, 39*(11), 1517–1524.

Porter, L. S., Keefe, F. J., Hurwitz, H., & Faber, M. (2005). Disclosure between patients with gastrointestinal cancer and their spouses. *Psycho-Oncology, 14*(12), 1030–1042.

Power, W. E., & Dell Orto, A. E. (2004). *Families living with chronic illness and disability: Interventions, challenges, and opportunities.* New York: Springer.

Puterman, J., & Cadell, S. (2008). Timing is everything: The experience of parental cancer for young adult daughters—A pilot study. *Journal of Psychosocial Oncology, 26*(2), 103–121.

Rait, D., & Lederberg, M. (1989). The family of the cancer patient. In Holland, J. (Ed.), *Handbook of psycho-oncology* (pp. 585–597). New York: Oxford University Press.

Rait, D. S., Ostroff, J. S., Smith, K., Cella, D. F., Tan, C., & Lesko, L. M. (1992). Lives in a balance: Perceived family functioning and the psychosocial adjustment of adolescent cancer survivors. *Family Process, 31*(4), 383–397.

Raveis, V. H., Karus, D., & Pretter, S. (1999). Factors associated with anxiety in adult daughter caregivers to a parent recently diagnosed with cancer. *Journal of Psychosocial Oncology, 17*(3/4), 1–26.

Rolland, J. S. (2004). Families and chronic illness: An integrative model. In Catherall, D. R. (Ed.), *Handbook of stress, trauma, and the family* (pp. 89–116). New York: Brunner-Routledge.

Rustad, L. (1984). Family adjustment to chronic illness and disability in midlife. In Eisenberg, M., Sutkin, L., & Jansen, M. (Eds.), *Chronic illness and disability through the life span: Effects on self and family* (pp. 222–242). New York: Springer.

Schnur, J. B., Valdimarsdottir, H. B., Montgomery, G. H., Nevid, J. S., & Bovbjerg, D. H. (2004). Social constraints and distress among women at familial risk for breast cancer. *Annals of Behavioral Medicine, 28*(2), 142–148.

Schulz, K. H., Schultz, H., Schultz, O., & Von Kerekjarto, M. (1996). Family structure and psychosocial stress in families of cancer patients. In Baider, L., Cooper, C. L., & De-Nou, A. K. (Eds.), *Cancer and the family* (pp. 225–255). New York: John Wiley & Sons.

Shakespeare-Finch, J., & Barrington, A. J. (2012). Behavioural changes add validity to the construct of posttraumatic growth. *Journal of Traumatic Stress, 25*(4), 433–439.

Shifren, K. (2008). Early caregiving: Perceived parental relations and current social support. *Journal of Adult Development, 15*(3-4), 160–168.

Silva, S. M., Moreira, H. C., & Canavarro, M. C. (2012). Examining the links between perceived impact of breast cancer and psychosocial adjustment: The buffering role of posttraumatic growth. *Psycho-Oncology, 21*(4), 409–418.

Singhal, S., Vachani, A., Antin-Ozerkis, D., Kaiser, L. R., & Abelda, S. M. (2005). Prognostic implications of cell cycle, apoptosis and angiogenesis and bio-markers in non-small cell lung cancer: A review. *Clinical Cancer Research, 11*(11), 3974–3986.

Soothill, K., Morris, S. M., Thomas, C., Harman, J. C., Francis, B., & McIllmurray, M. B. (2003). The universal, situational, and personal needs of cancer patients and their main carers. *European Journal of Oncology Nursing, 7*(1), 5–13.

Stephens, M. A., & Franks, M. M. (2009). All in the family: Providing care to chronically ill and disabled older adults. In Qualls, S. H., & Zarit, S. H. (Eds.), *Aging families and caregiving* (pp. 61–83). New Jersey: John Wiley & Sons.

Stetz, K. (2003). Quality of life in families experiencing cancer. In King, C., & Hinds, P. (Eds.), *Quality of life from nursing and patient perspectives. Theory, research & practice* (2nd ed., pp. 219–238). Burlington, MA: Jones and Bartlett Publishers.

Symister, P., & Friend, R. (2003). The influence of social support and problematic support on optimism and depression in chronic illness: A prospective study evaluating self-esteem as a mediator. *Health Psychology, 22*(2), 123–129.

Tansella, C. Z. (1995). Psychosocial factors and chronic illness in childhood. *European Psychiatry, 10*(6), 297–305.

Tebb, S. (1995). An aid to empowerment: A caregiver well-being scale. *Health & Social Work, 20*(2), 87–92.

Tedeschi, R. G., & Calhoun, L. G. (2004). Posttraumatic growth: Conceptual foundations and empirical evidence. *Psychological Inquiry, 15*(1), 1–18.

Teixeira, R. J., & Pereira, M. G. (2012). Psychological morbidity, burden, and the mediating effect of social support in adult children caregivers of oncological patients undergoing chemotherapy. *Psycho-Oncology*. doi: 10.1002/pon.3173

Teixeira, R. J., & Pereira, M. G. (2013). Factors contributing to posttraumatic growth and its buffering effect in adult children of cancer patients undergoing treatment. *Journal of Psychosocial Oncology*. doi: 10.1080/07347332.2013.778932.

Teixeira, R. J., & Pereira, M. G. (in press). Growth and the cancer caregiving experience: Psychometric properties of the Portuguese Posttraumatic Growth Inventory. *Families, Systems, & Health*.

Teixeira, R. J., & Pereira, M. G. (submitted a). Psychological morbidity and autonomic reactivity to emotional stimulus in parental cancer. *European Journal of Cancer Care*.

Teixeira, R. J., & Pereira, M. G. (submitted b). Family functioning and PTSD symptoms in adult children facing parental cancer. *Journal of Family Issues*.

Thomas, C., & Morris, S. M. (2002). Informal carers in contexts. *European Journal of Cancer Care, 11*, 178–182.

Thomas, C., Morris, S. M., & Harman, J. C. (2002). Companions through cancer: The care given by informal carers in cancer contexts. *Social Science & Medicine, 54*(4), 529–544.

Thornton, A. A., Perez, M. A., & Meyerowitz, B. E. (2004). Patient and partner quality of life and psychosocial adjustment following radical prostatectomy. *Journal of Clinical Psychology in Medical Settings, 11*(1), 15–30.

Uruk, A. C., Sayger, T. V., & Cogdal, P. A. (2007). Examining the influence of family cohesion and adaptability on trauma symptoms and psychological well-being. *Journal of College Student Psychotherapy, 22*(2), 51–63.

Vanderwerker, L., Laff, R., Kadan-Lottick, N., McColl, S., & Prigerson, H. (2005). Psychiatric disorders and mental health service use among caregivers of advanced cancer patients. *Journal of Clinical Oncology, 23*(28), 6899–6907.

Veach, T., & Nicholas, D. (1998). Understanding families of adults with cancer: Combining the clinical course of cancer and stages of family development. *Journal of Counseling and Development, 76*(2), 144–156.

Wagner, C. D., Bigatti, S. M., & Storniolo, A. M. (2006). Quality of life of husbands of women with breast cancer. *Psycho-Oncology, 15*(2), 109–120.

Walsh, F. (2003). Family resilience: A framework for clinical practice. *Family Process, 42*(1), 1–18.

Warren, K., Franklin, C., & Streeter, C. L. (1998). New directions in systems theory: Chaos and complexity. *Social Work, 43*(4), 357–372.

Weiss, T. (2002). Posttraumatic growth in women with breast cancer and their husbands: An intersubjective validation study. *Journal of Psychosocial Oncology, 20*(2), 65–80.

Wolff, J. L., & Kasper, J. D. (2006). Caregivers of frail elders: Updating a national profile. *The Gerontologist, 46*(3), 344–356.

Wong, M., Ratner, J., Gladstone, K. A., Davtyan, A., & Koopman, C. (2010). Children's perceived social support after a parent is diagnosed with cancer. *Journal of Clinical Psychology in Medical Settings, 17*(2), 77–86.

World Health Organization. (2012). Cancer: Fact sheet no 297. Retrieved from http://www.who.int/mediacentre/factsheets/fs297/en/index.html.

Yeh, S., Johnson, M., & Wang, S. (2002). The changes in caregiver burden following nursing home placement. *International Journal of Nursing Studies, 39*(6), 591–600.

Zakowski, S. G., Valdimarsdottir, H. B., Bovbjerg, D. H., Borgen, P., Holland, J., Kash, K., . . . Van Zee, K. (1997). Predictors of intrusive thoughts and avoidance in women with family histories of breast cancer. *Annals of Behavioral Medicine, 19*(4), 362–369.

Chapter 16

Interdependence of Breast Cancer Patients and Their Partners: The Shared Experience and Coping through It Together

Sam M. Dorros

An elderly gentleman who lost his first wife to advanced-stage breast cancer several decades ago recently described his experience dealing with her cancer as follows:

> It was like being on a treadmill, with chaos and destruction all around. It was as if *death* was always right behind you, on your heels, chasing you. The devastation around was trying to hold onto the life you once knew, and having to deal with doctors and tests everyday. And you kept trying to take steps forward but the steps got you nowhere. Because, ultimately, you would always fall steadily backwards . . . towards death.

His description of his ordeal with his wife's cancer is vivid and haunting. Although death is the sad reality for many women diagnosed with breast cancer, there are more survivors nowadays than ever before, thanks to improvements in early detection and treatments for cancer. The most recent data indicate that the survival rate at five years after diagnosis is 88 percent for women diagnosed with stage I breast cancer, followed by 81 percent and 74 percent for stage IIA and stage IIB, respectively (American Cancer Society, 2013). However, breast cancer remains the most frequently diagnosed cancer in women and is the second leading cause of cancer-related deaths in women (American Cancer Society, 2013).

The diagnosis and treatment of cancer has a number of features that represent substantial stressors for patients, and it affects the well-being of the cancer patient's larger social network (Weihs, Enright, Simmens, & Reiss, 2000). Above and beyond the fear of death and anxiety of the cancer spreading, there are a range of other concerns, including adjustments in social and family roles and changes in appearance or attractiveness (Manne et al., 2004). A large body of research illustrates the importance of close relationships in successful coping with illness and positive psychosocial adjustment. Social support, especially from family members or a spouse, is extremely beneficial and is associated with lower psychological distress in patients with breast cancer (Baider, Ever-Hadani, Goldzweig, Wygoda, & Peretz, 2003; Baider et al., 2004; Hoskins, 1995; Hoskins et al., 1996; Northouse, 1988, 1989; Northouse, Templin, & Mood, 2001).

Although social support is extremely beneficial for cancer patients, partners may have difficulty providing social support because of their own distress (Grunfeld et al., 2004; Manne et al., 2006; Manne, Taylor, Dougherty, & Kemeny, 1997; Northouse, Templin, Mood, & Oberst, 1998), given that approximately 30 percent of caregivers or partners experience significant emotional distress or some type of mood disturbance (Hagedoorn, Sanderman, Bolks, Tunistra, & Coyne, 2008; Pitceathly & Maguire, 2003). Indeed, Braun, Mikulincer, Rydall, Walsh, and Rodin (2007) found that 40 percent of cancer patients' spouses scored above the cutoff range for clinically significant levels of depression. Therefore a diagnosis of cancer does not solely affect that one individual; it impacts everyone in the family as well.

This chapter focuses on breast cancer patients and their partners' experience with cancer as it relates to negative affect, distress, and adjustment. In addition, this chapter will take a relational approach in describing the effects and outcomes for the patient and her partner. Research findings related to cross-over effects in distress and quality of life of couples coping with cancer will also be presented. In discussing aspects of interdependence and highlighting the shared experience of cancer, two important variables, social support and marital quality, will also be expanded upon. Finally, several positive coping strategies, such as emotional expression and communal coping, will be discussed.

EMOTIONAL DISTRESS AND HEALTH OUTCOMES

The diagnosis and treatment of cancer can be exceptionally taxing on patients' emotional and physical well-being, which has negative implications for overall health and quality of life (Michaelson et al., 2008; Helgeson, Snyder, & Seltman, 2004). For women with breast cancer, depression and fatigue are two of the most common distressing outcomes (Badger, Braden, & Mishel, 2001; Badger, Segrin, Meek, Lopez, & Bonham, 2004; McDaniel & Nemeroff, 1993; Newport & Nemeroff, 1998; Pasacreta, 1997). Approximately 10–25 percent of women with breast cancer are diagnosed with a major depressive disorder (Fann et al., 2008). Research has shown that psychological or emotional distress is a significant problem for cancer patients because it can negatively influence recovery from cancer (Alferi, Carver, Antoni, Weiss, & Duran, 2001; Han et al., 2005) and has implications for disease progression (Cousson-Gelie, Bruchon, Dilhuydy, & Jutand, 2007; Weihs, Enright, & Simmens, 2008).

For example, Weihs et al. (2000) found that negative affect (especially when concurrent with restriction of emotions) predicted shortened survival rate among women with breast cancer. Higher emotional distress predicted a shorter time interval from diagnosis to recurrence, and shortened survival time in women with breast cancer (Gilbar, 1996; Levy, Herberman, Maluish, Schlien, & Lippman, 1985). Not only can depression suppress a person's regular or healthy immune functioning (Carlson, Specca, Patel, & Goodey, 2003), but it can also negatively affect long-term survival rates if a person's depression is persistent and severe (Cousson-Gelie et al., 2007; Giese-Davis & Spiegel, 2003; Weihs et al., 2008). A reasonable explanation for these findings is that an individual's physical health suffers due to an increased activation of stress, which agitates normal physiological processes and creates disturbances in one's physical health (e.g., Sapolsky, 2004).

Past research shows that when events are experienced negatively, the immune system is suppressed and susceptibility to illness increases (Maddi, Bartone, & Puccetti, 1987; Sapolsky, 2004). The deleterious effects of stress are due in part to an increase in cortisol levels (Cohen & Williamson, 1991; Monjan & Collector, 1977). Cortisol suppresses immune system functioning by decreasing antibody production, T-cells, macrophages, and monocytes (Luecken & Compas, 2002). Further, Walker (2004) found that chronic stress has been found to suppress natural killer (NK) cell activity (a component of the immune system that plays a major role in destroying tumors and infected cells), which is associated with an increased risk of cancer progression. Therefore, not only does stress contribute to a host of infectious diseases (i.e., colds, herpes virus activation), but it could also play a role in the development, progression, or recurrence of cancer. Recent evidence is beginning to show a clear link between cortisol and the development and progression of tumors (Luecken & Compas, 2002). Given the negative physical health outcomes, special attention should be paid to help decrease patients' subjective experiences of depression, negative affect, and stress. In addition, positive psychological adjustment to cancer is critical, given that it has been linked to cancer recovery and length of survival (Greer, Morris, & Pettingale, 1979).

DYADIC INTERDEPENDENCE IN COUPLES

A major life event such as a cancer diagnosis and the ensuing treatment regimes (i.e., chemotherapy, radiation, surgery) often cause dramatic changes in relationships and roles, and affects both the cancer patients and their close family members (Weihs et al., 2000). Patients and their partners consistently report the negative effects that their cancer diagnosis and treatment have had on themselves and their family members, and they cite anxiety, stress, depression, and uncertainty as common problematic outcomes (Grunfeld et al., 2004). For example, Mellon and Northouse (2001) found that partners of men with prostate cancer reported a 63 percent decline in the family's overall quality of life after diagnosis of cancer. Given that cancer often affects the psychological and emotional well-being of the patient with cancer and his/her spouse or partner, it is commonly considered to be a relationship disease (Alferi et al., 2001).

There are a number of theories and concepts defined in the literature that explain the process of interdependence. Broadly, the *systems theory* concept of interdependence predicts that major events such as serious illness affect the larger family and social networks, and not just the ill individual (Bertalanffy, 1975; Broderick, 1993). Specifically, *family systems theory* predicts that close relational others (e.g., kin) experience increases in distress as the family member with cancer becomes more distressed, whereby affective states and overall well-being are interdependent among family members. In their book, *Family Communication,* Segrin and Flora (2011) describe a family system as being "open," "ongoing," "dynamic," and "emergent," which means that a family is affected by internal and external forces, that it is always evolving, and that members are more than the sum of their parts (pp. 26–27). Therefore, family members are mutually dependent on each other and, for better or worse, will affect and be affected by each other in a continual progression over time. Further, *emotional contagion* is another explanation for the occurrence of interdependence between a breast cancer patient's affect and quality of life and that of her partner (Hatfield, Cacioppo, & Rapson, 1992, 1994). According to the emotional contagion hypothesis, people "catch" the emotional states of those with whom they interact through largely unconscious interpersonal processes (e.g., nonverbal communication), such as mimicking and matching behaviors (Hatfield et al., 1992, 1994). Finally, Coyne's (1976a, 1976b) *interactional theory of depression* explains how people in a close relationship can come to share the same emotional state. According to Coyne (1976a, 1976b), people with depression induce a negative affective state in others, ultimately resulting in a downward spiral of interpersonal demand and withdrawal, and steadily increasing levels of negative affect in both dyad members.

Past research has documented that interdependence manifests in couples when applied to health contexts. For example, emotional distress and quality of life indicators are particularly interdependent in couples coping with cancer (Hagedoorn et al., 2008; Lewis & Hammond, 1992; Northouse et al., 2007; Northouse & Swain, 1987; Segrin et al., 2005; Segrin, Badger, Dorros, Meek, & Lopez, 2007). Segrin et al. (2007) illustrated that breast cancer patients' level of anxiety was significantly associated with that of their partners' anxiety over a period of 10 weeks. Kornblith et al. (2001) found that prostate cancer partners' psychological distress and well-being fluctuated in relation to the patients' physical and psychological well-being over a period of six months. Northouse et al. (2007) reported that prostate cancer patients and their spouses were significantly more alike than dissimilar on measures of physical, social, and emotional well-being. In a meta-analysis of the existing literature on interdependence and couples coping with cancer, Hagedoorn et al. (2008) found a moderate degree ($r = .29$) of interdependence.

Several studies have examined cross-over effects of interdependence on adjustment and well-being in married couples living with breast cancer (e.g., Dehle & Weiss, 2002; Northouse et al., 2001; Whisman, Uebelacker, & Weinstock, 2004). Dehle and Weiss (2002) found that husband's anxiety (but not wife's anxiety) predicted his own and his wife's subsequent marital adjustment. Whisman et al. (2004) showed that individuals' self-reported marital satisfaction was predicted by their own, but not their partners', levels of anxiety. Northouse et al. (2001) reported that although marital satisfaction was not significantly associated with adjustment among women with breast cancer, it was significantly associated with the adjustment of their husbands. Using structural equation analyses, Segrin et al. (2007) determined that partners' anxiety significantly influenced breast cancer patients' levels of anxiety, depression, fatigue, and symptom management. Further, Dorros, Card, Segrin, and Badger (2010) revealed a pattern of influence whereby the interaction of high levels of depression coupled with high levels of stress in women with breast cancer was associated with lowered emotional well-being in partners—including self-reports of the *physical* health of partners. Taken together, these findings suggest that relational interdependence has the potential for cross-over effects in distress and marital well-being in patients and partners living with cancer.

Although members of dyads with cancer experience similar levels of emotional distress, some research has found that partners experience even *higher* levels of emotional distress than the patients themselves (Grunfeld et al., 2004; Hagedoorn et al., 2008; Lewis, Cochrane, & Fletcher, 2005; Lewis, Fletcher, Cochrane, & Fann, 2008; Manne et al., 2006; Northouse et al., 1998; Pitceathly & Maguire, 2003; Segrin, Badger, Sieger, Meek, & Lopez, 2006). Partners often disregard their own needs and overextend themselves to assist their loved ones with cancer and thus are particularly vulnerable to stress and burnout; as a consequence, they often experience high levels of distress (du Pré, 2010). Indeed, Braun et al. (2007) found that 23 percent of spouses in their study had higher levels of depression than the patients with cancer. However, recent findings from Hagedoorn et al.'s (2008) meta-analysis revealed that it was gender, not role, that determined the levels of distress in couples coping with cancer. Specifically, women consistently reported higher levels of distress than did men, regardless of their role (i.e., patient or partner) (Hagedoorn et al., 2008).

Partners' emotional well-being is important because their distress can hinder effective communication and negatively influence marital adjustment and quality of life of both dyad members. For example, partners' emotional distress can contribute to ineffective communication with their spouses about important issues that need to be discussed (Hilton, 1994; Manne et al., 2003; Manne et al., 2004), which can affect how the dyad members cope with challenges as a couple (Walker, 1997). Further, a partner's depressed mood can strain the relationship and affect his or her ability to provide adequate support to the patient with cancer (Baider et al., 2003, 2004). In sum, a vicious cycle ensues in which partners' distress affects their ability to provide support to their spouses with cancer—and as a result, the patient with cancer is less able to obtain needed support from his/her partner, which has negative consequences for both dyad members. Wootten et al. (2007) found that dyadic adjustment and relationship satisfaction were negatively associated with cancer patients' emotional distress, which underscores the need for a partner's ability to provide support to the person with cancer.

CLOSE RELATIONSHIPS AND WELL-BEING

Social Support

Many women turn to their friends and family for support when dealing with breast cancer (Pistrang & Barker, 1995). Social support refers to "the general feeling of being adequately cared for or supported by others" (Rook, 1987, p. 1133). Social support is an important factor in psychosocial adjustment to breast cancer (Holland & Holahan, 2003; Holly, Kennedy, & Taylor, 2003) and as a buffer to the stress of the diagnosis and treatment (Cohen & Syme, 1985; Trunzo & Pinto, 2003). It is important to note that the *perception* of social support, (i.e., what the recipient sees in the support relationship, rather than what actually is done) is more important in the adjustment and coping process (Cohen, Gottlieb, & Underwood, 2000). Essentially, social support has the power to reduce the possibility of an individual developing a mental health disorder by alleviating anger, anxiety, or self-doubt, and it is thought to play a role in the recovery from illness (Cohen et al., 2000).

The *buffer hypothesis* suggests that individuals with higher levels of social support are relatively resistant to the negative mental health outcomes of distressing life events (Hudek-Knezevic, Kardum, & Pahljina, 2002; Rook, 1987). Research has consistently showed support for the buffering model in social support, particularly when there is a match between the specific needs and type of support provided (Cohen & Wills, 1985). The *main effect model* suggests that the powerful benefits of social support result from increases in positive affect, self-esteem, and feelings of belonging. Social support is thought to have a biological or behavioral adaptation that promotes positive effects on the immune system and limits stress-related endocrine functioning (Cohen, 1988; Spiegel, 1993). Indeed, social support has been found to be associated with longer survival among women with breast cancer (Maunsell, Brisson, & Deschenes, 1992).

The vitally important role that social support plays in one's physical and psychological well-being is especially associated with support garnered or received from one's spouse, intimate partner, and/or close family members (Baider et al., 2003; Picard, Dumont, Gagnon, & Lessard, 2006; Spiegel, 1997; Turner-Cobb, Sephton, Koopman, Blake-Mortimer, & Spiegel, 2000). Gotcher (1992) found that the most well-adjusted cancer patients were those who had the most frequent communication with, and received the most emotional support from, their family members. Having a network of friends and family members to provide social support or a spouse to confide in while coping with cancer has been associated with decreased risk of recurrence and mortality rates in women with breast cancer (Weihs et al., 2008; Maunsell, Brisson, & Deschenes, 1992; Weihs et al., 2008), and for survival rates in men with prostate cancer (Krongrad, Lai, Burke, Goodkin, & Lai, 1996). Social support is thought to have a biological or behavioral adaptation that promotes positive effects on the immune system and limits stress-related endocrine functioning (Cohen, 1988; Spiegel, 1993). For example, Turner-Cobb et al. (2000) found that among women with metastatic breast cancer, a greater quality of social support was associated with lower cortisol concentrations, the latter of which indicates a healthy (or at least healthier) neuroendocrine functioning. As a whole, these findings suggest that higher social integration and available support from a spouse, intimate partner, or other social network members is associated with positive psychosocial outcomes and increased survivability (e.g., Baider et al., 2003; Krongrad et al., 1996; Maunsell et al., 1992; Picard et al., 2006; Turner-Cobb et al., 2000; Weihs et al., 2008).

Satisfaction with the source of the support is also an important variable to consider. Neuling and Winefield (1988) found that patients who were satisfied with support from family members were significantly less depressed and anxious than those individuals who were not satisfied by the support from their family. Rodrigue and Park (1996) examined marital quality and cancer patients' psychological adjustment. They found that adults who reported greater marital satisfaction reported fewer symptoms of anxiety and depression and overall distress than did subjects with low marital quality (Rodrigue & Park, 1996).

Typically social support is understood as a multidimensional construct (Bloom, 1986). Bloom's (1986) concept of psychosocial support includes three key elements: informational support, instrumental or tangible support, and emotional support. *Informational support* provides useful information, advice, and guidance (Hudek-Knezevic et al., 2002). *Instrumental or tangible support* includes financial help, encouragement in decision making, material resources, and needed services (Cohen & Wills, 1985). *Emotional support* consists of affection, caring from others, the feeling of love, and the ability to talk about problems (Trunzo & Pinto, 2003). For example, in a study conducted by Dunkel-Schetter (1984) on breast cancer and colorectal cancer patients, these three types of social support, quantity of support, satisfaction with support from spouse, and overall strength of support, were associated with positive adjustment.

Which type of support is most helpful for cancer patients? Some research indicates that breast cancer patients prefer emotional support (Bloom & Spiegel, 1984; Trunzo & Pinto, 2003). Indeed, Gotcher (1993) found that emotional support was the best predictor of distress and adjustment. Other research has shown that women experiencing breast cancer report high needs for information, particularly as it relates to their specific situation (Chalmers, Marles, & Tataryn, 2003). For example, Neuling and Winefield (1988) found that women preferred empathetic support from family and friends, and informational support from surgeons. Typically cancer patients (in general) do not feel the need for information from nonmedical sources (Dunkel-Schetter, 1984). Further, the effectiveness of social support may depend on the relationship of the giver to the receiver. Therefore, spouses, family members, and friends may contribute different types of social support to an individual in need.

As far as the source of support, research shows that husbands, or life partners, may be depended upon the most (Neuling & Winefield, 1988; Primono, Yates, & Woods, 1990). Primono et al. (1990) found that breast cancer patients select their partners as the most important source of social support during the process. Primono et al. (1990) found that an individual's spouse, followed by family, provided more affective support than friends. Husbands may play a particularly important role in the recovery process (Northouse & Swain, 1987), and patients without partners may be especially vulnerable to higher levels of distress (Rodrigue & Park, 1996).

Family support is also extremely important. Perlman and Rook (1987) posit that family support is both widespread and beneficial. Family members, in particular, have been consistently found to be the most important source of instrumental support (e.g., help, money), and provide empathetic support more frequently than any other type of support (Neuling & Winefield, 1988). Indeed, in a study of social support in older adults' family relationships, family members were identified more often as sources of emotional support than were friends (Rook & Ituarte, 1999). Segrin (2003) found that middle-age to older adults showed a preference for social support from family members or kin, whereas young adults showed a preference for social support from friends.

Friends have been found to offer less instrumental support overall than family members (Crohan & Antonucci, 1989). Even though patients' friends provide less support of every kind than their families, patients report greater satisfaction from the support given by friends than family members (Neuling & Winefield, 1988). This might underscore the notion that family members' support is considered more "obligatory" while friend support is more "voluntary" (Adams & Blieszner, 1994). Indeed, Lawton (1983) found that family members helped to relieve negative affect, but it was friends who were able to encourage positive affect. Perhaps family members are important in reducing negative affect in order to protect against emotional distress, but successful adjustment is more impressive when the patient has some source of positive affect (e.g., through friends), which provides support for the main effect model.

Further, another source of social support is peer support groups. Research shows that support from peer groups for women with breast cancer improved the individual's ability to control pain (Spiegel & Bloom, 1983). It is thought that peer groups offer a chance for women to learn from each other and to interact with women who have successfully dealt with or overcome their disease, and they provide a solid sense of community for the individual (Tracy & Gussow, 1976).

As a final note on the issue of social support, some research has suggested that unsupportive responses from a partner have a stronger association than positive support to a patient's psychological distress (Manne et al., 1997). Rook (1990) described this phenomena as a "negativity effect," whereby negative interaction or strain with others may have a greater effect than support or positive interactions. For example, in their study on breast cancer and social support, Manne et al. (2003) found a link between patient distress and partner unsupportive behaviors for patients who had low levels of family and friend support. In particular, husbands' critical responses and avoidant responses were associated with psychological distress in women with breast cancer (Manne, Ostroff, Winkel, Grana, & Fox, 2005).

MARITAL QUALITY AND RELATIONSHIP SATISFACTION

Both marital status and quality of marriage are strongly tied to individuals' physical health and emotional well-being (Kiecolt-Glaser & Newton, 2001). In general, married people are healthier than people who are divorced, separated, or widowed (even after controlling for age and income). Marital status is also associated with lower rates of mortality from a number of chronic and acute health conditions (Ross, Mirowsky, & Goldsteen, 1990). Overall, men enjoy more health benefits from marriage than women do; but the negative effect of marital status on mortality (i.e., being single, separated, divorced, or widowed) is also considerably stronger for men (Kiecolt-Glaser & Newton, 2001; Krongrad et al., 1996). Even though men benefit more from being married, women are more affected by marital quality—especially if it is poor (Kiecolt-Glaser & Newton, 2001). The fact that relational well-being is more strongly linked to emotional well-being in women is most likely due to women's heightened sensitivity to relationship functioning (Segrin, Powell, Givertz, & Brackin, 2003).

Poor marital quality is associated with physiological changes, deteriorated health outcomes, and increased mortality rates (Kiecolt-Glaser & Newton, 2001). Coyne et al. (2001) found that marital quality predicted four-year survival rates and illness severity in patients coping with congestive heart failure. Further, observational studies of married couples' interactions showed that hostile behaviors (i.e., interrupting, criticizing) were more predictive of greater physiological responses (i.e., blood pressure, immune changes, and endocrine levels) than were positive interactions (i.e., providing support, general positivity) (Coyne et al., 2001).

Evidence has shown that there is a reciprocal nature between marriage and health/illness, and several bidirectional pathways have been proposed to explain how marriage affects individuals' health (Burman & Margolin, 1989; Kiecolt-Glaser & Newton, 2001). Stress and social support are two important factors known to directly affect marital quality, either in a protective or deleterious function (Burman & Margolin, 1989). The receipt of emotional support can buffer the effects of stress, while the exposure to marital conflict can exacerbate stress, both via direct physiological pathways (Gallo, Troxel, Matthews, & Kuller, 2003; Kiecolt-Glaser & Newton, 2001; Ryff & Singer, 2000). Conversely, a spouse's poor health or chronic illness can create stress in a marriage and negatively influence marital quality (Burman & Margolin, 1989). Overall, marital distress, depression, and immune function form a triad of mutual influence in marriage, such that: poor marital quality is associated with indicators of poorer immune function, poor marital quality is associated with greater depression, and depression is associated with poorer immune function (Kiecolt-Glaser & Newton, 2001).

Throughout the mental health literature it is clear that the *quality* of interpersonal relations affects the onset, course, and recovery from psychological problems (Segrin, 2001). Individuals who report greater marital satisfaction experience fewer symptoms of depression and anxiety when adjusting to cancer than those who report low marital quality (Rodrigue & Park, 1996). Northouse et al. (2001) found that marital satisfaction was significantly associated with adjustment among husbands of women with breast cancer. Involvement in a satisfying close relationship provides a sense of positive affect and of being valued and understood, along with a feeling of stability. For example, Pistrang and Barker (1992, 1995) found that breast cancer patients most often select their husbands or intimate partners as the most important source of social support during the cancer process. Thus, the fulfillment associated with satisfying relationships can provide a powerful counterbalance to the uncertainty and stress of a major negative life event, such as cancer diagnosis and treatment.

In addition, relationship satisfaction has implications for individuals' physical health outcomes. People with satisfying personal relationships exhibit better neuroendocrine functioning than people who are single or in distressed relationships (Kiecolt-Glaser, McGuire, Robles, & Glaser, 2002; Turner-Cobb et al., 2000). Rohrbaugh, Shoham, and Coyne (2006) found that a composite measure of marital quality was the best predictor of heart failure patients' survival over eight years, above and beyond baseline measures of illness severity. In their study, the two facets of the composite marital quality measure that most strongly predicted patients' health outcomes were: (1) the observed affective quality of the couple's actual interaction (i.e., positivity–negativity ratio); and (2) the reported frequency of their "useful discussions" about the patient's illness (i.e., indicative of communal coping) (Rohrbaugh et al., 2006).

COPING STRATEGIES AND HEALTH OUTCOMES

Emotional Expression

Past research indicates that emotional expression and avoidant coping have significant influences on an individual's psychological well-being, levels of distress, and health outcomes. Emotional expression refers to the outward, observable displays of emotion (Graves et al., 2005), and people vary both verbally and nonverbally in their overall levels of expressiveness (Graves et al., 2005). Females tend to use more positive emotion words, and are generally more emotionally expressive overall, than are males (Newman, Groom, Handelman, & Pennebaker, 2008). Emotionally expressive coping is defined as a person's efforts to identify, understand, and express his/her emotions (Stanton, Kirk, Cameron, & Danoff-Burg, 2000) and is positively related with improved psychological adjustment among patients with breast cancer (Stanton, Kirk et al., 2000). For example, Spiegel, Bloom, Kraemer, and Gottheil (1989) found that women with advanced breast cancer who were randomly assigned to a nonspecific group therapy condition lived 1.5 years longer on average than did the women in an information-only control group.

Results of textual analyses on emotional expression have shown that a greater use of positive emotion words (e.g., happy, joy, optimistic) and a moderate use of negative emotion words (e.g., angry, cried, sad) are associated with positive health outcomes (Chung & Pennebaker, 2007; Pennebaker & Chung, 2007). After a traumatic experience or distressing life event, an increase in an individual's use of positive emotion words predicts superior psychological and physical health outcomes (Chung & Pennebaker, 2007; Pennebaker & Chung, 2007). In a study of the expressive writing narratives of women with advanced breast cancer, Laccetti (2007) found a significant association in greater use of positive to negative words and enhanced emotional well-being in women with advanced breast cancer at a three-month follow-up. Low, Stanton, & Danoff-Burg (2006) investigated the specific mechanisms underlying these positive health effects from emotional expression in women with breast cancer. Results indicated that the beneficial health outcomes from expressive writing could be explained by a decrease in participants' autonomic arousal (i.e., heart rate) (Low et al., 2006). In terms of the expression of negative emotions, research indicates a curvilinear relationship whereby optimal benefits occur when individuals use a moderate number of negative emotion words because both extremes (very high or low amounts) are associated with poorer health outcomes (Pennebaker & Chung, 2007).

On the other hand, avoidant coping, or an individual's efforts to suppress or avoid intrusive thoughts, is associated with deteriorated psychological outcomes (Owen et al., 2006). In fact, Owen et al. (2006) found that avoidant coping was the most consistent predictor of psychological distress in women at one and four months after diagnosis with early stage breast cancer. Owen et al. (2006) also observed a significant interaction between emotional suppression and the use of cognitive words on breast cancer patients' psychological adjustment and mood disturbance. Further, Weihs et al. (2000) found that negative affect (especially when concurrent with restriction of emotions) predicted a shortened survival rate among women with breast cancer. Similar to Weihs et al.'s findings, Owen et al. (2006) found that women with recurrent breast cancer who exhibited low-grade anxiety coupled with high emotional constraint were at a greater risk of mortality. In general, men are less likely to disclose their feelings or express emotions when coping (Notarius & Johnson, 1982), which has gender implications for positive psychosocial adjustment to cancer and possible health outcomes.

In addition to emotional and physical well-being, emotional expressiveness is associated with relationship satisfaction and stability in romantic couples. For example, Slatcher, Vazire, and Pennebaker (2008) found that men's genuinely expressed positive emotion words, as measured in their daily instant messages (IMs) to their romantic partners, were positively related to their own satisfaction, their *partners'* satisfaction, and whether the relationship was still intact six months later. Simmons, Gordon, and Chambless (2005) found that partners' use of positive emotion words when discussing a problem-solving task was associated with relationship stability. Therefore, they hypothesized that greater expression of positive feelings (or positivity in general) can lead to improved relationship outcomes (Simmons et al., 2005). Further, the degree to which couples discuss emotional reactions to stress and/or stressful events with each other enhances dyad members' perceptions of closeness. Therefore, disclosure of emotions is related to better-perceived partner responsiveness, which in turn, positively influences the couple's feelings of intimacy (Lewis et al., 2005).

Yet, partners of people coping with cancer may be less willing and less likely to self-disclose to their spouses. Past research has shown that although partners have many fears and concerns about their loved ones' illness, they often hold back from talking about their concerns and obscure their own feelings (Lewis et al., 2005). This makes sense, given that partners most likely do not want to burden their spouses with cancer with their own worries and preoccupations, so partners will avoid negative self-disclosure and revealing the depth of their concerns in an effort to protect the cancer survivor. However, this is a problematic interpersonal consequence because a partner's avoidance of open communication about the cancer experience with his/her spouse is associated with increased distress in the spouse with cancer (Harrison & Maguire, 1994; Nordin, Berglund, Glimelius, & Sjödén, 2001). Research indicates that even additional or outside support is not able to mitigate the negative effects of a distant or emotionally unavailable spouse on a female patient's emotional well-being (Weihs, Enright, Howe, & Simmens, 1999), which highlights the centrality and importance of a viable and emotionally supportive relationship partner.

Communal Coping and "We-Talk"

Communication (or talk) between couples creates and shapes how members of a dyad define their health, marriage, and self (Lyons, Mickelson, Sullivan, and Coyne, 1998). Further, the words couples use in conversation are associated with their relationship satisfaction and relational outcomes. Past research suggests a paramount role for first-person plural pronouns ("we" and "us") because it is hypothesized to reflect a couple's cognitive commitment (i.e., "we-ness"). Initially labeled by Lyons et al. (1998), "communal coping" is an instrumental dimension of couple coping that suggests a cooperative problem-solving process whereby dyad members identify problems and address an issue or challenge as "our" issue, rather than "yours" or "mine" (Acitelli & Badr, 2005; Berg & Upchurch, 2007; Bodenmann, 2005; Lewis et al., 2006; Lyons et al., 1998). This cooperative "we-based" coping in couples is a larger reflection of the dyad members' shared identity and the couple's level of interdependence (Agnew, Van Lange, Rusbult, & Langston, 1998; Simmons et al., 2005). Specifically, greater use of first-person plural pronouns (i.e., "we," "us," "our") in a couple's communication with each other highlights positive relationship aspects such as: relational commitment, a shared identity, and effective problem solving (Agnew et al., 1998; Simmons et al., 2005).

When couples recounted their marital history in laboratory settings, judges' ratings of couple "we-ness" (based largely on partners' tendency to use "we," rather than "he," "she," or "I") correlated with concurrent positive interaction behavior and marital satisfaction, and predicted whether the couples divorced over the next four years (Gottman & Levenson, 1999). Gottman, Coan, Carrere, and Swanson (1998) also found that "we" talk in the interactions of newlywed couples predicted relationship satisfaction and marital stability. However, this finding has not been supported across all studies. For example, Simmons et al. (2005) did not find a significant association between couples' use of "we-talk" and relationship satisfaction; however, results showed that couples who engaged in more "we-talk" were more effective at generating mutually satisfying problem solutions. Further, Slatcher et al. (2008) did not find that couples' use of "we" in their daily instant messages (IMs) was associated with their relationship satisfaction or relationship stability. Finally, Rohrbaugh, Mehl, Shoham, Reilly, & Ewy (2008) found that partners' "we-talk" during open-ended interviews predicted positive changes in symptoms of patients with chronic heart failure over six months. However, the positive influence of "we-talk" on health outcomes was only evident in the language use of the spouse/partner, and not the patient with heart failure (Rohrbaugh et al., 2008). Thus, their results provide support for the positive benefits of a communal coping orientation (at least unidirectionally from partner to patient), as well as additional evidence of the occurrence of partner effects in health outcomes in couples (e.g., Ruiz, Matthews, Scheier, & Schulz, 2006; Rohrbaugh et al., 2008).

CONCLUSION

Breast cancer is a major life experience for the woman who is diagnosed and her partner. Cross-over effects are evident for psychological distress, emotional well-being, and adjustment. However, in coping with cancer, couples would be well advised to be emotionally expressive with each other and provide social support to each other, especially in the form of emotional acceptance and affirmation. Having a mind-set to approach challenges as a team and to work through this process "together" is extremely helpful in building solidarity as a couple and can have positive benefits psychologically, if not even physically. Finally, reducing stress, depression, and negative affect is a critical component in negotiating through the experience of cancer. However, having positivity in one's interpersonal interaction and general outlook is as important as minimizing negativity. In sum, no person is an island, and no relationship occurs in a vacuum. Communication is at the core of all interpersonal interactions, and close relationships are, by nature, interdependent. Therefore, dyad members simultaneously and mutually influence each another. Close relational partners affect each other's attitudes, behaviors, and outcomes. And when one person is diagnosed with cancer, that relational experience is no different. The key, perhaps, is to go at it together.

REFERENCES

Acitelli, L. K., & Badr, H. J. (2005). My illness or our illness? Attending to the relationship when one partner is ill. In Revenson, T. A., Kayser, K., & Bodenmann, G. (Eds.), *Couples coping with stress* (pp. 121–136). Washington, DC: American Psychological Association.

Adams, R. G., & Blieszner, R. (1994). An integrative conceptual framework for friendship research. *Journal of Social & Personal Relationships, 11,* 163–184. doi.org/10.1177/0265407594112001.

Agnew, C. R., Van Lange, P. A. M., Rusbult, C. E., & Langston, C. A. (1998). Cognitive interdependence: Commitment and the mental representation of close relationships. *Journal of Personality and Social Psychology, 74,* 939–954.

Alferi, S. M., Carver, C. S., Antoni, M. H., Weiss, S., & Duran, R. E. (2001). An exploratory study of social support, distress, and life disruption among low-income Hispanic women under treatment for early stage breast cancer. *Health Psychology, 20,* 41–46. doi.org/10.1037/0278-6133.20.1.41.

American Cancer Society. (2013). *Cancer facts & figures: 2013.* Atlanta, GA: American Cancer Society, Inc. Retrieved from http://www.cancer.org/acs/groups/cid/documents/webcontent/003090-pdf.pdf.

Badger, T. A., Braden, C. J., & Mishel, M. H. (2001). Depression burden, self-help interventions, and side effects experienced by women with breast cancer. *Oncology Nursing Forum, 28,* 567–574.

Badger, T. A., Segrin, C., Dorros, S., Meek, P., & Lopez, A. M. (2007). Depression and anxiety in women with breast cancer and their partners. *Nursing Research, 56,* 44–53. doi.org/10.1097/00006199-200701000-00006.

Badger, T. A., Segrin, C., Meek, P., Lopez, A. M., & Bonham, E. (2004). A case study of telephone interpersonal counseling for women with breast cancer and their partners. *Oncology Nursing Forum, 31,* 997–1003. doi.org/10.1188/04 .ONF.997-1003.

Badger, T. A., Segrin, C., Meek, P., Lopez, A. M., Bonham, E., & Sieger, A. (2005). Telephone interpersonal counseling with women with breast cancer: Symptom management and quality of life. *Oncology Nursing Forum, 32,* 273–279. doi .org/10.1188/05.ONF.273-279.

Baider, L., Andritsch, E., Goldzweig, G., Ever-Hadani, P., Hofman, G., Krenn, G., & Samonigg, H. (2004). Changes in psychological distress of women with breast cancer in long-term remission and their husbands. *Psychosomatics, 45,* 58–68.

Baider, L., Ever-Hadani, P., Goldzweig, G., Wygoda, M. R., & Peretz, T. (2003). Is perceived family support a relevant variable in psychological distress? A sample of prostate and breast cancer couples. *Journal of Psychosomatic Research, 55,* 453–460. doi.org/10.1016/S0022-3999(03)00502-6.

Berg, C. A., & Upchurch, R. (2007). A developmental–contextual model of couples coping with chronic illness across the adult life span. *Psychological Bulletin, 133,* 920–954.

Bertalanffy, L., von. (1975). *Perspectives on general systems theory: Scientific-philosophical studies.* New York: George Braziller.

Bloom, B. L. (1986). New possibilities in prevention. In Hough, R., & Gongla, P. A. (Eds.), *Psychiatric epidemiology and prevention: The possibilities.* Los Angeles: UCLA Neuropsychiatric Institute, 165–189.

Bloom, J. R., & Spiegel, D. (1984). The relationship of two dimensions of social support to the psychological well-being and social functioning of women with advanced breast cancer. *Social Science & Medicine, 19,* 831–837. doi .org/10.1016/0277-9536(84)90400-3.

Bodenmann, G. (2005). Dyadic coping and its significance for marital functioning. In Revenson, T. A., Kayser, K., & Bodenmann, G. (Eds.), *Couples coping with stress* (pp. 33–49). Washington, DC: American Psychological Association.

Braun, M., Mikulincer, M., Rydall, A., Walsh, A., & Rodin, G. (2007). Hidden morbidity in cancer: Spouse caregivers. *Journal of Clinical Oncology, 25,* 4829–4834. doi.org/10.1200/JCO.2006.10.0909.

Broderick, C. B. (1993). *Understanding family processes: Basics of family systems theory.* Newbury Park, CA: Sage.

Burman, B., & Margolin, G. (1989). Marriage and health. *Advances, 6,* 5–58.

Carlson, L. E., Specca, M., Patel, K. D., & Goodey, E. (2003). Mindfulness-based stress reduction in relation to quality of life, mood, symptoms of stress, and immune parameters in breast and prostate cancer outpatients. *Psychosomatic Medicine, 65,* 571–581. doi.org/10.1097/01.PSY.0000074003.35911.41.

Chalmers, K., Marles, S., & Tataryn, D. (2003). Reports of information and support needs of daughters and sisters of women with breast cancer. *European Journal of Cancer Care, 12,* 81–90. doi.org/10.1046/j.1365-2354.2003.00330.x.

Chung, C. K., & Pennebaker, J. W. (2007). The psychological functions of function words. In Fielder, K. (Ed.), *Frontiers in social psychology* (pp. 1–30). New York: Psychology Press.

Cohen, S. (1988). Psychosocial models of the role of social support in the etiology of physical disease. *Health Psychology, 7,* 269–297. doi.org/10.1037/0278-6133.7.3.269.

Cohen, S., Gottlieb, B. H., & Underwood, L. G. (2000). Social relationships and health. In Cohen, S., Underwood, L. G., and Gottlieb, B. H. (Eds.), *Social support measurement and intervention: A guide for health and social scientists* (pp. 3–25). New York: Oxford University Press.

Cohen, S., & Syme, S. L. (1985). *Social support and health.* San Diego, CA: Academic Press.

Cohen S., & Williamson, G. M. (1991). Stress and infectious disease in humans. *Psychological Bulletin, 109,* 5–24. doi.org/10.1037/0033-2909.109.1.5.

Cohen, S., & Wills, T. A. (1985). Stress, social support, and the buffering hypothesis. *Psychological Bulletin, 98,* 310–357. doi.org/10.1037/0033-2909.98.2.310.

Cousson-Gelie, F., Bruchon, M., Dilhuydy, J. M., & Jutand, M. A. (2007). Do anxiety, body image, social support, and coping strategies predict survival in breast cancer? A ten-year follow-up study. *Psychosomatics, 48,* 211–216. doi.org/10.1176/appi.psy.48.3.211.

Coyne, J. C. (1976a). Depression and the response of others. *Journal of Abnormal Psychology, 85,* 186–193.

Coyne, J. C. (1976b). Toward an interactional description of depression. *Psychiatry, 39,* 28–40.

Coyne, J. C., Rohrbaugh, M. J., Shoham, V., Sonnega, J. S., Nicklas, J. M., & Cranford, J. A. (2001). Prognostic importance of marital quality for survival of congestive heart failure. *American Journal of Cardiology, 88,* 526–529.

Crohan, S., & Antonucci, T. (1989). Friends as a source of social support in old age. In Adams, R., & Blieszner, R. (Eds.), *Older adult friendship: Structure and process.* Newbury Park, CA: Sage.

Dehle, C., & Weiss, R. L. (2002). Associations between anxiety and marital adjustment. *The Journal of Psychology, 136,* 328–338. doi.org/10.1080/00223980209604160.

Dorros, S., Card, N., Segrin, C., & Badger, T. A. (2010). Interdependence in women with breast cancer and their partners: An interindividual model of distress. *Journal of Consulting and Clinical Psychology, 78,* 121–125. doi.org/10.1037/a0017724.

Dunkel-Schetter, C. (1984). Social support and cancer: Findings based on patient interviews and their implications. *Journal of Social Issues, 40,* 77–98. doi.org/10.1111/j.1540-4560.1984.tb01108.x.

du Pré, A. (2010). *Communicating about health: Current issues and perspectives* (3rd ed.). New York: Oxford University Press.

Ell, K., Sanchez, K., & Vourlekis, B. (2005). Depression, correlates of depression, and receipt of depression care among low-income women with breast and gynecologic cancer. *Journal of Clinical Oncology, 23,* 3052–3060. doi.org/10.1200/JCO.2005.08.041.

Fann, J. R., Thomas-Rich, A. M., Katon, W. J., Cowley, D., Pepping, M., McGregor, B. A., & Gralow, J. (2008). Major depression after breast cancer: A review of epidemiology and treatment. *General Hospital Psychiatry, 30,* 112–126. doi .org/10.1016/j.genhosppsych.2007.10.008.

Gallo, L. C., Troxel, W. M., Matthews, K. A., & Kuller, L. H. (2003). Marital status and quality in middle-aged women: Associations with levels and trajectories of cardiovascular risk factors. *Health Psychology, 22,* 453–463.

Giese-Davis, J., & Spiegel, D. (2003). Emotional expression and cancer progression. In Davidson, R. J., Scherer, K. R., & Goldsmith, H. H. (Eds.), *Handbook of affective sciences* (pp. 1053–1082). New York: Oxford University Press.

Gilbar, O. (1996). The connection between the psychological condition of breast cancer patients and survival: A follow-up after eight years. *General Hospital Psychiatry, 18,* 266–270. doi.org/10.1016/0163-8343(96)00023-0.

Gotcher, J. M. (1992). Interpersonal communication and psychosocial adjustment. *Journal of Psychosocial Oncology, 10,* 21–39. doi.org/10.1300/J077V10N03_02.

Gotcher, J. M. (1993). The effects of family communication on psychosocial adjustment of cancer patients. *Journal of Applied Communication Research, 21,* 176–188. doi.org/10.1080/00909889309365365.

Gottman, J. M., Coan, J., Carrere, S., & Swanson, C. (1998) Predicting marital happiness and stability from newlywed interactions. *Journal of Marriage and the Family, 60,* 5–22.

Gottman, J. M., & Levenson, R. W. (1999). What predicts change in marital interaction over time? A study of alternative medicine. *Family Process, 38,* 143–158.

Graves, K. D., Schmidt, J. E., Bollmer, J., Fejfar, M., Langer, S., Blonder, L. X., & Andrykowski, M. (2005). Emotional expression and emotional recognition in breast cancer survivors: A controlled comparison. *Psychology and Health, 20,* 579–595.

Greer, S., Morris., T., & Pettingale, K. (1979). Psychological responses to breast cancer: Effect on outcome. *Lancet, 2,* 785–787. doi.org/10.1016/S0140-6736 (79)92127-5.

Grunfeld, E., Coyle, D., Whelan, T., Clinch, J., Reyno, L., Earle, C. C., . . . Glossop, R. (2004). Family caregiver burden: Results of a longitudinal study of breast cancer patients and their principal caregivers. *CMAJ: Canadian Medical Association Journal, 170,* 1795–1801. doi:10.1503/cmaj.1031205.

Hagedoorn, M., Sanderman, R., Bolks, H. N., Tuinstra, J., & Coyne, J. C. (2008). Distress in couples coping with cancer: A meta-analysis and critical review of role and gender effects. *Psychological Bulletin, 134,* 1–30.

Han, W. T., Collie, K., Koopman, J., Azarow, J., Classen, C., & Morrow, G. R. (2005). Breast cancer and problems with medical interactions: Relationships with traumatic stress, emotional self-efficacy, and social support. *Psycho-Oncology, 14,* 318–330. doi.org/10.1002/pon.852.

Harrison, J., & Maguire, P. (1994). Predictors of psychiatric morbidity in cancer patients. *The British Journal of Psychiatry, 165,* 593–598. doi.org/10.1192/ bjp.165.5.593.

Hatfield, E., Cacioppo, J. T., & Rapson, R. L. (1992). Primitive emotional contagion. In Clark, M. S. (Ed.), *Emotion and social behavior* (pp. 151–177). Newbury Park, CA: Sage.

Hatfield, E., Cacioppo, J. T., & Rapson, R.L. (1994). *Emotional contagion*. Paris: Cambridge University Press.

Helgeson, V. S., Snyder, P., & Seltman, H. (2004). Psychological and physical adjustment to breast cancer over 4 years: Identifying distinct trajectories of change. *Health Psychology, 23*, 3–15. doi.org/10.1037/0278-6133.23.1.3.

Hilton, B. A. (1994). Family communication patterns in coping with early breast cancer. *Western Journal of Nursing Research, 16*, 366–391. doi.org/10.1177/019394599401600403.

Holland, K. D., & Holahan, C. K. (2003). The relation of social support and coping to positive adaptation to breast cancer. *Psychology and Health, 18*, 15–29. doi.org/10.1080/0887044031000080656.

Holly, P., Kennedy, P., & Taylor, A. (2003). Immediate breast reconstruction and psychological adjustment in women who have undergone surgery for breast cancer: A preliminary study. *Psychology, Health & Medicine, 8*, 441–452. doi.org/10.1080/1354850310001604586.

Hoskins, C. N. (1995). Adjustment to breast cancer in couples. *Psychological Reports, 77*, 1017–1018. doi.org/10.2466/pr0.1995.77.3.1017.

Hoskins, C. N. (1997). Differences in adjustment between women with breast cancer and their partners: Implications for nursing interventions. *Clinical Effectiveness in Nursing, 1*, 105–111. doi.org/10.1016/S1361-9004(06)80012-9.

Hoskins, C. N., Baker, S., Sherman, D., Bohlander, J., Bookbinder, M., Budin, W., Ekstrom, D., Knauer, C., & Maislin, G. (1996). Social support and patterns of adjustment to breast cancer. *Research and Theory for Nursing Practice, 10*, 99–123.

Hudek-Knezevic, J., Kardum, I., & Pahljina, R. (2002). Relations among social support and negative affect in hospitalized and nonhospitalized cancer patients. *Journal of Psychosocial Oncology, 20*, 45–63. doi.org/10.1300/J077v20n02_03.

Kiecolt-Glaser, J. K., McGuire, L., Robles, T., & Glaser, R. (2002). Emotions, morbidity, and mortality: New perspectives from psychoneuroimmunology. *Annual Review of Psychology, 53*, 83–107. doi.org/10.1146/annurev.psych.53.100901.135217.

Kiecolt-Glaser, J. K., & Newton, T. L. (2001). Marriage and health: His and hers. *Psychological Bulletin, 127*, 472–503.

Kornblith, A. D., Herdon, J. E., Zuckerman, E., Goodley, P. A., Savarese, D., & Vogelzang, N. J. (2001). The impact of docetaxel, estramustine, and low dose hydrocortisone on quality of life of men with hormone refractory prostate cancer and their partners: A feasibility study. *Annals of Oncology, 12*, 633–641. doi.org/10.1023/A:1011102619058.

Krongrad, A., Lai, H., Burke, M. A., Goodkin, K., & Lai, S. (1996). Marriage and mortality in prostate cancer. *The Journal of Urology, 156*, 1696–1700.

Krumholz, H., Butler, J., & Miller, J. (1998). Prognostic importance of emotional support for elderly patients hospitalized with heart failure. *Circulation, 97*, 958–964. doi.org/10.1097/00005392-199611000-00041.

Laccetti, M. (2007). Expressive writing in women with advanced breast cancer. *Oncology Nursing Forum, 34*, 1019–1024. doi.org/10.1188/07.ONF.1019-1024.

Lawton, M. P. (1983). Environment and other determinants of well-being in older people. *Gerontologist, 23*, 349–357. doi.org/10.1093/geront/23.4.349.

Lewis, F. M., Cochrane, B. B., & Fletcher, K. A. (2005). Predictors of spousal depressed mood in women with breast cancer. *Oncology Nursing Forum, 32*, 165.

Lewis, F. M., Cochrane, B. B., Fletcher, K. A., Zahlis, E. H., Shands, M. E., Gralow, J. R., Wu, S. M., & Scmitz, K. (2008). Helping her heal: A pilot study of an educational counseling intervention for spouses of women with breast cancer. *Psycho-Oncology, 17*, 131–137. doi.org/10.1002/pon.1203.

Lewis, F. M, Fletcher K. A., Cochrane, B. B., & Fann, J. R. (2008). Predictors of depressed mood in spouses of women with breast cancer. *Journal of Clinical Oncology, 26*, 1289–1295.

Lewis, F. M., & Hammond, M. A. (1992). Psychosocial adjustment of the family to breast cancer: A longitudinal analysis. *Journal of American Medical Women's Association, 47*, 194–200.

Lewis, M. A., McBride, C. M., Pollak, K. I., Puleo, E., Butterfield, R. M., & Emmons, K. M. (2006). Understanding health behavior change among couples: An interdependence and communal coping approach. *Social Science and Medicine, 62*, 1369–1380.

Levy, S., Herberman, R., Maluish, A., Schlien, B., & Lippman, M. (1985). Prognostic risk assessment in primary breast cancer by behavioral and immunological parameters. *Health Psychology, 4*, 99–113. doi.org/10.1037/0278-6133.4.2.99.

Low, C. A., Stanton, A. L., & Danoff-Burg, S. (2006). Expressive disclosure and benefit-finding among breast cancer patients: Mechanisms for positive health effects. *Health Psychology, 25*, 181–189. doi.org/10.1037/0278-6133.25.2.181.

Luecken, L. J., & Compas, B. E. (2002). Stress, coping, and immune function in breast cancer. *Annals of Behavioral Medicine, 24*, 336–344. doi.org/10.1207/S15324796ABM2404_10.

Lyons, R. F., Mickelson, K. D., Sullivan, M. J. L., & Coyne, J. C. (1998). Coping as a communal process. *Journal of Personal and Social Relationships, 15*, 579–605.

Maddi, S. R., Bartone, P. T., & Puccetti, M. C. (1987). Stressful events are indeed a factor in physical illness: Reply to Schroeder and Costa (1984). *Journal of Personality and Social Psychology, 52*, 833–843. doi.org/10.1037/0022-3514.52.4.833.

Manne, S. L., Ostroff, J. S., Norton, T. R., Fox, K., Goldstein, L., & Grana, G. (2006). Cancer-related relationship communication in couples coping with early stage breast cancer. *Psycho-Oncology, 15*, 234–247. doi.org/10.1002/pon.941.

Manne, S. L., Ostroff, J., Sherman, M., Glassman, M., Ross, S., & Goldstein, L. (2003). Buffering effects of family and friend support on associations between partner unsupportive behaviors and coping among women with breast cancer. *Journal of Social and Personal Relationships, 20*, 771–792. doi.org/10.1177/0265407503206004.

Manne, S. L., Ostroff, J. S., Sherman, M., Heyman, R. E., Ross, S., & Fox, K. (2004). Couples' support-related communication, psychological distress, and relationship satisfaction among women with early stage breast cancer. *Journal of Consulting and Clinical Psychology, 72,* 660–670. doi.org/10.1037/0022-006X.72.4.660.

Manne, S. L., Ostroff, J., Winkel, G., Grana, G., & Fox, K. (2005). Partner unsupportive responses, avoidant coping, and distress among women with early stage breast cancer: Patient and partner perspectives. *Heath Psychology, 24,* 635–641. doi.org/10.1037/0278-6133.24.6.635.

Manne, S. L., Taylor, K. L., Dougherty, J., & Kemeny, N. (1997). Supportive and negative responses in the partner relationship: Their association with psychological adjustment among individuals with cancer. *Journal of Behavioral Medicine, 20,* 101–125. doi.org/10.1023/A:1025574626454.

Maunsell, E., Brisson, J., & Deschenes, L. (1992). Psychological distress after initial treatment of breast cancer: Assessment of potential risk factors. *Cancer, 70,* 120–125. doi.org/10.1002/1097-0142(19920701)70:1<120::AID-CNCR2820700120>3.0.CO;2-U.

McDaniel, J. S., & Nemeroff, C. B. (1993). Depression in the cancer patient: Diagnostic, biological and treatment aspects. In Chapman, C. R., & Foley, K. M. (Eds.), *Current and emerging issues in cancer pain: Research and practice* (pp. 1–19). New York: Raven.

Mellon, S., & Northouse, L. L. (2001). Family survivorship and quality of life following a cancer diagnosis. *Research in Nursing and Health, 24,* 446–459. doi.org/10.1002/nur.10004.

Michaelson, M. D., Cotter, S. E., Gargollo, P. C., Zietman, A. L., Dahl, D. M., & Smith, M. R. (2008). Management of complications of prostate cancer treatment. *CA: A Cancer Journal for Clinicians, 58,* 196–213. doi.org/10.3322/CA.2008.0002.

Monjan, A. A., & Collector, M. (1977). Stress-induced modulations of the immune response. *Science, 196,* 307–308. doi.org/10.1126/science.557841.

Neuling, S. J., & Winefield, H. R. (1988). Social support and recovery after surgery for breast cancer: Frequency and correlates of supportive behaviors by family, friends and surgeons. *Social Science & Medicine, 27,* 385–392. doi.org/10.1016/0277-9536(88)90273-0.

Newman, M. L., Groom, C. J., Handelman, L. D., & Pennebaker, J. W. (2008). Gender differences in language use: An analysis of 14,000 text samples. *Discourse Processes, 45,* 211–236. doi.org/10.1080/01638530802073712.

Newport, D. J., & Nemeroff, C. B. (1998). Assessment and treatment of depression in the cancer patient. *Journal of Psychosomatic Research, 45,* 215–237. doi.org/10.1016/S0022-3999(98)00011-7.

Nordin, K., Berglund, G., Glimelius, B., & Sjödén, P. O. (2001). Predicting anxiety and depression among cancer patients—A clinical model. *European Journal of Cancer, 37,* 376–384. doi.org/10.1016/S0959-8049(00)00398-1.

Northouse, L. L. (1988). Social support in patients' and husbands' adjustment to breast cancer. *Nursing Research, 37,* 91–95. doi.org/10.1097/00006199 -198803000-00008.

Northouse, L. L. (1989). A longitudinal study of the adjustment of patients and husbands to breast cancer. *Oncology Nursing Forum, 16,* 511–516.

Northouse, L. L., Mood, D. W., Montie, J. E., Sandler, H. M., Forman, J. D., & Hussain, M. (2007). Living with prostate cancer: Patients' and spouses' psychological status and quality of life. *Journal of Clinical Oncology, 25,* 4171–4177. doi.org/10.1200/JCO.2006.09.6503.

Northouse L. L., & Swain, M. A. (1987). Adjustment of patients and husbands to the initial impact of breast cancer. *Nursing Research, 36,* 221–225. doi.org/10.1097/ 00006199-198707000-00009.

Northouse, L. L., Templin, T., & Mood, D. (2001). Couples' adjustment to breast disease during the first year following diagnosis. *Journal of Behavioral Medicine, 24,* 115–136. doi.org/10.1023/A:1010772913717.

Northouse, L. L., Templin, T., Mood, D., & Oberst, M. (1998). Couples' adjustment to breast cancer and benign breast disease: A longitudinal analysis. *Psycho-Oncology, 7,* 37–48. doi.org/10.1002/(SICI)1099-1611(199801/02) 7:1<37::AID-PON314>3.3.CO;2-R.

Notarius, C., & Johnson, J. (1982). Emotional expression in husbands and wives. *Marriage and the Family, 44,* 483–489. doi.org/10.2307/351556.

Owen, J. E., Giese-Davis, J., Cordova, M., Kronenwetter, C., Golant, M., & Spiegel, D. (2006). Self-report and linguistic indicators of emotional expression in narratives as predictors of adjustment to cancer. *Journal of Behavioral Medicine, 29,* 335–345. doi.org/10.1007/s10865-006-9061-8.

Pasacreta, J. V. (1997). Depressive phenomena, physical symptom distress, and functional status among women with breast cancer. *Nursing Research, 46,* 214–221. doi.org/10.1097/00006199-199707000-00006.

Pennebaker, J. W., & Chung, C. K. (2007). Expressive writing, emotional upheavals, and health. In Friedman, H., & Silver, R. (Eds.), *Handbook of health psychology* (pp. 263–284). New York: Oxford University Press.

Perlman, D., & Rook, K. S. (1987). Social support, social deficits, and the family: Toward the enhancement of well-being. *Applied Social Psychology Annual, 1,* 17–44.

Picard, L., Dumont, S., Gagnon, P., & Lessard, G. (2006). Coping strategies among couples adjusting to primary breast cancer. *Journal of Psychosocial Oncology, 23,* 115–136. doi.org/10.1300/J077v23n02_08.

Pistrang, N., & Barker, C. (1992). Clients' beliefs about psychological problems. *Counselling Psychology Quarterly, 5,* 325–335.

Pistrang, N., & Barker, C. (1995). The partner relationship in psychological response to breast cancer. *Social Science and Medicine, 40,* 789–797. doi.org/ 10.1016/0277-9536(94)00136-H.

Pitceathly, C., & Maguire, P. (2003). The psychological impact of cancer on patients' partners and other key relatives: A review. *European Journal of Cancer, 39,* 1517–1524. doi.org/10.1016/S0959-8049(03)00309-5.

Primono, J., Yates, B. C., & Woods, N. F. (1990). Social support for women during chronic illness: The relationship among sources and types to adjustment. *Research in Nursing and Health, 13,* 153–161. doi.org/10.1002/nur.477 0130304.

Rodrigue, J. R., & Park, T. L. (1996). General and illness-specific adjustment to cancer: Relationship to marital status and marital quality. *Journal of Psychosomatic Research, 40,* 29–36. doi.org/10.1016/0022-3999(95)00540-4.

Rohrbaugh, M. J., Mehl, M. R., Shoham, V., Reilly, E. S., & Ewy, G. A. (2008). Prognostic significance of spouse *we* talk in couples coping with heart failure. *Journal of Consulting and Clinical Psychology, 76,* 781–789. doi.org/10.1037/a0013238.

Rohrbaugh, M. J., Shoham, V., & Coyne, J. C. (2006). Effects of marital quality on 8-year survival of patients with heart failure. *American Journal of Cardiology, 98,* 1069–1072.

Rook, K. (1987). Social support versus companionship: Effects on life stress, loneliness, and evaluations by others. *Journal of Personality and Social Psychology, 52,* 1132–1147. doi.org/10.1037/0022-3514.52.6.1132.

Rook, K. (1990). Stressful aspects of older adults' social relationships: Current theory and research. In Stephens, A. P., Crowther, J. H., Hobolt, S. E., & Tennenbaum, D. L. (Eds.), *Stress and coping in later-life families* (pp. 173–192). New York: Hemisphere.

Rook, K., & Ituarte, P. (1999). Social control, social support, and companionship in older adults' family relationships and friendships. *Personal Relationships, 6,* 199–211. doi.org/10.1111/j.1475-6811.1999.tb00187.x.

Ross, C., Mirowsky, J., & Goldsteen, K. (1990). The impact of the family on health: The decade in review. *Journal of Marriage and the Family, 52,* 1059–1078.

Rude, S. S., Gortner, E. M., & Pennebaker, J. W. (2004). Language use of depressed and depression-vulnerable college students. *Cognition & Emotion, 18,* 1121–1133. doi.org/10.1080/02699930441000030.

Ruiz, J. M., Matthews, K. A., Scheier, M. F., & Schulz, R. (2006). Does who you marry matter for your health? Influence of patients' and spouses' personality on their partners' psychological well-being following coronary artery bypass surgery. *Journal of Personality and Social Psychology, 91,* 255–267.

Ryff, C. D., & Singer, B. (2000). Interpersonal flourishing: A positive health agenda for the new millennium. *Personality and Social Psychology Review, 4,* 30–44.

Sapolsky, R. M. (2004). *Why zebras don't get ulcers* (3rd ed.). New York: Henry Holt.

Segrin, C. (2001). *Interpersonal processes in psychological problems.* New York: Guilford Press.

Segrin, C. (2003). Age moderates the relationship between social support and psychosocial problems. *Human Communication Research, 29,* 317–342. doi.org/10.1111/j.1468-2958.2003.tb00842.x.

Segrin, C., Badger, T., Dorros, S., Meek, P., & Lopez, A. M. (2007). Interdependent anxiety and psychological distress in women with breast cancer and their partners. *Psycho-Oncology, 16,* 634–643. doi.org/10.1002/pon.1111.

Segrin, C., Badger, T. A., Meek, P., Lopez, A. M., Bonham, E., & Sieger, A. (2005). Dyadic interdependence on affect and quality of life trajectories among women with breast cancer and their partners. *Journal of Personal and Social Relationships, 22*, 673–690. doi.org/10.1177/0265407505056443.

Segrin, C., Badger, T. A., Sieger, A., Meek, P., & Lopez, A. (2006). Interpersonal well-being and mental health among male partners of women with breast cancer. *Issues in Mental Health Nursing, 27*, 1–19. doi.org/10.1080/01612840600569641.

Segrin, C., & Flora, J. (2011). *Family Communication* (2nd ed.). New York: Routledge.

Segrin, C., Powell, H. L., Givertz, M., & Brackin, A. (2003). Symptoms of depression, relational quality, and loneliness in dating relationships. *Personal Relationships, 10*, 25–36. doi.org/10.1111/1475-6811.00034.

Simmons, R., Gordon, P. C., & Chambless, D. (2005). Pronoun use in marital interaction: What do "you" and "I" say about marital health? *Psychological Science, 16*, 932–936.

Slatcher, R. B., Vazire, S., & Pennebaker, J. W. (2008). Am "I" more important than "we"? Couples' word use in instant messages. *Personal Relationships, 15*, 407–424. doi.org/10.1111/j.1475-6811.2008.00207.x.

Spiegel, D. (1993). Psychosocial intervention in cancer. *Journal of National Cancer Institute, 85*, 1198–1205. doi.org/10.1093/jnci/85.15.1198.

Spiegel, D. (1997). Psychosocial aspects of breast cancer treatment. *Seminars in Oncology, 1*, 36–47.

Spiegel, D., & Bloom J. R. (1983). Pain in metastic breast cancer. *Cancer, 52*, 149–153. doi.org/10.1002/1097-0142(19830715)52:2<341::AID-CNCR2820520227>3.0.CO;2-G.

Spiegel, D., Bloom, J. R., Kraemer, H. C., & Gottheil, E. (1989). Effect of psychosocial treatment on survival of patients with metastatic breast cancer. *Lancet ii*, 888–891. doi.org/10.1016/S0140-6736(89)91551-1.

Stanton, A. L., Danoff-Burg, S., Cameron, C. L., Bishop, M., Collins, C. A., & Kirk, S. B. (2000). Emotionally expressive coping predicts psychological and physical adjustment to breast cancer. *Journal of Consulting and Clinical Psychology, 68*, 875–882.

Stanton, A., Kirk, S., Cameron, C., & Danoff-Burg, S. (2000). Coping through emotional approach: Scale construction and validation. *Journal of Personality and Social Psychology, 78*, 1150–1169.

Tracy, G., & Gussow, Z. (1976). Self-help groups: A grass-roots response to a need for services. *Journal of Application and Behavioral Science, 12*, 381–396. doi.org/10.1177/002188637601200309.

Trunzo, J. J., & Pinto, B. M. (2003). Social support as a mediator of optimism and distress in breast cancer survivors. *Journal of Consulting and Clinical Psychology, 71*, 805–811. doi.org/10.1037/0022-006X.71.4.805.

Turner-Cobb, J. M., Sephton, S. E., Koopman, C., Blake-Mortimer, J., & Spiegel, D. (2000). Social support and salivary cortisol in women with metastatic breast cancer. *Psychosomatic Medicine, 62*, 337–345.

Walker, B. L. (1997). Adjustment of husbands and wives to breast cancer. *Cancer Practice, 5*, 92–98.

Walker, L. G. (2004). Hypnotherapeutic insights and interventions: A cancer odyssey. *Contemporary Hypnosis, 21*, 35–45.

Weihs, K. L., Enright, T. M., Howe, G., & Simmens, S. J. (1999). Marital satisfaction and emotional adjustment after breast caner. *Journal of Psychosocial Oncology, 17*, 33–49. doi.org/10.1300/J077v17n01_03.

Weihs, K. L., Enright, T. M., & Simmens, S. J. (2008). Close relationships and emotional processing predict decreased mortality in women with breast cancer: Preliminary evidence. *Psychosomatic Medicine, 70*, 117–124. doi.org/10.1097/PSY.0b013e31815c25cf.

Weihs, K. L., Enright, T. M., Simmens, S. J., & Reiss, D. (2000). Negative affectivity, restriction of emotions, and site of metastases predict mortality on recurrent breast cancer. *Journal of Psychosomatic Research, 49*, 59–68. doi.org/10.1016/S0022-3999(00)00143-4.

Weissman, M. M., & Markowitz, J. C. (1998). An overview of interpersonal psychotherapy. In Markowitz, J. C. (Ed.). *Interpersonal psychotherapy* (pp. 1–33). Washington, DC: American Psychiatric Press.

Weissman, M. M., Markowitz, J. C., & Klerman, G. L. (2000). *Comprehensive guide to interpersonal psychotherapy*. New York: Basic Books.

Whisman, M. A., Uebelacker, L. A., & Weinstock, L. M. (2004). Psychopathology and marital satisfaction: The importance of evaluating both partners. *Journal of Consulting and Clinical Psychology, 72*, 830–838. doi.org/10.1037/0022-006X.72.5.830.

Wootten, A., Burney, S., Foroudi, F., Frydenberg, M., Coleman, G., & Ng, K.T. (2007). Psychological adjustment of survivors of localized prostate cancer: Investigating the role of dyadic adjustment, cognitive appraisal, and coping style. *Psycho-Oncology, 16*, 994–1002. doi.org/10.1002/pon.1159.

Chapter 17

The Experience and Construction of Changes in Women's Sexuality after Breast Cancer: A Material-Discursive-Intrapsychic Analysis

Janette Perz, Jane M. Ussher, and Emilee Gilbert[1]

INTRODUCTION

Breast cancer is the most common cancer in women and the second lead-ing cause of cancer deaths in women globally (World Health Organiza-tion, 2009). It is now recognized that changes to sexual well-being can be the most problematic aspect of life post–breast cancer, with the impact lasting for many years after successful treatment (Andersen, 2009; Bertero & Wilmoth, 2007), often associated with serious physical and emotional side effects (Langellier & Sullivan, 1998). Indeed, research has shown that when compared with healthy same-aged women, women with breast can-cer experience lower levels of sexual satisfaction and have more difficulty maintaining their sexual lives (Speer et al., 2005). Until recently, research examining the impact of breast cancer on sexuality was primarily con-ducted from a positivist-realist paradigm (Wilmoth, 2001), privileging the physical and material aspects of women's experience, and focusing on levels of sexual "dysfunction" post–breast cancer, where functional sexu-ality is conceptualized as penile/vaginal intercourse (Fobair et al., 2006).

Recent research has shown, however, that engaging in sexual intercourse may not be positioned as women's primary focus of sexual adjustment and satisfaction after a breast cancer diagnosis, and engagement in sexual intercourse does not necessarily equate to sexual satisfaction (Wilmoth, 2001). Moreover, the primary focus on the physical effects of breast cancer or breast cancer treatment on sexual behavior assumes that a woman's experience of sexuality is limited to its corporeal dimensions, negating the influence of the social construction of sexuality and illness (Meyerowitz et al., 1999) and the ways in which the meaning of sex is negotiated by individuals and within relationships (Gilbert, Ussher, & Perz, 2010a).

As a counterpoint to the primacy of positivism and realism, research from a social constructionist paradigm has provided insight into women's lived experiences of changes to sexuality after breast cancer (Archibald, Lemieux, Byers, Tamlyn, & Worth, 2006), and the ways in which sociocultural discourses shape the experience and interpretation of sexuality (Young, 1992). As Judith Butler (1990) has argued, our understanding of sexual subjectivity is confined within a heterosexual matrix, within which masculinity and femininity are performed through engagement in normative sexual practices, described as the "coital imperative" (Gavey, McPhillips, & Braun, 1999), with failure to perform coitus positioned as dysfunction, and other practices as not "real sex" (Few, 1997). These social and cultural discourses teach us about what is normal and abnormal, and profoundly impact how we come to construct our understanding of sexuality, and explain why many heterosexual couples who cannot physically engage in sexual intercourse following diagnosis and treatment of cancer cease all expression of sexual intimacy. However, within a social constructionist paradigm, intrapsychic and intersubjective aspects of women's experiences are often ignored, and the physical body is either positioned as the passive object of cultural constructions, or it is absent from explorations of lived experiences of sexuality after breast cancer. In other words, the physical dimension of illness can get neglected by social constructionists, who tend to explore the constructions and meanings ascribed to symptoms rather than the materiality of the illness, the functioning of the body, and the impact this has on a person's life (Ussher, 2008).

In order to address the limitations of both realism and constructionism, this chapter will adopt a material-discursive-intrapsychic perspective (Ussher, 2000), which acknowledges the materiality of sexual changes following breast cancer, women's intrapsychic experience of such changes within a relational context, and the influence of the discursive construction of femininity and sexuality. In this vein, we will review the available research on breast cancer and sexuality, and then examine a recently completed Australian study of sexual well-being after breast cancer as an illustrative case example.

MATERIALITY: CHANGES TO THE BODY AND SEXUAL FUNCTIONING FOLLOWING DIAGNOSIS AND TREATMENT

Research with Western women has found that embodied changes and disturbances to sexual functioning frequently reported following the diagnosis and treatment of breast cancer include: dyspareunia (Speer et al., 2005); fatigue (Fobair et al., 2006); vaginal dryness (Ganz, Greendale, Petersen, Kahn, & Bower, 2003; Ganz, Rowland, Desmond, Meyerowitz, & Wyatt, 1998); decreased sexual interest or desire (Avis, Crawford, & Manuel, 2004); decreased sexual arousal (Knobf, 2001); numbness in previously sensitive breasts (Wilmoth, 2001); difficulty achieving orgasm (Fobair et al., 2006; Speer et al., 2005); and lack of sexual pleasure (Meyerowitz et al., 1999). Research in non-Western cultures has yielded similar results, with diminished sexual desire, decreased orgasm, vaginal dryness, coital pain, decreased sexual activity, deterioration of the sexual relationship, a loss of interest in sexual partners, and sexual dissatisfaction reported by Iranian, Turkish, and Chinese women after breast cancer (Alicikus et al., 2009; Can et al., 2008; Garrusi & Faezee, 2008; Zee et al., 2008).

A considerable amount of research has investigated the relationship between breast cancer treatment and changes to sexual well-being, with women who undergo chemotherapy being reported to be at higher risk of reporting sexual difficulties after treatment than those who have not received such treatment (Avis et al., 2004; Ganz, Desmond, Belin, Meyerowitz, & Rowland, 1999; Ganz et al., 1998; Thors, Broeckel, & Jacobsen, 2001). Chemotherapy is also associated with problems of arousal, lubrication, orgasm, and sexual pain (Alder et al., 2008), issues that are particularly common shortly after treatment (Burwell, Case, Kaelin, & Avis, 2006). However, while research has found that radiation is associated with feeling medically invaded (Langellier & Sullivan, 1998), it is not as likely to be associated with decreased sexual desire as chemotherapy (Takahashi et al., 2008). Yet the impact of chemically induced menopause (CIM) on sexuality has also been associated with decreased sexual desire; pain during intercourse; vaginal dryness; decreased sexual arousal; a severe or complete loss of pleasurable sexual sensations; and decreased frequency or intensity of orgasms (Archibald et al., 2006).

The combination of loss of sexual function, premature menopause, and the associated symptoms of vaginal dryness tends to be particularly severe (Ganz et al., 1998), and can be devastating for young women who may also be concerned with loss of reproductive opportunity (Ganz et al., 2003). However, the evidence of a link between hormonal treatment with tamoxifen, an estrogen antagonist, and sexual functioning is somewhat contentious. Ganz et al. (1998) found no difference in sexual functioning between women treated with or without tamoxifen, while Mortimer et al. (1999) found that some women treated with tamoxifen complained of pain, burning, or discomfort with intercourse; vaginal tightness; hot flashes; and negative feelings during intercourse. There has also been much recent research examining the impact of breast cancer surgery on the sexual functioning of women, though the results are mixed. Some have found that women who received breast-conserving surgery report fewer problems associated with sexual interest than women who had a mastectomy (Ganz et al., 1999; Markopoulos et al., 2009), and that women who have had a mastectomy experience difficulty relaxing and enjoying sex and difficulty reaching orgasm (Burwell et al., 2006), as well as a decreased frequency of sex post-surgery (Takahashi et al., 2008). However, others provide little evidence of a link between type of surgical treatment and sexual functioning (Rogers & Kristjansen, 2002; Thors et al., 2001).

The fertility of women with breast cancer can also be compromised because of the disease itself or resulting from gonadal damage secondary to chemotherapy, or radiotherapy, which can produce early menopause or uterine damage (Camp-Sorrell, 2009; Tschudin & Bitzer, 2009). While there have been significant advances in strategies to preserve fertility, these interventions are not always risk free and can result in ovarian stimulation and surgical damage to ovaries, as well as risks from delaying commencement of cancer treatment (Stern, 2010).

INTRAPSYCHIC EXPERIENCES: EMOTIONS AND BODY IMAGE

While some women experience the changes to their sexuality after breast cancer positively (Archibald et al., 2006; Ganz et al., 1998; Langellier & Sullivan, 1998), the majority of evidence shows that women with breast cancer experience a range of serious negative emotional changes as a result of disturbances to their sexuality, including fear of loss of fertility, negative body image, feelings of sexual unattractiveness (Bertero & Wilmoth, 2007), loss of femininity (Wilmoth, 2001), and depression and anxiety (Garrusi & Faezee, 2008), as well as alterations to their sexual self-concept (Wilmoth, 2001). Having to adjust to the removal of the breast or to the alteration in appearance of the breast, loss of bodily hair, loss of menstruation and childbearing capacity, feeling old before their time (Wilmoth, 2001), concern about weight gain or loss, and a partner's difficulty understanding a woman's feelings (Fobair et al., 2006) can exacerbate these negative emotional changes. Although some researchers have argued that such changes are more prevalent in women with preexisting anxiety, depression, or sexual dysfunction (Can et al., 2008; Fobair et al., 2006), the potential emotional impact of disturbances to sexuality is an issue for a large proportion of women with breast cancer. Women who report negative changes to their sexuality can also report worrying about what causes these sexual changes, how long the changes will last, the extent to which the changes may impact their intimate relationship, and how they can cope with the sexual changes (Gilbert, Ussher, Perz, 2010b).

Equally, the consequences of infertility following cancer have been described as "devastating," resulting in distress, fear, and feeling "broken hearted" (Tschudin et al., 2010, p. 615). Conversely, being fertile is a predictor of good quality of life post-cancer (Rudberg, Nilsson, & Wikblad, 2000). Researchers have also reported that fertility concerns can result in depression, anxiety, and low self-esteem, as well as changes to body image and gender identity in cancer survivors (Carter et al., 2005; Connell, Patterson, & Newman, 2006; Crawshaw & Sloper, 2010; Gurevich, Bishop, Bower, Malka, & Nyhof-Young, 2004; Reis, Beji, & Coskun, 2010; Rosen, Rodriguez-Wallberg, & Rosenzweig, 2009).

Although the physical pain of breast cancer and treatment diminishes with time, the experience of emotional pain may persist as women grieve the loss of fertility or of their breast, or feel as though a part of them has died (Langellier & Sullivan, 1998). In this vein, breasts are often positioned as such a significant part of women's sense of self that those who undergo a mastectomy feel like "half a woman" (Manderson & Stirling, 2007). Research also shows that the strongest consistent predictor of sexual problems after breast cancer is lower perceived sexual attractiveness (Burwell et al., 2006), and that women who have a poor body image after breast cancer have lower rates of sexual satisfaction and are more dissatisfied with their sexual relationship than those with a positive body image (Speer et al., 2005). Overall, however, it is suggested that body image and sexuality are most significantly affected by breast cancer during the first year of survivorship, and that body image is more likely to be affected by mastectomy compared to breast-conserving treatment or breast reconstruction (Fobair et al., 2006; Ganz et al., 1998). For example, studies have shown that mastectomy patients are more likely than women who have received breast-conserving surgery or reconstruction to dislike their appearance without clothes (Alicikus et al., 2009), avoid looking at themselves in mirrors (Langellier & Sullivan, 1998), and feel embarrassed, ugly, or self-conscious (Manderson & Stirling, 2007). Women who receive breast-conserving surgery also report fewer problems with dressing, body image, and being naked, than do women who have had a mastectomy (Markopoulos et al., 2009).

SOCIOCULTURAL AND DISCURSIVE CONSTRUCTS: THE CONSTRUCTION AND EXPERIENCE OF BREASTS, SEXUALITY, AND FERTILITY

Research that has taken a social constructionist approach to the issue of sexuality and breast cancer has been largely concerned with the ways in which sociocultural and medico-scientific discourses shape a woman's construction and experience of her illness and her body. For example, Langellier and Sullivan (1998) examined how these discourses are embedded in women's breast talk, and found that women talk about four different, but highly interrelated, types of breasts. The medicalized breast, constructed as a physical body part with disease; the functional breast, constructed as a symbol of women's emotional abilities to nurture others; the gendered breast, constructed as a symbol of femininity, beauty, and sexual desirability; and the sexualized breast, which incorporates the look and feel of the breast. These types of breasts are positioned in women's talk as belonging not only to themselves, but also to their children, husbands, and lovers. This is exemplified in Thomas-MacLean's (2005) interview study, where women who had undergone a mastectomy described feeling a loss of bodily symmetry post–breast cancer surgery that led them to manage appearances or hide their "deformity" from others. Women have also reported wearing a prosthesis to appear normal to those in public, and to avoid being viewed as asymmetrical or less than whole by husbands, male partners, or children (Manderson & Stirling, 2007). It has been argued that this is because within patriarchal culture there is a focus on the breast as a "daily visible and tangible signifier" of a woman's femininity for both herself and for others (Young, 1992, p. 215). A particular type of breast is both privileged and normalized—the breast that is round, firm, and not sagging or medically mutilated. The woman with breast cancer is thus potentially positioned outside normal femininity (Spence, 1995), which can have serious implications for women's sense of self, body image, psychological well-being, and sexuality.

Equally, when an individual is diagnosed with cancer and comes to be seen as ill, a different set of norms emerge for "acceptable" behavior within their illness state (Wellard, 1998, 53), including the notion that people with cancer have either limited sexual needs or are asexual (D'Ardenne, 2004). Schildrick (2005) has argued that people with a disability or serious illness are "disqualified" from normative discourses of sexuality, as "proper" sexuality is associated only with able-bodied, healthy, and usually young individuals, which "legitimates a denial of sexual desire and pleasure" (p. 334). This disqualification and denial is also associated with the prominence of the "coital imperative" in medical, social, and legal discourse (Gavey et al., 1999, p. 37), wherein individuals who cannot perform sexual intercourse *properly* are positioned as dysfunctional (Tiefer, 1996, 2001). It is thus not surprising that intercourse has been found to be strongly connected with feelings of acceptance, intimacy, and love, and absence of intercourse with feelings of self-doubt (Gavey et al., 1999). However, as Schildrick comments, (2005, p. 332), "'proper' sexuality is inevitably contested by those whose atypical morphology literally frustrates the performance of conventional paradigms and normative certainties," in their renegotiation of sex outside of the coital imperative.

The discursive construction of fertility and motherhood is also central to experiences of sexuality after breast cancer, in light of the pronatalism in Western culture (Morell, 2000). Non-mothers often feel stigmatized and perceive that they are positioned as less than whole, pitiable, and desperate (Letherby & Williams, 1999). Infertility following cancer can thus impact a woman's "sexual self," including sexual functioning, desire, and body image (Carpentier & Fortenberry, 2010; Carter et al., 2005; Reis et al., 2010), as well as erode self-confidence in romantic relationships (Carpentier & Fortenberry, 2010; Crawshaw & Sloper, 2010; Zebrack, Casillas, Nohr, Adams, & Zetler, 2004).

At the same time, for intimate partners who are also the carer of a person with cancer, renegotiating a sexual relationship may be particularly problematic given the discursive construction of the good carer and the social construction of appropriate or taboo sexual conduct for those in the role of carer. Carers may come to consider their partners purely as patients and as dependent upon them for their basic needs—needs that are often antithetical to the expression of sexuality within the relationship (Gilbert, Ussher, & Hawkins, 2009). For example, Manderson (2005) found that people with a stoma and their carers find it difficult to sexualize a body on which there is now attached a bag containing, in a very visual way, urinary fluid and defecation. Similarly, in the study we present below, a number of women with breast cancer reported that their partners were disgusted by, and could no longer sexualize, their breasts.

RELATIONSHIP CONTEXT AND SEXUAL RENEGOTIATION

One of the most important and consistent predictors of sexual health in women with breast cancer is the quality of their partnered relationship (Archibald et al., 2006; Ganz et al., 1999; Garrusi & Faezee, 2008). In fact, the quality of a woman's relationship is a stronger predictor of sexual satisfaction, sexual functioning, and sexual desire after breast cancer than is the physical or chemical damage to the body after treatment (Alder et al., 2008; Speer et al., 2005; Zee et al., 2008). Research has shown that if women can renegotiate their sexual practices when the type of sex they had pre-cancer is no longer desirable or possible, then they are more able to manage the changes to their sexual relationship (Gilbert et al., 2010a). The inability to renegotiate sexuality and intimacy post-cancer has been reported to be associated with difficulties in communicating about sexual matters (Arrington, 2003; Foy & Rose, 2001; Holmberg, Scott, Alexy, & Fife, 2001), often for fear of creating feelings of guilt in the person with cancer (Kuyper & Wester, 1998). However, there is a distinct lack of research that examines sexuality after cancer from a relational perspective. This negates the ways in which the experience of sexuality is shaped by the relationship context, including how a woman positions her partner post-cancer, how the partner positions the woman post-cancer, whether sex is positioned as a taboo in the context of cancer, and whether sex is openly communicated about.

CHANGES TO SEXUAL WELL-BEING AFTER BREAST CANCER: A STUDY OF AUSTRALIAN WOMEN

In order to illustrate the material-discursive-intrapsychic experience and construction of changes to sexuality after breast cancer, we will now present a case example drawing on the findings of a recent research study conducted with Australian women. The purpose of this study was to examine the lived experience of sexual well-being and couple intimacy in a large sample of individuals with breast cancer living in Australia, using a mixed method approach (see Ussher, Perz, & Gilbert, 2012, 2013).

Study Outline and Participants

The participants were 1,999 individuals drawn from the membership of a national organization for Australians affected by breast cancer, Breast Cancer Network Australia (BCNA). Participants ranged from 18 to 84 years, with an average age of 54.1. The sample was predominately female (99.8%), self-identified as Anglo-Australian (89.1%), and had further tertiary education and/or training (60.7%). The majority of participants were partnered (85.3%), heterosexual (98.0%), and had children (84.2%). On average, it had been 3.9 years since participants received their diagnosis of breast cancer, with 74.6 percent having been diagnosed with early stage breast cancer. At the time of the study, 45.6 percent had finished their treatment, and 45.5 percent were still receiving treatment. Menstruation had ceased for 77.8 percent of the sample, who described themselves as postmenopausal.

The study involved a survey that was available for online completion for a 14-day period in December 2010, involving a combination of closed and open-ended items. In the quantitative analysis presented below, percentages for frequency data were calculated on the number of participants who completed each item, rounded up for readability. For items with multiple options, percentages do not total 100, as participants could choose more than one response. Thematic analysis (Braun & Clarke, 2006) was used to analyze the open-ended responses. This involved independent reading of responses to each question by two members of the research team in order to ascertain the major themes that emerged and to develop a coding frame, based on notions of consistency, commonality, and the function and effects of specific themes. Demographic information is provided for longer quotes, which are omitted to enhance readability from shorter quotes.

In the analysis presented below, we examine accounts of changes to sexual well-being and relationships; what was perceived to cause such changes; avenues of coping; and impact on partners.

The Impact of Breast Cancer on Sexual Well-Being and Relationships

In answer to a question on the impact of breast cancer or breast cancer treatment on sexual well-being, the majority of 1,956 participants reported a decrease in frequency of sex (78%), energy for sex (76%), sexual arousal (74%), feeling desirable (73%), interest in sex (71%), sexual pleasure (64%), satisfaction with sex (62%), and intimacy (60%). (See Table 17.1.) No change was reported by the majority of participants in the areas of "partner interest in sex" (64%) and "communication with partner about sexual needs" (51%); however, a considerable proportion of the sample also reported decreases in these areas. Only 7 percent of the sample noted an increase in the area of "communication with partner about sexual needs," this being the largest recorded increase.

Table 17.1 The impact of breast cancer or breast cancer treatment on sexual well-being (*n*=1,956)

| | Percentage (*n*) | | |
Area	Decreased	No change	Increased
Frequency of sex	77.9% (1,427)	20.3% (372)	1.8% (33)
Energy for sex	76.0% (1,379)	22.4% (407)	1.5% (28)
Sexual arousal	73.6% (1,344)	24.2% (442)	2.2% (40)
Feeling desirable	73.4% (1,385)	25.1% (473)	1.6% (30)
Interest in sex	71.4% (1,308)	26.1% (479)	2.5% (45)
Sexual pleasure	64.2% (1,151)	33.8% (607)	2.0% (36)
Satisfaction with sex	61.9% (1,096)	35.6% (630)	2.5% (44)
Intimacy	60.4% (1,090)	34.5% (623)	5.1% (93)
Communication with partner about sexual needs	42.4% (746)	50.5% (889)	7.2% (126)
Partner interest in sex	32.4% (565)	64.3% (1,120)	3.3% (58)

Of 1,956 participants who described which aspects of breast cancer or breast cancer treatment were perceived to have affected sexual well-being (see Table 17.2), the most frequent responses were: tiredness (71%), vaginal dryness (63%), hot flushes (51%), and feeling unattractive (51%).

When asked what had been tried to deal with changes to sexual well-being after the onset of breast cancer, the most common response, reported by 61 percent of 1,598 respondents, was talking to partner/husband, followed by lubricant (57%), exercise (45%), reading information booklets/leaflets (31%), talking to a health professional (26%), antidepressants (20%), psychotherapy/counseling (16%), sex aids (14%), medications (11%), and books (11%).

The majority of 1,999 respondents reported that breast cancer had affected their sexual relationship, with 24 percent of respondents saying it was affected *dramatically*, 26 percent *considerably*, 32 percent *somewhat*, and only 15 percent *not at all*. Of the 1,348 participants who answered a question asking whether their partners had experienced any negative consequences as a result of their breast cancer, the most common reports were: fear of hurting me during sex (52%), lack of interest in sex (37%), difficulties in communication (34%), tiredness (28%), and change in role (seeing me as a patient) (20%). The pattern of these proportions in all of the above items did not differ according to age, relationship status, sexual orientation, or current stage of cancer treatment.

More than 400 participants (*n*=413) responded to an item inquiring into the influence of cancer upon their ability to enter into a new relationship, with 57 percent indicating that it had an impact. The most frequently identified issues were related to feelings around appearance and the perceptions of others, with *body image/attractiveness concerns* noted by 77 percent of the sub-sample, followed by *lack of confidence* (67%), *not feeling desirable* (65%), and *fear of rejection* (47%). Of these concerns, *not feeling desirable* and *fear of rejection* were more commonly reported by women seeking new heterosexual relationships (64 percent and 46 percent, respectively) compared to women seeking a new same-sex relationship (14 percent and 0 percent, respectively). The most common physical effects reported were *fatigue* (47%), *vaginal dryness* (43%), and *upper body or other pain* (23%).

The Subjective Experience of Changes to Sexual Well-Being after Breast Cancer

One thousand two hundred and fifty nine participants, all women, provided answers to an open-ended question asking about the subjective experience of changes to sexual well-being after breast cancer. The most common responses related to 1) negative emotional consequences, 2) physical changes, 3) feeling unattractive or lacking femininity, 4) reconciliation of self to changes, 5) concerns about impact on partner or relationship, and 6) partner support and relationship improvement.

Table 17.2 Aspects of breast cancer or breast cancer treatment that have affected sexual well-being (*n*=1,956)

Item	Percentage (*n*)
Tiredness	71.0% (1,387)
Vaginal dryness	63.3% (1,237)
Hot flushes	51.2% (1,000)
Feeling unattractive	50.8% (993)
Weight gain	48.8% (953)
Difficulty being aroused	45.8% (894)
Feeling uncomfortable exposing my body	44.0% (860)
Medication side effects	39.0% (762)
Loss of confidence in myself	38.4% (751)
Depression/anxiety	37.8% (738)
Change in size or shape of breast	37.6% (734)
Difficulty reaching orgasm	35.9% (701)
Loss of sensation	35.8% (700)
Reduced nipple sensation	35.4% (692)
Pain during intercourse	33.4% (653)
Anxiety about sex	28.6% (558)
Early menopause	28.1% (550)
Appearance changes (e.g., hair loss)	27.0% (527)
Pain in upper body	26.9% (525)
Relationship changes	22.8% (446)
Fear	21.4% (418)
Loss of identity	17.0% (332)
Anger	16.3% (319)
Lymphodema	16.3% (318)
Guilt	12.6% (246)
Feelings of shame	10.2% (200)
Other[a]	36.9% (722)
Erectile difficulties (for men with breast cancer)	100.0% (5)

[a] Each less than 10%—increased sensitivity (9.9%, *n*=193); thrush (8.4%, *n*=164); vaginal discharge (8.0%, *n*=157); irregular menstruation (6.1%, *n*=120); weight loss (3.9%, *n*=76); more energy (0.6%, *n*=12).

Negative Emotional Consequences: Devastation, Depression, and Sadness

Over a third of participants (*n*=439) described negative emotional consequences of changes to sexual well-being post–breast cancer. The most commonly reported feelings were *devastating* and *depressing,* with other descriptors including *confusing, disturbing, soul destroying, shocking and unexpected, frustrating, traumatic,* and *demoralizing.* For the majority of women, these feelings were associated with a loss of interest in sex, or not experiencing pleasure during sex, as is illustrated by the following accounts: "I find that I have no desire for sex. When I have sex I find that it was not enjoyable which then made me feel guilty" (47-year-old woman, locally advanced breast cancer, two years post-diagnosis); "Very upsetting. I love my husband very much and our relationship is very good. My physical body does not arouse or respond like it used to" (51-year-old woman, early breast cancer, three years post-diagnosis); "It's very upsetting but I have no interest in sex at all, couldn't care if I never have sex again!!!" (49-year-old woman, early breast cancer, two years post-diagnosis).

A significant proportion of women reported sadness and loss as a result of sexual changes, with one saying, "I feel a sense of loss, as if part of me has died," and another saying, "I felt like my heart had been ripped out. Very empty." Many women also told us that they "miss the sexual aspect of my life":

> I feel as if an integral part of my life is no longer well within my reach. Although I am getting older and therefore might be expected to lose interest in sex to a certain degree, sex has been an important component of my life until I started receiving treatment for breast cancer. I worry about my loss of interest in sex and I miss the sexual aspect of my life. (65-year-old woman, early breast cancer, three years post-diagnosis)

A substantial number of women told us that they experienced feelings of loss because of the changes in their relationships with their partners, feeling that a "door was being closed," and they could not always discuss it: "Sad as I love my husband dearly, but this has changed our intimate relationship" (46-year-old woman, early breast cancer, five years post-diagnosis). The "totally unexpected" nature of changes to sexual well-being were also a source of distress for many participants, who told us that they had been given no information about what to expect: "Terrible! I am young and had not expected the side effects sexually that come from menopause and treatments . . . very sad" (26-year-old woman, early breast cancer, three years post-diagnosis); "Devastating. A complete shock, no one tells you that it ruins your sex life" (61-year-old, secondary breast cancer, three years post-diagnosis); "It was totally unexpected as nobody seemed to mention sexual dysfunction as a result of treatment. It made me feel that I had lost something very precious. I just wanted to be normal again" (56-year-old woman, early breast cancer, three years post-diagnosis).

Physical Changes to Sexual Well-Being; Painful Sex and Absence of Desire

Approximately one-quarter of respondents (*n*=249) described the changes to sexual well-being after breast cancer in terms of physical changes, including vaginal dryness; absence of sexual desire, arousal, or orgasm; and absence of breast sensitivity or breast tenderness: "Enjoy the sexual experience but very conscious of my breast and the fact they have no feeling. Weight put on the breast can be painful" (48-year-old woman, early breast cancer, two years post-diagnosis); "Main problem is lack of interest and vaginal dryness. Husband VERY supportive but doesn't initiate sex as often because he doesn't want to be pushy as he knows I just can't be bothered a lot of the time" (50-year-old woman, early breast cancer, three years post-diagnosis); "Due to not having an oestrogen my vagina has basically closed up, shrunk in other words. . . . I have a prolapse as well which doesn't help" (55-year-old woman, locally advanced breast cancer, three years post-diagnosis).

Vaginal dryness, or vaginal prolapse, can lead to painful coital sex. This was an experience commonly reported by women, which can sometimes lead to avoidance of sex: "Sexual intercourse is very painful. We can get pleasure from mutual masturbation but penetration for me is very, very painful. It is almost like my husband is wearing a condom with cut glass attached to it" (65-year-old woman, early breast cancer, six years post-diagnosis); "I do not lubricate, the skin external and internal to the vagina is very delicate, tearing easily. So sex is now painful for me regardless of the type of lubricants we use" (31-year-old woman, locally advanced breast cancer, three years post-diagnosis). A number of women gave accounts of dealing with these physical changes by renegotiating coital sexual activity after breast cancer, primarily through the use of lubricants. In some instances this was positioned positively, as an effective solution: "Breast cancer diagnosed Oct 2008. Met new partner (widower) Jan 09 and commenced sexual relationship Feb 09. No probs except dryness due to Arimidex (use lubricant)" (67-year-old woman, early breast cancer, three years post-diagnosis).

In other instances lubrication was described as "messy" and as interrupting the spontaneity of sex: "The only way to have sex is with lubrication, which is messy, and I find it extremely frustrating and annoying for not only me but for my husband as the first thing I reach for is my bottle of lubricant" (38-year-old woman, early breast cancer, nine years post-diagnosis). Masturbation was also described as a solution, with one 75-year-old woman with locally advanced breast cancer, one year post-diagnosis, telling us: "As a still attractive older woman, no sexual partner means masturbation is an option on occasion." These accounts of renegotiation were in the minority, however, with the majority of women reporting that they had ceased sexual activity, or endured uncomfortable or painful sex to please their partners. As one woman commented, "There is physical and emotional pain involved in having sex—I worry that I am only doing it to keep him happy, not at all for myself."

Women also reported that the physical consequences of cancer or cancer treatment, including tiredness, nausea, feeling "sore" or "uncomfortable," as well as weight gain, had an impact on their sexual well-being: "Forced menopause and feeling overweight impact on feeling 'sexy,' and less desirable" (48-year-old woman, early breast cancer, three years post-diagnosis); "Sex is the last thing on your mind when your chest hurts, you lose all your hair, you are tired and feel very unattractive—you just want to survive and get through" (35-year-old woman, secondary breast cancer, two years post-diagnosis).

In contrast, a very small number of women reported increased sexual pleasure or desire, "increased libido," or that sex was a way of feeling "real and alive" during treatment: "I went from not feeling a desirable woman, to feeling the more sexually interested and excited I have ever been" (50-year-old woman, early breast cancer, two years post-diagnosis); "I am shocked that my libido has increased" (35-year-old woman, early breast cancer, two years post-diagnosis). These cases may be in the minority, but they suggest that detrimental effects of breast cancer on sexual well-being cannot be assumed to be the case for all women.

Feeling Unattractive and Lacking in Femininity: I Am Not Really a Woman Anymore

Approximately one-fifth of respondents (*n*=212*)* reported feeling unattractive or lacking in femininity after breast cancer, and as a consequence, told us that they felt that this had an impact on their sexual well-being. Thus, women described themselves as being distressed because of "negative feelings about my body," or because "I don't feel attractive at all anymore."

When first diagnosed, I was alone, so sex not important; now it is naturally more important, and having no breasts now sometimes makes me feel less feminine considering my fiancé was always a "boob" man (41-year-old woman, early breast cancer, six years post-diagnosis)

Other women provided more pejorative comments about themselves, feeling *old and ugly, maimed, grotesque, mutilated,* a *freak, damaged goods, like an old has-been, undesirable, deformed,* feelings that were associated with breast scars, reconstruction, hair loss, and weight gain: "I feel my body is not my own. I do not like my 'fake' breasts. I feel old now and ugly" (55-year-old woman, early breast cancer, three years post-diagnosis); "I hate to look at myself. I can't look in the mirror. I can't even touch myself to see if the lump is still there. I can't stand to be looked at or touched. A hug is all I can bear" (48-year-old woman, locally advanced breast cancer, one year post-diagnosis). These feelings led many women to hide their bodies from their partners, saying "I don't want my husband to see or touch my breast," or "I don't feel like exposing my breast and have partner touching it and seeing it." Many women also reported feeling "like I was a different person," "my femininity was ripped off overnight," "not really a woman," "less womanly," "less of a person," or "an inadequate partner":

> Horrible!! I'm 28 and have been married for 9 months and have had sex probably 4 times in that time. . . . I used to enjoy it very much and now have no physical pleasure from it and barely ever do it . . . this has impacted on my identity as a woman and as a wife, has made me consider my partner having an affair because I am not able to satisfy him sexually. (29-year-old woman, early breast cancer, one year post-diagnosis)

In some instances, this feeling was associated with partner rejection, which confirmed the woman's fears, as is illustrated in the following accounts: "Husband avoided my reconstructed breast, which made me feel it wasn't a 'normal' thing" (58-year-old woman, early breast cancer, two years post-diagnosis); "devastating, don't feel like a whole person anymore, partner won't look at chest anymore so sex is just not worth it" (48-year-old woman, early breast cancer, two years post-diagnosis); "he says I have 'mutilated my body.' It isn't a pretty sight, and I don't like it either, but I'm stuck with it" (48-year-old woman, locally advanced breast cancer, two years post-diagnosis). In contrast, other women described partner support as alleviating their fears about being "unattractive" or "deformed," or of their partners helping to address their lack of "confidence in body image": "Took time for me to accept myself as I am. My partner, to his credit, loves me how I am" (53-year-old woman, early breast cancer, diagnosed 1996). "Initially, I felt that I was unattractive, even deformed. I worried that my husband wouldn't love my body as before. He tells me over and over that he loves me even more now so. . . . I have to get over it and just believe him" (60-year-old woman, early breast cancer, one year post-diagnosis).

Partner support or acceptance did not always alleviate women's negative feelings about their body or femininity, however, as illustrated in the following accounts: "I know it is me and not my husband as he has been wonderful, telling me constantly that in his eyes I am still the same to him. But I feel ugly with these scars" (68-year-old woman, locally advanced breast cancer, two years post-diagnosis); "Although my husband says he has no problem with my body as it now . . . I have a problem with it! . . . I just can't get passed [*sic*] this feeling. This affects our intimacy greatly!" (47-year-old woman, early breast cancer, two years post-diagnosis).

No Change or Reconciling Self to Changes in Sexual Well-Being: It Really Hasn't Worried Me

Approximately one-tenth of participants (*n*=123) described having experienced no change in sexual well-being or having reconciled themselves to such changes since the diagnosis of breast cancer: "No change after breast cancer diagnosis"; "It really hasn't worried me all that much"; "It has not really changed me. I feel the same"; "Not very important for me"; "This is something we have both come to terms with and manage accordingly"; "I was too tired to care." Others positioned changes in sexual well-being as temporary and looked forward to improvements in the future: "I hope I will 'get back to normal' after I finish treatment. I feel the need to conserve my energy for healing at this time" (40-year-old woman, early breast cancer, one year post-diagnosis).

At the same time, for a small number of participants, the cessation of sexual activity was welcomed: "Now I have a reason to say no"; "In some ways a relief"; "Being over 70 and never very partial to sex it was fine"; "Couldn't care less whether I had sex ever again." For other women, sex was positioned as unimportant, or as less important than other aspects of health since the diagnosis of breast cancer, which meant that changes to sexual well-being were accepted: "Other things seem more important and my partner has been so caring that sex seems quite unimportant"; "Find I am focused on how my health is rather than sex"; "Too many other things to worry about because of the absolute shock of the diagnosis and the treatment process." A few women commented that sex had never been important: "Sex was never an issue with us and haven't done so for about over 20 years prior to diagnosis and we are very happy"; "After so many years of marriage we have become very good friends, so sex is not that important"; "Did not have sex before and not having it now"; "The need for sex was no longer part of my life."

Concerns about Impact on Partner or Relationship: Letting My Partner Down

For approximately one-fifth of the sample (*n*=190), the impact of changes in sexual well-being for their partner was their major concern. Thus, a 52-year-old woman with locally advanced breast cancer, three years post-diagnosis, told us: "It made me feel as though I was neglecting my husband but I just don't feel the same about sex as I used to." Other women described their concern as "Letting my partner down"; "I know he would like more from me"; "I feel he is missing out"; or "I feel terrible about this and the impact it has on my partner."

> I'd say I've had less than 5 orgasms in 12 months and I am not even bothered, which is not how I used to be. I worry about how my partner must feel as I struggle to appear interested when we have sex. We are close but I know he would like more from me. (34-year-old woman, early breast cancer, one year post-diagnosis)

Approximately 10 percent of respondents ($n=126$) told us that their relationship had experienced difficulty, or broken down, as a result of changes to their sexual well-being after breast cancer. Comments included: "It was all very difficult, and placed a big strain on my relationship"; "My husband had affairs behind my back . . . our marriage is all but finished although we are still together"; "Devastating and almost ended my marriage"; "Ex husband made me feel like a leper"; "the diagnosis brought about the end of my marriage"; "I did not realize the impact on my marriage until it was too late"; "My husband did not react well and subsequently left." A number of women also told us that existing relationship difficulties had been exacerbated by the occurrence of breast cancer: "He does not seem interested anymore in sex at all. It had been a bit of a problem previous to my diagnosis and has got much worse since"; "My diagnosis just exacerbated problems that already existed in my marriage. A noncommunicative relationship just got worse."

The majority of respondents attributed these relationship changes or breakdown to their own disinterest in sex: "I went from a high libido to no libido or interest at all; my husband replaced me in less than two months"; "It is very frustrating for my partner, my interest in sex has declined, therefore creating tension in the marriage"; "Pre-diagnosis sex was fun but now I have no desire. My relationship with husband is strained and stressed. He still wants sex but I am not aroused." For other women, these relationship changes were attributed to their partners becoming a "carer," "brother," or "housemate" and thus no longer their lovers: "I feel the relationship with my husband has become like housemates rather than husband and wife"; "My partner is now my carer—and I think it is this fact which has altered our sexual relationship." Difficulties in communication were also described as causing relationship tension: "Devastating, had good relationship before, very loving, as soon as I had the first operation he didn't communicate at all"; "Very hard to come to terms with since my partner isn't good at communicating and in denial about my health issues"; "Devastating, communication became very strained for the first time in our relationship."

Partner Support and Relationship Improvement: We're Closer Now

A small proportion of women, approximately one-tenth, described feeling closer, or experiencing greater intimacy, with their partners since the diagnosis of breast cancer: "Whilst the act of sex has decreased, the intimacy between us has increased in other ways"; "Our relationship has moved to another level of loving without sex"; "I actually feel more secure in my relationship post diagnosis"; "The BC experience has brought us together and improved intimacy considerably"; "We stopped taking our sex life for granted and made an effort to maintain intimacy and our sex life."

Breast cancer was also described as offering an opportunity to renegotiate intimacy in order to meet a woman's needs, often addressing needs that had been there prior to breast cancer. One woman described this as "freedom" from sex, while another described increased "communication, flirtiness and warmth," which resulted in a richer relationship with her husband, with whom she had developed "a deep unspoken bond that is much richer than the earlier sexual moments." Better communication since diagnosis was also reported by a number of women participants: "Much closer to partner and more open"; "We communicate our needs much better than before my diagnosis"; "I found that we communicated better regarding issues during treatment and since." Having a supportive partner who accepted the changes the woman was experiencing, and who exerted "no pressure" for sex, or was "willing to wait until I'm willing," was also described as "the most important thing" by a number of women:

> At diagnosis we were both so devastated, and I felt that I would never be able to have sex again, but as time goes on and acceptance happens our sex life has improved, thanks mainly to my partner's attitude that he loves me and does not find anything different about me. (65-year-old woman, early breast cancer, one year post-diagnosis)

Having a secure relationship before breast cancer was described as important for a number of women, allowing the couple to cope with changes in sexual desire or activity: "We are very secure in our relationship and agreed that intercourse was not high on the list of needs. Support, sharing conversations, and just being together was more important" (54-year-old woman, early breast cancer, two years post-diagnosis). Equally, a number of women described new relationships developing since diagnosis and treatment for breast cancer, sometimes after a previous relationship had ended post-cancer: "I have found a very considerate amazing beautiful partner. I also still feel sexy and whole and goddess like"; "Marriage breakdown prior to diagnosis—no sexual relationship for six months or more—new relationship after treatment finished."

When I was first diagnosed, I went through a terrible time of feeling undesirable, fearing disfigurement and seeking affirmation. I felt very needy. I sought reassurance and was firmly rejected. Although upsetting at the time, this was paradoxically helpful in forcing me to face up to my future independently and take ownership of what was happening to me. The effect of the surgery was much less disfiguring than I'd feared, and my confidence has returned. I've since had an affirming sexual relationship. (62-year-old woman, early breast cancer, one year post-diagnosis)

These accounts suggest that relationship difficulty or breakdown does not mean the end of sexual relationships for women with breast cancer, as new relationships can develop and be rewarding, both emotionally and sexually.

The End of Fertility: A Double Trauma for Women with Breast Cancer

The question "has breast cancer had an effect on your fertility?" was answered by 1,830 participants, 83 percent of the sample; 24.6 percent (n=452) of these 1,830 participants reported that cancer had had an effect on their fertility, with 21.3 percent (n=391) reporting that they did not know, and 54 percent (n=987) reporting that it had not had an effect. Three hundred and eighty-one women provided information in open-ended questions about the ways in which breast cancer had affected their fertility. A substantial number of participants gave accounts that confirmed previous reports that infertility post-cancer is a "double trauma" (Carter et al., 2010), which can be as painful as facing cancer itself (Nieman et al., 2006; Schover, 2005). Participants described being "angry," "desperate" for children, and "very upset" about their changed fertility status: "Can't have children because they had to bring on menopause. Very angry" (45-year-old woman, secondary breast cancer, six years post-diagnosis); "I was oestrogen positive so I can't have any more children which I desperately wanted, it's too much risk, also my ovaries stopped producing eggs on my fourth round of chemotherapy" (39-year-old woman, locally advanced breast cancer, one year post-diagnosis). One participant described infertility, and the associated changes to sexual well-being, as the most significant long-lasting effect of her breast cancer:

This is a very, very important issue as breast cancer survivors are constantly reminded of their fight with the cancer in their daily life due to the impact it has on the sexual relationship with your partner. The cancer changes everything anyway, but this impact lasts the longest and is a constant in the relationship and is a very important part of trying to return to a "normal" life after treatment and the disappointments that infertility as a result of the cancer has left in the relationship. (49-year-old woman, early breast cancer, 14 years post-diagnosis)

Uncertainty about fertility status post-cancer can also be difficult for women (Zebrack et al., 2004) and can exacerbate anxiety related to disclosure of fertility status post-cancer to a new partner (Crawshaw & Sloper, 2010; Zebrack et al., 2004), or be a source of anxiety for those who are already parents but desire more children in the future (Del Pup et al., 2006), as is illustrated by the following account: "I assume treatments have made me infertile, but don't know for sure. That's difficult" (40-year-old woman, locally advanced breast cancer, three years post-diagnosis). A number of women also reported that they had been trying to get pregnant through IVF before breast cancer, but that this was not an option for them in the future: "I was on unsuccessful IVF treatment before breast cancer diagnosis. Breast cancer and menopause ended that" (43-year-old woman, early breast cancer, three years post-diagnosis); "now menopausal but have five frozen embryos, but five years post-chemo I will be old (45)" (42-year-old woman, early breast cancer, three years post-diagnosis). These accounts suggest that uncertainty about fertility, or current fertility status, is not a static or fixed experience for women with breast cancer and may change over time, depending on responses to cancer treatment, fertility preservation, or other health-related factors (Connell et al., 2006).

CONCLUSION

The findings presented in this study of Australian women support and extend previous research that reports significant changes in sexual well-being after diagnosis and treatment for breast cancer. In a previous survey of 863 women that examined self-reported changes to sexual functioning after breast cancer, it was found that one-third reported that cancer had a negative impact on their sexuality (Meyerowitz et al., 1999). In the present study, the largest study of sexual well-being in the context of breast cancer published to date (see Gilbert et al., 2010a), the proportion was far greater, suggesting that one-third may be a significant underestimate. Decreases in frequency of sex; sexual arousal, interest, and desire; as well as in sexual pleasure, satisfaction, and intimacy were attributed to a range of factors, including tiredness and pain, psychological distress and body image, and medically induced menopausal changes such as vaginal dryness, hot flushes, and weight gain. However, accounts of material changes to the body and relationships, as well as intrapsychic consequences, cannot be separated from discursive constructions of illness, femininity, and (hetero)sexuality, which give meaning to the experience of sexual well-being after breast cancer: a material-discursive-intrapsychic interaction (Ussher, 2005). For example, the focus on vaginal dryness experienced by women with breast cancer as a major cause of sexual difficulty, and the paucity of accounts of renegotiating sexual activity when coital sex was painful or difficult, illustrates the dominance of the coital imperative in the construction and experience of heterosexuality (Gavey et al., 1999). Challenging the coital imperative through the exploration of noncoital sexual practices should thus be central to professional advice and support for individuals with breast cancer.

While some individuals experience the changes to their sexuality after breast cancer positively (Archibald et al., 2006; Ganz et al., 1998; Langellier & Sullivan, 1998), the majority of evidence shows that people with breast cancer experience a range of serious negative emotional changes as a result of disturbances to their sexuality and fertility, confirmed and elaborated upon by the findings of the present study. Having to adjust to the removal of a breast or to the alteration in appearance of the breast, loss of bodily hair, feeling "old" before one's time (Wilmoth, 2001), concern about weight gain or loss, and a partner's greater difficulty in understanding one's feelings (Fobair et al., 2006) can exacerbate these negative emotional changes, as was found in the present study. As Archibald and colleagues (2006) showed in their interview study with 30 women with breast cancer, 62 percent of those who reported experiencing negative changes to their sexual well-being also reported that the changes had an adverse impact on them emotionally. These women were worried about what was causing sexual changes, how long the changes would last, the extent to which the changes would impact their intimate relationships, and how they could cope with the sexual changes, as well as feeling that their sexual pleasure or functioning was no longer under their control, and guilt over how the sexual changes would affect their relationships with their partners. The findings of the present study confirm these reports in a larger sample of individuals with breast cancer and provide further insight into the nature of these effects.

Partners play a key role in women's experiences of the changed body after breast cancer, illustrating the intersubjective nature of the construction and experience of sexuality in the context of breast cancer—the importance of relationship context and partner reaction, as well as the complexity of the woman's own response. While partner rejection was consistently associated with women's feelings of negativity about the body or femininity, partner support did not always alleviate these negative feelings. The way the woman felt about herself, and her ability to accept the changes to her body, also impacted the way she positioned her body after breast cancer, allowing herself to still feel like a sexual woman, or conversely, to feel "neutered," as one participant described herself. At the same time, accounts of relationship change after breast cancer confirm previous research reports that the diagnosis of cancer can change the relational dynamics between people with cancer and their life partners, which can have an impact on their ability to cope (Ussher, Wong, & Perz, 2011). It has been reported that partners of people with cancer assume new roles in the household (Ben-Zur, Gilbar, & Lev, 2001), in addition to providing physical and emotional support, which can have an impact on the sexual relationship (Gilbert et al., 2009). Couples living with cancer have also reported communication problems (Zahlis & Shandis, 1991) or increased conflict (Badr & Carmack Taylor, 2006), and in some instances have attributed relationship breakdown to cancer (Kornblith, Anderson, & Cella, 1990), as was found in the present study. Conversely, it has been argued that couples living with cancer are no more likely to separate than are couples in the general community (Schover, 2004), and that cancer can have a positive effect on couple relationships (Badr & Carmack Taylor, 2006), bringing people with cancer and their partners closer together (Dorval et al., 2005), through creating greater intimacy (Manne et al., 2004). These conflicting findings have led Hagedoorn, Sanderman, Bolks, Tuinstra, and Coyne (2008) to conclude, in their meta-analysis of distress in couples coping with cancer, that further research is needed on "just how much cancer intrudes upon and organizes the daily lives of couples confronted with the disease" (p. 24). The findings of the present study make a substantial contribution to addressing this plea, through exploring both negative and positive accounts of the impact of cancer on sexual relationships.

While the experiences of partners are often neglected in research on sexuality and intimacy post-cancer (Reichers, 2004), there is growing acknowledgment of their unmet needs in this area (De Groot et al., 2005). Reported disruptions include decreases in their own sex drive; fear of initiating sex with their partners; difficulty regaining a level of "normality" within the sexual relationship; and feeling unwanted and unattractive because of cessation of sex (Harden et al., 2002; Hawkins et al., 2009a; Sanders, Pedro, Bantum, & Galbraith, 2006). Many of these findings have been confirmed and extended by the findings of the present study, which reported on partner experiences from the perspective of the person with breast cancer. This reinforces the need to include partners, as well as people with cancer, in future research in cancer and sexuality. At the same time, the accounts of individuals who are not in a relationship highlight the importance of sexual well-being for those with breast cancer who are currently single, and the need for support, if requested, to alleviate fears or concerns about entering a new relationship. Sexuality is not only a relational issue; changes in sexual well-being, and in sexual desire and arousal, can also have an impact on those who are not in a relationship.

A significant proportion of participants also reported distress associated with infertility, uncertainty about fertility status, and changes to sexual well-being resulting from premature menopause, which had implications for fertility. This confirms previous reports that infertility and premature menopause are a significant cause of anxiety for women with breast cancer (Schover, 2005), compromising attempts at normality and dominating recovery (Crawshaw & Sloper, 2010), as well as serving to disrupt the life course (Exley & Letherby, 2001).

The research reviewed in this chapter, and the findings outlined in this study, are of significance to clinicians, as sexual well-being is central to psychological well-being and quality of life (World Health Organization, 1995), and sexual intimacy has been found to make the experience of cancer more manageable and assist in the recovery process (Schultz & Van de Wiel, 2003). Health professionals can play an important role in ameliorating concerns surrounding sexual well-being and fertility after breast cancer (Can et al., 2008), offering specific suggestions related to sexual enhancement products (Herbenick, Reece, Hollub, Satinsky, & Dodge, 2008) and emotional adjustment to sexual changes (Archibald et al., 2006), as well as information for partners (Gilbert et al., 2009). Equally, clinical guidelines (Lee et al., 2006) and researchers (Davis, 2006; Maltaris, Weigel, & Dittrich, 2009) recommend that fertility information should be provided at the point of diagnosis, and as infertility can be a late effect of cancer (Loscalzo & Clark, 2007), information is also needed after treatment has ended.

However, the finding that only 25 percent of participants in the present study had discussed sexual well-being or fertility with a health professional, despite the high levels of distress reported, is a matter of concern. This appears to confirm previous findings that few health professionals engage in discussions of sexual well-being with people with cancer, even in areas where it might be expected, such as breast cancer (Hawkins et al., 2009b; Hordern & Street, 2007). Further education and training of health professionals is also required, in order that they will be able to advise couples affected by breast cancer on issues of sexual well-being and fertility, and address unmet needs in this arena.

In conclusion, the analysis in this chapter has demonstrated that there is compelling evidence that breast cancer can have a significant impact on a woman's sexuality, both physically and psychologically, influenced by the discursive construction of "normal" sexuality and femininity, as well as a woman's relationship context. While each of these areas has been considered separately, reflecting the existing research in this field, it is important to acknowledge that they are irrevocably connected. The physical body cannot be conceptualized independently from women's intrapsychic negotiation, her relational context, and the discursive constructions of sexuality and femininity in a particular sociocultural context: a material-discursive-intrapsychic (MDI) interaction.

NOTE

1. The study discussed in this chapter was commissioned and funded by Breast Cancer Network Australia (BCNA), in the form of a research contract with the University of Western Sydney. Thanks are offered to Michelle Marven and Astrid Keir from BCNA for their advice on the survey and the interpretation of the data, and to Caroline Joyce, Emma Hurst, and Lauren Kadwell for research assistance and support. Finally, we thank all of the individuals with breast cancer who completed the survey and shared their personal stories of sexual well-being after breast cancer with us.

An earlier version of this chapter was published as:

Ussher, J. M., Perz, J., & Gilbert, E. (2013). The experience and construction of changes to women's sexuality after breast cancer. In Castaneda, D. (Ed.), *The essential handbook of women's sexuality* (Vol. 2, pp. 171–196). Santa Barbara, CA: Praeger.

Portions of this chapter were adapted, with permission from Wolters Kluwer, from:

Ussher, J. M., Perz, J., & Gilbert, E. (2012). Changes to sexual well-being and intimacy after breast cancer. *Cancer Nursing, 35*(6), 456–465.

Ussher, J. M., Perz, J., Gilbert, E., Wong, W. K. T., & Hobbs, K. (2013). Renegotiating sex and intimacy after cancer: Resisting the coital imperative. *Cancer Nursing, 36*(6), 454–462.

REFERENCES

Alder, J., Zanetti, R., Wight, E., Urech, C., Fink, N., & Bitzer, J. (2008). Sexual dysfunction after premenopausal stage I and II breast cancer: Do androgens play a role? *Journal of Sexual Medicine, 5,* 1898–1906.

Alicikus, Z. A., Gorken, I. B., Sen, R. C., Kentil, S., Kinay, M., Alanyali, H., et al. (2009). Psychosexual and body image aspects of quality of life in Turkish breast cancer patients: A comparison of breast conserving treatment and mastectomy. *Tumori, 95,* 212–218.

Andersen, B. L. (2009). In sickness and in health: Maintaining intimacy after breast cancer recurrence. *The Cancer Journal, 15*(1), 70–73.

Archibald, S., Lemieux, S., Byers, E. S., Tamlyn, K., & Worth, J. (2006). Chemically-induced menopause and the sexual functioning of breast cancer survivors. *Women & Therapy, 29*(1/2), 83–106.

Arrington, M. I. (2003). "I don't want to be an artifical man": Narrative reconstruction of sexuality among prostate cancer survivors. *Sexuality and Culture, 7*(2), 30–58.

Avis, N. E., Crawford, S., & Manuel, J. (2004). Psychosocial problems among young women with breast cancer. *Psycho-Oncology, 13,* 295–308.

Badr, H., & Carmack Taylor, C. L. (2006). Social constraints and spousal communication in lung cancer. *Psycho-Oncology, 15*(8), 673–683.

Ben-Zur, H., Gilbar, O., & Lev, S. (2001). Coping with breast cancer: Patient, spouse, and dyad models. *Psychosom Med, 63*(1), 32–39.

Bertero, C., & Wilmoth, M. C. (2007). Breast cancer diagnosis and its treatment affecting the self. *Cancer Nursing, 30*(3), 194–202.

Braun, V., & Clarke, V. (2006). Using thematic analysis in psychology. *Qualitative Research in Psychology, 3,* 77–101.

Burwell, S. R., Case, D. L., Kaelin, C., & Avis, N. E. (2006). Sexual problems in younger women after breast cancer surgery. *Journal of Clinical Oncology, 24*(18), 2815–2821.

Butler, J. P. (1990). *Gender trouble: Feminism and the subversion of identity.* New York: Routledge.

Camp-Sorrell, D. (2009). Cancer and its treatment effect on young breast cancer survivors. *Seminars in Oncology Nursing, 25*(4), 251–258.

Can, G., Oskay, U., Durna, Z., Aydiner, A., Saip, P., Disci, R., et al. (2008). Evaluation of sexual function of Turkish women with breast cancer receiving systemic treatment. *Oncology Nursing Forum, 35*(3), 471–476.

Carpentier, M. Y., & Fortenberry, J. D. (2010). Romantic and sexual relationships, body image, and fertility in adolescent and young adult testicular cancer survivors: A review of the literature. *Journal of Adolescent Health, 47*(2), 115–125.

Carter, J., Raviv, L., Applegarth, L., Ford, J. S., Josephs, L., & Grill, E. (2010). A cross-sectional study of the psychosexual impact of cancer-related infertility in women: Third-party reproductive assistance. *Journal of Cancer Survivorship, 4*(3), 236–246.

Carter, J., Rowland, K., Chi, D., Brown, C., Abu-Rustum, N., Castiel, M., et al. (2005). Gynecologic cancer treatment and the impact of cancer-related infertility. *Gynecologic Oncology, 97*(1), 90–95.

Connell, S., Patterson, C., & Newman, B. (2006). A qualitative analysis of reproductive issues raised by young Australian women with breast cancer. *Health Care for Women International, 27*(1), 94–110.

Crawshaw, M., & Sloper, P. (2010). "Swimming against the tide"—the influence of fertility matters on the transition to adulthood or survivorship following adolescent cancer. *European Journal of Cancer Care, 19*(5), 610–620.

D'Ardenne, P. (2004). The couple sharing long-term illness. *Sexual and Relationship Therapy, 19*(3), 291–308.

Davis, M. (2006). Fertility considerations for female adolescent and young adult patients following cancer therapy: A guide for counseling patients and their families. *Clinical Journal of Oncology Nursing, 10*(2), 213–219. doi: 10.1188/06 .CJON.213-219.

De Groot, J. M., Mah, K., Fyles, A., Winton, S., Greenwood, S., & De Petrillo, A. D. (2005). The psycho-social impact of cervical cancer among affected women and their partners. *International Journal of Gynecological Cancer, 15,* 918–925.

Del Pup, L., Campagnutta, E., Giorda, G., De Piero, G., Sopracordevole, F., & Sisto, R. (2006). Fertility preservation methods for female neoplastic patients. *Radiology and Oncology, 40*(3), 175–181.

Dorval, M., Guay, S., Mondor, M., Masse, B., Falardeau, M., & Robidoux, A. (2005). Couples who get closer after breast cancer: Frequency and predictors in a prospective investigation. *Journal of Clinical Oncology, 23*, 3588–3596.

Exley, C., & Letherby, G. (2001). Managing a disrupted lifecourse: Issues of identity and emotion work. *Health, 5*(1), 112–132.

Few, C. (1997). The politics of sex research and constructions of female sexuality: What relevance to sexual health work with young women? *Journal of Advanced Nursing, 25*, 615–625.

Fobair, P., Stewart, S. L., Chang, S., D'Onofrio, C., Banks, P. J., & Bloom, J. R. (2006). Body image and sexual problems in young women with breast cancer. *Psycho-Oncology, 15*, 579–594.

Foy, S., & Rose, K. (2001). Men's experiences of their partner's primary and recurrent breast cancer. *European Journal of Oncology Nursing, 5*(1), 42–48.

Ganz, P. A., Desmond, K., Belin, T. R., Meyerowitz, B. E., & Rowland, J. H. (1999). Predictors of sexual health in women after a breast cancer diagnosis. *Journal of Clinical Oncology, 17*(8), 2371–2380.

Ganz, P. A., Greendale, G. A., Petersen, L., Kahn, B., & Bower, J. E. (2003). Breast cancer in younger women: Reproductive and late health effects of treatment. *Journal of Clinical Oncology, 21*(22), 4184–4193.

Ganz, P. A., Rowland, J. H., Desmond, K., Meyerowitz, B. E., & Wyatt, G. E. (1998). Life after breast cancer: Understanding women's health-related quality of life and sexual functioning. *Journal of Clinical Oncology, 16*(2), 501–514.

Garrusi, B., & Faezee, H. (2008). How do Iranian women with breast cancer conceptualise sex and body image? *Sex and Disability, 26*, 159–165.

Gavey, N., McPhillips, K., & Braun, V. (1999). Interruptus coitus: Heterosexuals account for intercourse. *Sexualities, 2*(1), 35–68.

Gilbert, E., Ussher, J. M., & Hawkins, Y. (2009). Accounts of disruptions to sexuality following cancer: The perspective of informal carers who are partners of a person with cancer. *Health: An Interdisciplinary Journal, 13*(5), 523–541.

Gilbert, E., Ussher, J. M., & Perz, J. (2010a). (Re)negotiating the sexual relationship in the context of cancer care: Informal carers' experiences of caring and gender practices in couple relationships. *Archives of Sexual Behaviour 39*(4), 998–1009.

Gilbert, E., Ussher, J. M., & Perz, J. (2010b). Sexuality after breast cancer: A review. *Mauritius, 66*, 397–407.

Gurevich, M., Bishop, S., Bower, J., Malka, M., & Nyhof-Young, J. (2004). (Dis)embodying gender and sexuality in testicular cancer. *Social Science and Medicine, 58*(9), 1597–1607.

Hagedoorn, M., Sanderman, R., Bolks, H. N., Tuinstra, J., & Coyne, J. C. (2008). Distress in couples coping with cancer: A meta-analysis and critical review of role and gender effects. *Psychological Bulletin, 134*(1), 1–30.

Harden, J., Schafenacker, A., Northouse, L., Mood, D., Pienta, K., Hussain, M., et al. (2002). Couples' experience with prostate cancer: A focus group. *Oncology Nursing Forum, 29*(4), 701–709.

Hawkins, Y., Ussher, J. M., Gilbert, E., Perz, J., Sandoval, M., & Sundquist, K. (2009a). Changes in sexuality and intimacy after the diagnosis of cancer. The experience of partners in a sexual relationship with a person with cancer. *Cancer Nursing, 34*(4), 271–280.

Hawkins, Y., Ussher, J. M., Gilbert, E., Perz, J., Sandoval, M., & Sundquist, K. (2009b). Changes in sexuality and intimacy following the diagnosis and treatment of cancer: The experience of informal cancer carers. *Cancer Nursing, 32*(4), 271–298.

Herbenick, D., Reece, M., Hollub, A., Satinsky, S., & Dodge, B. (2008). Young female breast cancer survivors. Their sexual function and interest in sexual enhancement products and services. *Cancer Nursing, 31*(6), 417–425.

Holmberg, S. K., Scott, L., Alexy, W., & Fife, B. L. (2001). Relationship issues of women with breast cancer. *Cancer Nursing, 24*(1), 53–60.

Hordern, A. J., & Street, A. F. (2007). Communicating about patient sexuality and intimacy after cancer: Mismatched expectations and unmet needs. *Medical Journal of Australia, 186*(5), 224–227.

Knobf, T. M. (2001). The menopausal symptom experience in young mid-life women with breast cancer. *Cancer Nursing, 24*(3), 201–211.

Kornblith, A. B., Anderson, J., & Cella, D. F. (1990). Quality of life assessment of Hodgkin's disease survivors: A model for comparative care. *Oncology 4*, 93–101.

Kuyper, M. B., & Wester, F. (1998). In the shadow: The impact of chronic illness on the patient's partner. *Qualitative Health Research, 8*(2), 237–253.

Langellier, K. M., & Sullivan, C. F. (1998). Breast talk in breast cancer narratives. *Qualitative Health Research, 8*(1), 76–94.

Lee, S. J., Schover, L. R., Partridge, A. H., Patrizio, P., Wallace, W. H., Hagerty, K., et al. (2006). American Society of Clinical Oncology recommendations on fertility preservation in cancer patients [Consensus Development Conference Practice Guideline]. *Journal of Clinical Oncology: Official Journal of the American Society of Clinical Oncology, 24*(18), 2917–2931.

Letherby, G., & Williams, C. (1999). Non-motherhood: Ambivalent autobiographies. *Feminist Studies, 25*(3), 719–728.

Loscalzo, M. J., & Clark, K. L. (2007). The psychosocial context of cancer-related infertility [Review]. *Cancer treatment and research, 138*, 180–190.

Maltaris, T., Weigel, M., & Dittrich, R. (2009). Cancer and fertility preservation in females: Where we stand and where we are heading. *Expert Review of Endocrinology & Metabolism, 4*(1), 79–89.

Manderson, L. (2005). Boundary breaches: The body, sex, and sexuality after stoma surgery. *Social Science Medicine, 61*, 405–415.

Manderson, L., & Stirling, L. (2007). The absent breast: Speaking of the mastectomied body. *Feminism and Psychology, 17*(1), 75–92.

Manne, S., Ostroff, J., Rini, C., Fox, K., Goldstein, L., & Grana, G. (2004). The interpersonal process model of intimacy: The role of self-disclosure, partner disclosure, and partner responsiveness in interactions between breast cancer patients and their partners. *Journal of Family Psychology, 18*(4), 589–599.

Markopoulos, C., Tsaroucha, A. K, Kouskos, E., Mantas, D., Antonopoulou, Z., & Karvelis, S. (2009). Impact of breast cancer sugery on the self esteem and sexual life of female patients. *The Journal of International Medical Research, 37*, 182–188.

Meyerowitz, B. E., Desmond, K., Rowland, J. H., Wyatt, G. E., & Ganz, P. A. (1999). Sexuality following breast cancer. *Journal of Sex & Marital Therapy, 25*, 237–250.

Morell, C. (2000). Saying no: Women's experiences with reproductive refusal. *Feminism & Psychology, 10*(3), 313–322.

Mortimer, J. E., Boucher, L., Baty, J., Knapp, D. L., Ryan, E., & Rowland, J. H. (1999). Effect of tamoxifen on sexual functioning in patients wih breast cancer. *Journal of Clinical Oncology, 17*(5), 1488–1492.

Nieman, C. L., Kazer, R., Brannigan, R. E., Zoloth, L. S., Chase-Lansdale, P. L., Kinahan, K., et al. (2006). Cancer survivors and infertility: A review of a new problem and novel answers. *Journal of Supportive Oncology, 4*(4), 171–178.

Reichers, E. A. (2004). Including partners into the diagnosis of prostate cancer: A review of the literature to provide a model of care. *Urologic Nursing, 24*(1), 22–38.

Reis, N., Beji, N. K., & Coskun, A. (2010). Quality of life and sexual functioning in gynecological cancer patients: Results from quantitative and qualitative data. *European Journal of Oncology Nursing, 14*(2), 137–146.

Rogers, M., & Kristjansen, L. J. (2002). The impact on sexual functioning of chemotherapy-induced menopause in women with breast cancer. *Cancer Nursing, 25*(1), 57–65.

Rosen, A., Rodriguez-Wallberg, K. A., & Rosenzweig, L. (2009). Psychosocial distress in young cancer survivors. *Seminars in Oncology Nursing, 25*(4), 268–277.

Rudberg, L., Nilsson, S., & Wikblad, K. (2000). Health-related quality of life in survivors of testicular cancer 3 to 13 years after treatment. *Journal of Psychosocial Oncology, 18*(3), 19–31.

Sanders, S., Pedro, L. W., Bantum, E. O., & Galbraith, M. E. (2006). Couples surviving prostate cancer: Long-term intimacy needs and concerns following treatment. *Clinical Journal of Oncology Nursing, 10*(4), 503–508.

Schildrick, M. (2005). Unreformed bodies: Normative anxiety and the denial of pleasure. *Women's Studies, 34*, 327–344.

Schover, L. R. (2004). Myth-busters: Telling the true story of breast cancer survivorship. *Journal of the National Cancer Institute, 96*, 1800–1801.

Schover, L. R. (2005). Motivation for parenthood after cancer: A review. *JNCI Monographs, 34*, 2–5.

Schultz, W. C. M., & Van de Wiel, H. B. M. (2003). Sexuality, intimacy and gynaecological cancer. *Journal of Sex and Marital Therapy, 29(s)*, 121–128.

Speer, J. J., Hillenberg, B., Sugrue, D. P., Blacker, C., Kresge, C. L., Decker, V. B., et al. (2005). Study of sexual functioning determinants in breast cancer survivors. *The Breast Journal, 11*(6), 440–447.

Spence, J. (1995). *Cultural sniping: The art of transgression.* London: Sage.

Stern, K. (2010). Protection and preservation of fertility for young women with cancer. *Obstetrics and Gynaecology, 12*(3), 22–25.

Takahashi, M., Ohno, S., Inoue, H., Kataoka, A., Yamaguchi, H., Uchida, Y., et al. (2008). Impact of breast cancer diagnosis and treatment on women's sexuality: A survey of Japanese patients. *Psycho-Oncology, 17,* 901–907.

Thomas-MacLean, R. (2005). Beyond dichotomies of health and illness: Life after breast cancer. *Nursing Inquiry, 12*(3), 200–209.

Thors, C. L., Broeckel, J. A., & Jacobsen, P. (2001). Sexual functioning in breast cancer survivors. *Cancer Control, 8*(5), 442–448.

Tiefer, L. (1996). The medicalization of sexuality: Conceptual, normative, and professional issues. *Annual Review of Sex Research, 7,* 252–282.

Tiefer, L. (2001). The selling of "female sexual dysfunction." *Journal of Sex and Marital Therapy, 27*(5), 625–628.

Tschudin, S., & Bitzer, J. (2009). Psychological aspects of fertility preservation in men and women affected by cancer and other life-threatening diseases. *Human Reproduction Update, 15*(5), 587–597.

Tschudin, S., Bunting, L., Abraham, J., Gallop-Evans, E., Fiander, A., & Boivin, J. (2010). Correlates of fertility issues in an internet survey of cancer survivors. *Journal of Psychosomatic Obstetrics & Gynecology, 31*(3), 150–157.

Ussher, J. M. (2000). Women's madness: A material-discursive-intrapsychic approach. In Fee, D. (Ed.), *Psychology and the postmodern: Mental illness as discourse and experience* (pp. 207–230). London: Sage.

Ussher, J. M. (2005). Unravelling women's madness: Beyond positivism and constructivism and towards a material-discursive-intrapsychic approach. In Menzies, R., Chunn, D. E., & Chan, W. (Eds.), *Women, madness, and the law: A feminist reader* (pp. 19–40). London: Glasshouse Press.

Ussher, J. M. (2008). Reclaiming embodiment within critical psychology: A material-discursive analysis of the menopausal body. *Social and Personality Psychology Compass, 2*(5), 1781–1798.

Ussher, J. M., Perz, J., & Gilbert, E. (2012). Changes to sexual well-being and intimacy after breast cancer. *Cancer Nursing, 35*(6), 456–464.

Ussher, J. M., Perz, J., & Gilbert, E. (2013). Information needs associated with changes to sexual well-being after breast cancer. *Journal of Advanced Nursing, 69*(3), 327–337.

Ussher, J. M., Wong, W. K. T., & Perz, J. (2011). A qualitative analysis of changes in relationship dynamics and roles between people with cancer and their primary informal carer. *Health: An Interdisciplinary Journal, 15*(6), 650–667.

Wellard, S. (1998). Constructions of chronic illness. *International Journal of Nursing Studies, 35,* 49–55.

Wilmoth, M. C. (2001). The aftermath of breast cancer: An altered sexual self. *Cancer Nursing, 24*(4), 278–286.

World Health Organization. (1995). The world health organisation quality of life assessment (WHOQOL) position paper. *Social Science and Medicine, 41,* 1403–1409.

World Health Organization. (2009). Breast cancer prevention and control.

Young, I. M. (1992). Breasted experience: The look and the feeling. In Leder, D. (Ed.), *The body in medical thought and practice* (pp. 215–232). Dordrecht, Netherlands: Kluwer Academic Publishers.

Zahlis, E. H., & Shandis, M. E. (1991). Breast cancer: Demands of the illness of the patient's partner. *Journal of Psychosocial Oncology, 9*(1), 75–93.

Zebrack, B. J., Casillas, J., Nohr, L., Adams, H., & Zetler, L. K. (2004). Fertility issues for young adult survivors of childhood cancer. *Psycho-Oncology, 13*(10), 689–699.

Zee, B., Huang, C., Mak, S., Wong, J., Chan, E., & Yeo, W. (2008). Factors related to sexual health in Chinese women with breast cancer in Hong Kong. *Asia-Pacific Journal of Clinical Oncology, 4*, 218–226.

Chapter 18

Exploring the Role of Stress and Neuroticism in Negative Health Outcomes: Can Stress and Personality Predict the Progression and Recurrence of Cancer?

Sam M. Dorros

Being diagnosed with cancer is understandably a very distressing event. There may be stress associated with adjustments in social and family roles, worries about changes in appearance or attractiveness, and anxiety about the recurrence or spread of cancer, and fears of death (Manne et al., 2003). One in eight women will develop breast cancer in their lifetime, as breast cancer is the second most common type of cancer in women, apart from skin cancer (American Cancer Society, 2013). The American Cancer Society (2013) estimates that 232,340 new cases of invasive breast cancer will be diagnosed, and 39,620 deaths from breast cancer this year. Research has shown that women suffer physically and psychologically as a consequence of the diagnosis and treatment of breast cancer (Badger, Braden, & Mishel, 2001).

Depending on the level of anxiety or depression in an individual, the diagnosis and treatment of cancer may have immunological consequences (Tjemsland, Soreide, Matre, & Malt, 1997). Stress has been correlated with lower natural killer (NK) cells in women with breast cancer (Levy, Herberman, Lippman, & D'Angelo, 1987). NK cells are important in destroying tumor cells (as well as virus-infected cells) and in fighting against new and abnormal growth (Brittenden, Heys, Ross, & Eremin, 1996). Therefore, positive psychological adjustment to cancer is critical, given that it has been linked with length of survival (Greer, Morris, & Pettingale, 1979).

In studies on negative affect and recurrence of breast cancer, researchers have found that higher emotional distress predicted shorter time from diagnosis to recurrence among those who recurred (e.g., Levy, Herberman, Maluish, Schlien, & Lippman, 1985) and shortened survival time (Gilbar, 1996). For example, Weihs, Enright, Simmens, & Reiss (2000) found that negative affectivity (especially when it was concurrent with restriction of emotions) predicted shortened survival rate. However, negative affectivity is not shown to predict whether breast cancer recurs (Levy et al., 1985). Therefore, future research needs to examine recurrence stress and neuroticism in more detail as any significant findings would be invaluable to the scientific community and breast cancer patients. This chapter will take an in-depth look at the role of stress and personality in influencing health outcomes and will survey the existing literature to determine whether such a link exists.

STRESS

Effects of Stress

Past research shows that when events are experienced negatively, the immune system is suppressed (Dienstbier, 1989; Sapolsky, 2004) and susceptibility to illness increases (Maddi, Bartone, & Puccetti, 1987). The deleterious effects of stress are due in part to an increase in cortisol levels (Cohen & Williamson, 1991; Monjan & Collector, 1977). Cortisol suppresses immune system functioning by decreasing antibody production, T-cells, macrophages, and monocytes (Luecken & Compas, 2002). Specifically, chronic stress is predictive of increased vulnerability to upper respiratory infections (Herbert & Cohen, 1993; Kemeny, 2003; Sapolsky, 2004). A meta-analysis of 38 studies on stress and immunity revealed that stress was significantly related to the number and percent of circulating white blood cells, immunoglobulin levels, and antibody titers to herpes viruses (Herbert & Cohen, 1993). Extreme cases of stress can result in hippocampal atrophying, which manifests as memory loss (Kemeny, 2003; McEwen, 2000).

Further, Walker (2004) found that chronic stress has been found to suppress natural killer (NK) cell activity (a component of the immune system that plays a major role in destroying tumors and infected cells), which is associated with an increased risk of cancer progression. Therefore, not only does stress contribute to a host of infectious diseases (i.e., colds, herpes virus activation), but it could also play a role in the development, progression, or recurrence of cancer. Recent evidence is beginning to show a clear link between cortisol and the development and progression of tumors (Luecken & Compas, 2002). Given the negative physical health outcomes of stress, more research needs to be dedicated to understanding individual vulnerability factors that increase subjective experiences of stress.

Predisposing factors to stress include long-standing behavioral patterns (e.g., childhood experiences, stable personality characteristics) that may alter the susceptibility of the individual to illness (Rabkin & Strening, 1976). Neuroticism (N) is one personality variable that has been studied extensively in its role in physical health and stress, and it is traditionally measured as a mediator of stress (e.g., Rabkin & Strening, 1976). However, some researchers view N as a confounding variable in the stress-illness link (e.g., Costa & McCrae, 1987). This notion has led to a debate among scholars as to whether N actually causes physical illness, or if N creates a bias in self-reporting and symptom recall (e.g., Costa & McCrae, 1987). Taking into account the past research, it seems as if both arguments have merit. Given that the personality dimension of N includes perceiving the world in a negative light (Costa & McCrae, 1987; Wiebe & Smith, 1997), high-N individuals are also likely to perceive daily hassles, challenges, and life events in a negative manner as well. However, it is possible that N can also influence the occurrence or progression of illness through increased physiological reactions to stress.

Perhaps a third argument could be made, such that: N is not a confound in stress research, nor a mediator of stress, but a *direct contributor* to increased levels of stress through the process of negative cognitive appraisals of stressful events. As evidenced in the stress literature, the harmful physiological reactions of stress occur when the individual perceives challenges as threatening (Lazarus & Folkman, 1984). Research has yet to examine personality as a predictor of stress and illness. It seems reasonable that neuroticism could cause more negative appraisals of stress, which would increase physiological arousal, and thereby decrease immune system functioning. Therefore, Lazarus and Folkman's (1984) cognitive-appraisal theory of stress and coping will be described in more detail to guide the discussion of the role of N and increased susceptibility of illness. This investigation explores the neuroticism and health debate, and asserts that neuroticism can impact physical health outcomes through increased levels of stress (i.e., cortisol) and a decreased immune system.

Studies have empirically shown that stress is a factor in predicting physical illness (e.g., Maddi, Bartone, & Puccetti, 1987). However, some researchers view the stress-illness link as being rife with confounding variables like neuroticism (e.g., Maddi et al., 1987) and weak relations between stress and illness due to individual differences in susceptibility to stress (Rabkin & Strening, 1976); but those studies have been criticized because of substantial findings that authenticate the significant link between stress and both current and prospective illness (Maddi et al., 1987).

A lowered immune system has been associated with an increased risk of disease, specifically infectious diseases and cancer (Herbert & Cohen, 1993; Sapolsky, 2004). The deleterious effects of stress in decreasing immune system functioning (due to an increase in cortisol levels) have been documented in humans (Cohen & Williamson, 1991; Monjan & Collector, 1977), and the suppression of immunity in animals has been found to promote the growth of cancer (Sklar & Anisman, 1981). Walker (2004) found that chronic stress in particular has been found to suppress natural killer (NK) cell activity. Therefore it seems plausible that N could play a role in the development, progression, or recurrence of cancer.

A Background of Stress

In 1929 Cannon initially identified the "fight or flight" response to a stressor. A stressor is a situation that is likely to lead to appraisals of threat by a person (Dienstbier, 1989). Folkman and Lazarus (1985) described threat as "potential harm or loss" (p. 152). According to Lazarus and Folkman (1984), it is when an event is perceived as threatening and the consequent demands cannot be met that psychological stress and physiological arousal occur. According to Seyle (1956) frequent or prolonged periods of stress strain the body, which eventually leads to illness. Two terms common to stress research are allostasis and allostatic load. Allostasis refers to the process of adapting to challenges, and allostatic load refers to the price the body pays for being forced to adapt to adverse situations (McEwen, 2000).

Stress activates both the sympathetic and neuroendocrine systems (Wiebe & Smith, 1997). One of the physiological responses to stress that was first assessed by Seyle (1956) is called the pituitary-adrenal-cortical arousal or pathway. The pituitary gland releases adrenocorticotropin (ACTH), which stimulates the adrenal cortex to release cortisol (Dienstbier, 1989). Cortisol suppresses immune-system functioning by restricting the secretion of lymphokines and helper T-cells (Calabrese, Kling, & Gold, 1987). High levels of cortisol are also associated with neuroticism, depression, and anxiety (Anisman & LaPierre, 1982).

For example, in a stressful situation glucocorticoids are activated. From an evolutionary standpoint (e.g., running away from a lion), the fight or flight response is an adaptive function of the stress response (Seyle, 1956). However, today's stressors tend to be psychological in nature (although the same physiological responses in the body occur); therefore, nature's adaptive fight or flight response is ultimately harmful to us over the long term. Chronically elevated levels of glucocorticoids contribute to increased insulin levels, promote body fat, and increase plaque in the coronary arteries (McEwen, 2000). Further, in cases of elevated glucocorticoids and extreme stress (e.g., holocaust survivors), the human brain shows atrophy as a result of these hormones (McEwen, 2000). In particular, the hippocampus is sensitive to these hormones and shows greater changes than other brain areas. Hippocampal atrophying results in cognitive functions such as memory loss (Kemeny, 2003).

It is important to note that some social disruption stressors are acute (e.g., bereavement) and some are chronic (e.g., loneliness, marital distress). Of all the stressors most likely to cause HPA activation and cortisol release, chronic stress, depression, and social deprivation top the list (O'Leary, 1990).

Overview of Lazarus and Folkman's (1984) Theory

One of the most influential and prominent theories of stress ever developed is Lazarus and Folkman's (1984) cognitive-appraisal theory of stress and coping (Milgram & Tenne, 2000; Slavin, Rainer, McCreary, & Gowda, 1991; Sweet, Savoie, & Lemyre, 1999). Essentially, their theory examines the link between an individual's subjective stress appraisals and his/her health outcomes (e.g., depression, sleep disturbances) (Mak, Blewitt, & Heaven, 2004). This theory emphasizes the cognitive interpretation of events in one's environment (Slavin et al., 1991) and the available resources to cope with the stressor (Milgram & Tenne, 2000). According to the theory, people assess whether a given situation or task poses a threat to them, and whether they have the resources to deal effectively with the threat (Milgram & Tenne, 2000).

Stress is experienced when people perceive the event/stressor to strain or exceed their current resources, or as a threat to their well-being (Gowan, Riordan, & Gatewood, 1999; Slavin et al., 1991; Sweet et al., 1999). Consequently, people then experience negative emotional and somatic reactions (Gowan et al., 1999). For example, when college students perceive their resources to be inadequate to deal with academic stress/work, they experience anxiety or other aversive emotions, which leads to behavioral consequences such as trying to escape from the situation by putting off the task as long as possible (i.e., procrastination) (Milgram & Tenne, 2000). Therefore, this process involves the interaction among perception, cognition, affect, and coping (Costa & McCrae, 1990), and appraisals affect emotional, physiological, and behavioral responses to events (Tomaka, Blascovich, Kelsey, & Leitten, 1993). As we will see, cognitive appraisals and coping are both mediators of the stress response (Sweet et al., 1999).

Lazarus and Folkman's (1984) model of the stress process consists of five major elements: (1) the occurrence of the stressor, (2) primary cognitive appraisal, (3) secondary cognitive appraisal, (4) coping strategies, and (5) health outcomes (Slavin et al., 1991). *The occurrence of a potentially stressful event* includes both major life events (e.g., death, divorce) and minor events (e.g., daily hassles) (Slavin et al., 1991). The *anticipation* of a stressful event, or something harmful in the future, can also create stress reactions (Lazarus, 1963). In the face of some stressors, some people develop depression and others anxiety. Finlay-Jones and Brown (1981) suggested that the type of stressor determined which of the two psychopathologies would dominate. For example, if the stressor involved a loss (e.g., death, retirement), then depression is a more likely consequence; however, if the stressor involves threat (e.g., being a crime victim), then anxiety would more likely ensue (Finlay-Jones & Brown, 1981).

Primary cognitive appraisal is when the event/circumstance is evaluated in order to determine whether or not it presents a threat (i.e., potential harm and benefits) (Stanton & Schneider, 1993; Tomaka et al., 1993). Primary appraisals of a threat can be perceived to be: (a) irrelevant, (b) benign/positive, or (c) stressful (Slavin et al., 1991). Therefore appraisals either threaten or challenge the individual. A threat appraisal occurs when the individual anticipates future danger or harm and believes his/her coping resources to be inadequate, which evokes worry or fear, and the individual will likely avoid the danger (Mak et al., 2004). Beliefs or expectations about events (based on past experiences, or present stressor novelty) can determine whether the stressor will be perceived as threatening (Lazarus, 1963). Threat appraisals are associated with more negative emotional reactions such as anxiety, and threatened individuals will be less task focused (Tomaka et al., 1993). On the other hand, challenge appraisals occur when the individual has adequate coping resources and anticipates a positive outcome or an opportunity for positive gain or personal growth. This type of appraisal is associated with positive emotions such as eagerness and excitement, so that the individual is energized to perform and focus on the task (Mak et al., 2004; Tomaka et al., 1993).

Secondary cognitive appraisal is when an individual evaluates his/her resources and abilities/options for handling the event (Stanton & Schneider, 1993; Tomaka et al., 1993). These consist of either internal resources (e.g., intelligence) or external resources (e.g., social support) (Slavin et al., 1991). Secondary appraisals include three main dimensions: perceived impact (e.g., how much will this affect current life or future aspirations), perceived mastery (e.g., personal competence and control), and perceived uncertainty (e.g., ambiguous and unfamiliar or predictable and familiar) (Sweet et al., 1999). The controllability of the stressor (i.e., a changeable stressor or fixed/static stressor) is also appraised at this time and affects responses to the stressor. Subjects who appraised a stressor as unchangeable used more emotion-focused coping strategies (e.g., escape-avoidance), whereas subjects who perceived a stressor as changeable used more task-focused coping strategies (e.g., problem-solving) (Folkman, Lazarus, Dunkel-Schetter, DeLongis, & Gruen, 1986).

Depending on resources and options, the events are further appraised as: (a) events involving harm or loss, (b) events presenting a threat (of future harm), or (c) events presenting a challenge (Slavin et al., 1991). Given that the individual simultaneously reappraises the stressor and environmental demands over time as well as his/her personal resources (Mak et al., 2004; Sweet et al., 1999), cognitive appraisal is a dynamic and perpetual process (Tomaka et al., 1993).

Coping strategies are those that an individual employs (either cognitive or behavioral) to cope with the stressor (Slavin et al., 1991). Coping includes thoughts, actions, or feelings to modify or eliminate the source of stress (Sweet et al., 1999) and are either focused on the problem at hand or on the emotions one is experiencing. Problem-focused coping consists of active efforts to change the situation in some way (e.g., seeking guidance or help, planning, problem solving) (Slavin et al., 1991). Emotion-focused coping includes efforts to control one's emotions and may either be adaptive (e.g., using relaxation techniques, positive reinterpretation) or maladaptive (e.g., denial, escape/avoidance by using drugs or alcohol) (Slavin et al., 1991). Coping efforts that draw attention toward the stressor are considered approach-type strategies, while efforts that draw attention away from the stressor are considered avoidant-type strategies (Sweet et al., 1999). Research has shown that avoidant-type coping strategies are associated with higher levels of psychological distress and physical symptoms, whereas approach-type strategies have decreased levels of negative symptoms (Sweet et al., 1999).

Physical and mental health outcomes of stress encompass all dimensions of well-being, including psychological, behavioral, and physical problems, and somatic illness. For example, negative emotions (Folkman & Lazarus, 1988) and/or depression are common psychological reactions to stressful events. Behavioral issues include memory problems and lower sleep quality (Willette-Murphy, Todero, & Yeaworth, 2006). Somatic complaints and health problems such as the flu, sore throat, headaches, and backaches are significantly associated with daily stress (DeLongis, Folkman, & Lazarus, 1988). A lowered immunity frequently occurs due to the release of cortisol during stressful events (Gaab, Rohleder, Nater, & Ehlert, 2005).

Lazarus and Folkman's (1984) model of stress is cyclical, in that poor health outcomes and the taxing of a person's coping resources can increase vulnerability to stress and further precipitate stressful events (Slavin et al., 1991). Therefore, stress and coping in this model is truly a dynamic process (Costa & McCrae, 1990).

NEUROTICISM

Neuroticism and Stress

It is assumed that negative mental health is related to aversive physical symptoms, but could it actually predict disease? Costa and McCrae (1987) showed that physiological disturbance (i.e., sweating, trembling hands, and diarrhea) is strongly tied to emotional arousal; but what about more serious diseases like cancer? Can a negative state of mind play a role in the development and disease progression of a tumor, or the recurrence of cancer? Most researchers would agree that there is a link between an individual's mental state and his/her experience of certain physical symptoms, but they would not go so far as to say that personality in itself could predict illness. However, Cohen and Williamson (1991) reason that the argument between actual disease development and exaggerated somatic complaints with high N individuals is still up for debate, given that there have been a limited number of well-designed studies that examine the objective measures of illness.

Personality traits are believed to influence or exacerbate the perception of events or stimuli as threatening, which affects the extent of physiological arousal (Wiebe & Smith, 1997). Therefore, it seems likely that a high N personality would tend to experience greater stress (possibly to objectively less stressful events or situations) than low N personality types. Further, negative individuals may create stressful situations, interpersonal conflicts, or interpersonal rejection (e.g., depression), which could perpetuate the stress cycle even more (Wiebe & Smith, 1997). With a transactional approach to personality, it seems that either way it is examined, high N individuals will probably perceive more frequent and severe stressors in their daily lives.

Neuroticism has been defined as "a broad dimension of individual differences in the tendency to experience negative, distressing emotions and to possess associated behavioral and cognitive traits" (Costa & McCrae, 1987, p. 301). Traits associated with neuroticism include fearfulness, irritability, low self-esteem, social anxiety, poor inhibition of impulses, and helplessness (Costa and McRae, 1987). Despite objective reality, individuals who score high on neuroticism tend to hold negative views of themselves and the world (Wiebe & Smith, 1997). Negative affect (or affectivity) has also been closely related to neuroticism (Watson & Clark, 1984). Neuroticism as a personality trait appears to be quite stable across the life span (Costa et al., 1986); therefore it is distinguishable from periods of depression or anxiety (Costa & McRae, 1987).

It is important to note that it is *the subjective appraisal* of events that activates the sympathetic and neuroendocrine systems, not *the objective events* per se (Lazarus & Folkman, 1984; Wiebe & Smith, 1997). Therefore individuals who are high N may have a tendency to perceive events as more threatening, negative, and out of their control (e.g., helplessness) and consequently experience a greater physiological stress response. Indeed, sympathetic nervous system (SNS) arousal was found to be associated with N personality type (Dienstbier, 1989). Further, negative individuals may tend to create stressful situations, interpersonal conflicts, or experience interpersonal rejection (i.e., Coyne's [1976] interactional theory of depression), which could perpetuate the stress cycle even more (Wiebe & Smith, 1997). With a transactional approach to personality and stress, it seems that, from either direction stress and personality are examined, a high N individual would probably perceive, and experience, more frequent and severe stressors in their daily lives.

Neuroticism and Health: The Debate

Neuroticism (N) has been studied in past research as to its role in physical health and illness. Researchers have debated whether N actually causes physical illness or if the N-symptom correlation is actually a bias in self-reporting of high N individuals (Costa & McCrae, 1987). The majority of researchers in this area believe in the latter of the two (e.g., Costa & McCrae, 1987; Watson & Pennebaker, 1989). Most of the literature shows that N is linked to higher levels of somatic complaints, illness behavior, poorer health habits, and exaggerated levels of self-reported physical illness (Costa & McCrae, 1987; Watson & Pennebaker, 1989). Watson and Pennebaker (1989) explain that high N individuals are more likely to notice aches, pains, and symptoms and perceive them as indicators of illness, and therefore complain about them (i.e., symptom reporting). Further, Larsen (1992) found that high N individuals are likely to encode and recall selective symptoms. Cohen et al. (1995) measured negative affect and subjective symptoms in participants infected with a respiratory viral infection. The authors concluded that trait and state negative affect were associated with more disease-specific health complaints. In another study, higher N individuals complained more of chest pains yet were objectively shown to have healthy arteries, compared to patients with the actual disease (Costa, Fleg, McCrae, & Lakatta, 1982). Therefore N is associated with cardiac symptom reporting but not with the development of cardiac disease (Wiebe & Smith, 1997).

"We conclude from these studies that . . . neuroticism influences perceptions of health, but not health itself" (Costa & McCrae, 1985, p. 24). Therefore, from this research it would seem likely to be the case that N is a factor only in the reporting of illness, not a causal agent in the development of disease. However, some methodological limitations inherent to the majority of studies performed on stress and N need to be addressed before the case is closed on this important personality and health debate.

Methodological Issues in Neuroticism & Stress Research

There are three main methodological issues germane to the study of neuroticism and physical illness: (1) the use of retrospective data, (2) examining vague or nonspecific diseases, and (3) limiting health outcomes to participants' subjective reports of illness. The first methodological issue is that most studies rely on retrospective reports of illness. High N individuals may be more biased to recall prior illnesses because these individuals are prone to remember these negative states (Cohen et al. 1995; Larsen, 1992). Only a few studies have documented N and current illness (e.g., Cohen et al., 1995; Costa, Fleg, McCrae, & Lakatta, 1982). Therefore, more studies should examine current illness as well as include physiological reactions.

Another methodological problem is that many studies used measures of vague and nonspecific symptoms (i.e., stomachaches, muscle aches, backaches, faintness, dizziness, cold spells) but not a specific disease (Cohen et al., 1995). The only exception was a study in which the researchers infected participants with a respiratory viral infection (e.g., Cohen et al., 1995). However, research needs to focus on specific diseases to avoid this type of vague and nonspecific symptom reporting that high N individuals tend toward (Costa & McCrae, 1987; Watson & Pennebaker, 1989).

Finally, subjective measures of health and illness (e.g., self-report symptom checklists) are frequently used in health psychology research instead of also obtaining objective health data (Wiebe & Smith, 1997). There have only been a handful of studies that have included objective measures of illness and pathology in addition to subjective symptom reporting (e.g., Cohen et al., 1995; Costa, Fleg, McCrae, & Lakatta, 1982). Therefore, it is absolutely critical that research on N and physical illness include objective measures of health/illness to avoid exaggerated symptom reporting (Watson & Pennebaker, 1989).

When studies of N and stress have been well controlled and designed, physiological effects have been detected. For example, Ursin et al. (1984) found that schoolteachers who were high N individuals and had high job stress had lower levels of three salivary immunoglobulins than did individuals who scored low in both N and job stress. These three salivary immunoglobulins are the main defense mechanisms in protecting against respiratory infection (Ursin et al., 1984). Depression (one of the facets of N) is also associated with decreased immune system functioning and an increased susceptibility to illness (Calabrese et al., 1987; Sklar & Anisman, 1981). Therefore, further research on the physiological outcomes of neuroticism and stress is warranted.

NEGATIVE LIFE EVENTS AND CHANGES IN N

Neuroticism as a personality trait appears to be quite stable across the life span (Costa et al., 1986). Most of the literature on Neuroticism (N) and illness concludes that N does not directly impact physical health. Instead, the majority of researchers assert that high N individuals complain more and engage in increased somatization about physical health symptoms, which produces an artificial connection to personality and health. Therefore, it is possible that N individuals, by nature of their personality, have greater negative appraisals of the world and life events, thereby increasing levels of stress. Past studies have shown the deleterious effects of increased cortisol on immune system functioning and susceptibility to illness. And indeed, sympathetic nervous system (SNS) arousal was found to be associated with N (Dienstbier, 1989). The physiological reactions to the experienced stress (i.e., increased cortisol and decreased immune system functioning) will lead to a greater susceptibility to illness, specifically cancer.

Given that the personality dimension of N includes perceiving the world in a negative light (Costa & McCrae, 1987; Wiebe & Smith, 1997), high N individuals are also likely to perceive daily hassles, challenges, and life events in a negative manner as well. Researchers have yet to examine the role of N in creating additional perceptions of stress in daily life, which would cause an increase in cortisol levels and thereby decrease immune system functioning. As shown in the stress literature, the harmful physiological reactions of stress occur when the individual *perceives* challenges as threatening (Lazarus and Folkman, 1984). Therefore, it is possible that neuroticism could be a predictor of negative health outcomes due to increased levels of stress and decreased immune system functioning.

REFERENCES

Abela, J. R. Z., Aydin, C., & Auerbach, R. P. (2006). Operationalizing the "vulnerability" and "stress" components of the hopelessness theory of depression: A multi-wave longitudinal study. *Behaviour Research and Therapy, 44*, 1565–1583. Retrieved from http://dx.doi.org/10.1016/j.brat.2005.11.010 PMid:16458851.

American Cancer Society. (2013). *Cancer facts & figures: 2013*. Atlanta, GA: American Cancer Society, Inc. Retrieved from http://www.cancer.org/acs/groups/cid/documents/webcontent/003090-pdf.pdf.

Anisman, H., & LaPierre, Y. (1982). Neurochemical aspects of stress and depression: Formulations and caveats. In Neufeld, R. W. (Ed.), *Psychological stress and psychopathology* (pp. 179–217). New York: McGraw-Hill.

Badger, T. A., Braden, C. J., & Mishel, M. H. (2001). Depression burden, self-help interventions, and side effects experienced by women with breast cancer. *Oncology Nursing Forum, 28*, 567–574.

Brittenden, J., Heys, S., Ross, J., & Eremin, O. (1996). Natural killer cells and cancer. *Cancer, 77*, 1226–1243. Retrieved from http://dx.doi.org/10.1002/(SICI)1097-0142(19960401)77:7<1226::AID-CNCR2>3.0.CO;2-G.

Calabrese, J. R., Kling, M. A., & Gold, P. W. (1987). Alterations in immunocompetence during stress, bereavement, and depression: Focus on neuroendocrine regulation. *American Journal of Psychiatry, 144*, 1123–1134. doi: PMid:3307461.

Cannon, W. B. (1929). *Bodily changes in pain, hunger, fear, and rage*. Boston: Branford.

Cohen, F. (1979). Personality, stress, and the development of physical illness. In Stone, G. C., Cohen, F., & Adler, N. E. (Eds.), *Health Psychology: A handbook* (pp. 77–111). San Francisco: Jossey-Bass.

Cohen, S., Doyle, W. J., Skoner, D. P., Fireman, P., Gwaltney, J. M., & Newsom, J. T. (1995). State and trait negative affect as predictors of objective and subjective symptoms of respiratory viral infections. *Journal of Personality and Social Psychology, 68,* 159–169. http://dx.doi.org/10.1037/0022-3514.68.1.159 PMid:7861312.

Cohen S., & Williamson, G. M. (1991). Stress and infectious disease in humans. *Psychological Bulletin, 109,* 5–24. Retrieved from http://dx.doi.org/10.1037/0033-2909.109.1.5 PMid:2006229.

Costa, P. T., Fleg, J. L., McCrae, R. R., & Lakatta, E. G. (1982). Neuroticism, coronary artery disease, and chest pain complaints: Cross-sectional and longitudinal studies. *Experimental Aging Research, 8,* 37–44.

Costa, P. T., & McCrae, R. R. (1985). Hypochondriasis, neuroticism, and aging: When are somatic complaints unfounded? *American Psychologist, 40,* 19–28. Retrieved from http://dx.doi.org/10.1037/0003-066X.40.1.19 PMid:3977166.

Costa, P .T., & McCrae, R. R. (1987). Neuroticism, somatic complaints, and disease: Is the bark worse than the bite? *Journal of Personality, 52,* 299–316. Retrieved from http://dx.doi.org/10.1111/j.1467-6494.1987.tb00438.x.

Costa, P. T., & McCrae, R. R. (1990). Personality: Another "hidden factor" in stress research. *Psychological Inquiry, 1,* 22–24. Rertrieved from http://dx.doi.org/10.1207/s15327965pli0101_5.

Costa, P. T., McCrae, R. R., Zoderman, A. B., Barbano, H. E., Lebowitz, B., & Larson, D. M. (1986). Cross-sectional studies of personality in a national sample: Stability in neuroticism, extraversion, and openness. *Psychology and Aging, 1,* 144–149. Retrieved from http://dx.doi.org/10.1037/0882-7974.1.2.144 PMid:3267391.

Coyne, J. (1976). Toward an interaction description of depression. *Psychiatry, 39,* 28–40.

Daugherty, T. K., & Lawrence, J. W. (1996). Short-term effects of research participation on college men. *The Journal of Psychology, 30,* 71–77. Retrieved from http://dx.doi.org/10.1080/00223980.1996.9914989 PMid:8618214.

De Beurs, E., Comijs, H., Twisk, J. W. R., Sonnenberg, C., Beekman, A. T. F., & Deeg, D. (2005). Stability and change of emotional functioning in late life: Modelling of vulnerability profiles. *Journal of Affective Disorders, 84,* 53–62. Retrieved from http://dx.doi.org/10.1016/j.jad.2004.09.006 PMid:15620385.

DeLongis, A., Folkman, A., & Lazarus, R. S. (1988). The impact of daily stress on health and mood: Psychological and social resources as mediators. *Journal of Personality and Social Psychology, 54,* 486–495. Retrieved from http://dx.doi.org/10.1037/0022-3514.54.3.486 PMid:3361420.

Dienstbier, R. A. (1989). Arousal and physiological toughness: Implications for mental and physical health. *Psychological Review, 96,* 84–100. Retrieved from http://dx.doi.org/10.1037/0033-295X.96.1.84 PMid:2538855.

Finlay-Jones, R., & Brown, G. (1981). Types of stressful life events and onset of anxiety and depression disorders. *Psychological Medicine, 11,* 813–815.

Folkman, S., & Lazarus, R. S. (1985). If it changes it must be a process: Study of emotion and coping during three stages of a college examination. *Journal of Personality and Social Psychology, 48,* 150–170. Retrieved from http://dx.doi .org/10.1037/0022-3514.48.1.150.

Folkman, S., & Lazarus, R. S. (1988). Coping as a mediator of emotion. *Journal of Personality and Social Psychology, 54,* 466–473. Retrieved from http://dx.doi .org/10.1037/0022-3514.54.3.466 PMid:3361419.

Folkman, S., Lazarus, R. S., Dunkel-Schetter, C., DeLongis, A., & Gruen, R. (1986). Dynamics of a stressful encounter: Cognitive appraisal, coping, and encounter outcomes. *Journal of Personality and Social Psychology, 50,* 992–1003. Retrieved from http://dx.doi.org/10.1037/0022-3514.50.5.992 PMid:3712234.

Gaab, J., Rohleder, N., Nater, U. M., & Ehlert, U. (2005). Psychological determinants of the cortisol stress response: The role of anticipatory cognitive appraisal. *Psychoeuroendocinology, 30,* 599–610. Retrieved from http://dx.doi .org/10.1016/j.psyneuen.2005.02.001 PMid:15808930.

Gilbar, O. (1996). The connection between the psychological condition of breast cancer patients and survival: A follow-up after eight years. *General Hospital Psychiatry, 18,* 266–270. doi: org/10.1016/0163-8343(96)00023-0.

Gowan, M. A., Riordan, C. M., & Gatewood R. D. (1999). Test of a model of coping with involuntary job loss following a company closing. *Journal of Applied Psychology, 84,* 75–86. Retrieved from http://dx.doi.org/10.1037/ 0021-9010.84.1.75.

Greer, S., Morris., T., & Pettingale, K. (1979). Psychological responses to breast cancer: Effect on outcome. *Lancet, 2,* 785–787. doi: org/10.1016/S0140-6736 (79)92127-5.

Herbert, T. B., & Cohen, S. (1993). Stress and immunity: A meta-analytic review. *Psychosomatic Medicine, 55,* 364–379. doi: PMid:8416086.

Huang, C., Musil, C. M., & Zauszniewski, J. A. (2006). Effects of social support and coping of family caregivers of older adults with dementia in Taiwan. *International Journal of Aging & Human Development, 63,* 1–25. Retrieved from http://dx.doi.org/10.2190/72JU-ABQA-6L6F-G98Q PMid:16986648.

Kemeny, M. E. (2003). The psychobiology of stress. *Current Directions in Psychological Science, 12,* 124–129. Retrieved from http://dx.doi.org/10.1111/ 1467-8721.01246.

Larsen, R. J. (1992). Neuroticism and selective encoding and recall of symptoms: Evidence from a combined concurrent retrospective study. *Journal of Personality and Social Psychology, 62,* 480–488. Retrieved from http://dx.doi .org/10.1037/0022-3514.62.3.480 PMid:1560338.

Lazarus, R. S. (1963). A laboratory approach to the dynamics of psychological stress. *Administrative Science Quarterly, 8,* 192–213.

Lazarus, R. S., & Folkman, S. (1984). *Stress, appraisal and coping.* New York: Springer.

Lazarus, R. S., Opton, E., & Nomikos, M. S. (1965). The principle of short-circuiting of threat: Further evidence. *Journal of Personality, 33,* 622–635. Retrieved from http://dx.doi.org/10.1111/j.1467-6494.1965.tb01408.x PMid:5841349.

Levy, S., Herberman, R., Lippman, M., & D'Angelo, T. (1987). Correlation of stress factors with sustained depression of natural killer cell activity and predicted prognosis in patients with breast cancer. *Journal of Clinical Oncology, 5,* 348–353. doi: PMid:3546612.

Levy, S., Herberman, R., Maluish, A., Schlien, B., & Lippman, M. (1985). Prognostic risk assessment in primary breast cancer by behavioral and immunological parameters. *Health Psychology, 4,* 99–113. doi: org/10.1037/0278-6133.4.2.99.

Luecken, L. J., & Compas, B. E. (2002). Stress, coping, and immune function in breast cancer. *Annals of Behavioral Medicine, 24,* 336–344. Retrieved from http://dx.doi.org/10.1207/S15324796ABM2404_10 PMid:12434945.

Maddi, S. R., Bartone, P. T., & Puccetti, M. C. (1987). Stressful events are indeed a factor in physical illness: Reply to Schroeder and Costa (1984). *Journal of Personality and Social Psychology, 52,* 833–843. Retrieved from http://dx.doi.org/10.1037/0022-3514.52.4.833.

Magnus, K., Diener, E., & Fujita, F. (1993). Extraversion and neuroticism as predictors of objective life events: A longitudinal analysis. *Journal of Personality and Social Psychology, 65,* 1046–1053. Retrieved from http://dx.doi.org/10.1037/0022-3514.65.5.1046 PMid:8246112.

Mak, A. S., Blewitt, K., & Heaven, P. C. L. (2004). Gender and personality influences in adolescent threat and challenge appraisals and depressive symptoms. *Personality and Individual Differences, 36,* 1483–1496. Retrieved from http://dx.doi.org/10.1016/S0191-8869(03)00243-5.

Manne, S., Ostroff, J., Sherman, M., Glassman, M., Ross, S., & Goldstein, L. (2003). Buffering effects of family and friend support on associations between partner unsupportive behaviors and coping among women with breast cancer. *Journal of Social and Personal Relationships, 20,* 771–792. doi: org/10.1177/0265407503206004.

McEwen, B. S. (2000). The neurobiology of stress: From serendipity to clinical relevance. *Brain Research, 88,* 172–189. Retrieved from http://dx.doi.org/10.1016/S0006- 8993(00)02950-4.

Milgram, N., & Tenne, R. (2000). Personality correlates of decisional and task avoidant procrastination. *European Journal of Personality, 14,* 141–156. Retrieved from http://dx.doi.org/10.1002/(SICI)1099-0984(200003/04)14:2<141::AID-PER369>3.0.CO;2-V.

Monjan, A. A., & Collector, M. (1977). Stress-induced modulations of the immune response. *Science, 196,* 307–308. Retrieved from http://dx.doi.org/10.1126/science.557841 PMid:557841.

O'Leary, A. (1990). Stress, emotion, and human immune function. *Psychological Bulletin, 108,* 363–382. Retrieved from http://dx.doi.org/10.1037/0033-2909.108.3.363 PMid:2270233.

Rabkin, J. G., & Strening, E. H. (1976). Life events, stress, and illness. *Science, 194,* 1013–1020. Retrieved from http://dx.doi.org/10.1126/science.790570 PMid: 790570.

Sapolsky, R. M. (2004). Social status and health in humans and other animals. *Annual Review of Anthropology, 33,* 393–418. Retrieved from http://dx.doi .org/10.1146/annurev.anthro.33.070203.144000.

Segrin, C. (2001). *Interpersonal processes in psychological problems.* New York: Guilford.

Segrin, C., & Flora, J. (2000). Poor social skills are a vulnerability factor in the development of psychosocial problems. *Human Communication Research, 26,* 489–514. Retrieved from http://dx.doi.org/10.1111/j.1468-2958.2000 .tb00766.x.

Seyle, H. (1956). *The stress of life.* New York: McGraw-Hill.

Sklar, L. S., & Anisman, H. (1981). Stress and cancer. *Psychological Bulletin, 89,* 369–406. Retrieved from http://dx.doi.org/10.1037/0033-2909.89.3.369 PMid: 6114507.

Slavin, L. A., Rainer, K. L., McCreary, M. L., & Gowda, K. K. (1991). Toward a multicultural model of the stress process. *Journal of Counseling & Development, 70,* 156–163. Retrieved from http://dx.doi.org/10.1002/j.1556-6676.1991 .tb01578.x.

Stanton, A. L., & Schneider, P. R. (1993). Coping with a breast cancer diagnosis: A prospective study. *Health Psychology, 12,* 16–23. Retrieved from http:// dx.doi.org/10.1037/0278-6133.12.1.16 PMid:8462494.

Sweet, L., Savoie, J. A., & Lemyre, L. (1999). Appraisals, coping, and stress in breast cancer screening: A longtitudinal investigation of causal structure. *Canadian Journal of Behavioural Science, 31,* 240–253. Retrieved from http://dx.doi .org/10.1037/h0087093.

Tjemsland, L., Soreide, J. A., Matre, R., & Malt, U. F. (1997). Properative psychological variables predict immunological status in patients with operable breast cancer. *Psycho-Oncology, 6,* 311–320. Retrieved from http://dx.doi .org/10.1002/(SICI)1099-1611(199712)6:4<311::AID-PON285>3.0.CO;2-C.

Tomaka, J., Blascovich, J., Kelsey, R. M., & Leitten, C. L. (1993). Subjective, physiological, and behavioral effects of threat and challenge appraisal. *Journal of Personality and Social Psychology, 65,* 248–260. Retrieved from http://dx.doi .org/10.1037/0022-3514.65.2.248.

Ursin, H., Mykletun, R., Tonder, O., Vaernes, R., Relling, G., Isaksen, E., & Murison, R. (1984). Psychological stress-factors and concentrations of immunoglobulns and complement components in humans. *Scandinavian Journal of Psychology, 25,* 340–347. Retrieved from http://dx.doi.org/10.1111/j.1467-9450 .1984.tb01026.x PMid:6528261.

Walker, L. G. (2004). Hypnotherapeutic insights and interventions: A cancer odyssey. *Contemporary Hypnosis, 21,* 35–45. Retrieved from http://dx.doi .org/10.1002/ch.286.

Watson, D., & Clark, L. A. (1984). Negative affectivity: The disposition to experience aversive emotional states. *Psychological Bulletin, 96,* 465–490. Retrieved from http://dx.doi.org/10.1037/0033-2909.96.3.465 PMid:6393179.

Watson, D., and Pennebaker, J. (1989). Health complaints, stress, and distress: Exploring the central role of negative affectivity. *Psychological Review, 96,* 234–254. Retrieved from http://dx.doi.org/10.1037/0033-295X.96.2.234 PMid: 2710874.

Weihs, K. L., Enright, T. M., Simmens, S. J., & Reiss, D. (2000). Negative affectivity, restriction of emotions, and site of metastases predict mortality on recurrent breast cancer. *Journal of Psychosomatic Research, 49,* 59–68. Retrieved from http://dx.doi.org/10.1016/S0022-3999(00)00143-4.

Wiebe, D. J., & Smith, T. W. (1997). Personality and health: Progress and problems in psychosomatics. In Hogan, R., Johnson, J. A., & Briggs, S. R. (Eds.), *Handbook of personality psychology* (pp. 891–918). New York: Academic Press. Retrieved from http://dx.doi.org/10.1016/B978-012134645-4/50035-4.

Willette-Murphy, K., Todero, C., & Yeaworth, R. (2006). Mental health and sleep of older wife caregivers for spouses with Alzheimer's disease and related disorders. *Issues in Mental Health Nursing, 27,* 837–852. Retrieved from http://dx.doi.org/10.1080/01612840600840711 PMid:16938787.

Chapter 19

Managing Cancer from Diagnosis to Recovery: Advice for Employers

Katie L. Pustolka

Cancer is a frightening disease—one that has the potential to be so debilitating and deadly, yet is a disease so prevalent and commonplace in today's day and age. The statistics are staggering—with half of all men and one-third of women developing cancer during their lifetime, nearly everyone will be touched by cancer in some way. Not surprisingly, a cancer diagnosis has a profound impact on patients' lives, but also on the personal and professional lives of their loved ones, caregivers, and colleagues. Cancer, from diagnosis to recovery, poses a difficult administrative and supportive task for employers and human resources professionals.

According to the American Cancer Society, cancer is the general name for a group of more than 100 diseases. All cancers begin due to abnormal cell growth, and untreated cancers can cause serious illness and death. Of the more than 1 million Americans diagnosed with some form of cancer each year, 40 percent are working-age adults (Griffiths, 2011). Earlier detection and more sophisticated treatment options are providing more and more cancer patients and survivors the ability to remain at, and return to, work. Human resources personnel must be versed in how to manage and support the needs of employees facing cancer diagnosis or treatment, including those who are caregivers of patients.

Some of the most obvious but integral details that human resources departments need to be aware of are relevant laws and regulations, especially those specific to women's cancers. Human resources staff should be vigilant in staying up to date on legislation such as the Americans with Disabilities Act (ADA), the Family and Medical Leave Act (FMLA), the Women's Health & Cancer Rights Act, and state disability regulations, which are applicable based on employer size. It is important to note that the ADA does not contain a list of medical conditions that constitute disabilities. Rather, the ADA provides a general definition of disability, and each case must be examined individually. The ADA's definition on disability is also used in determining whether an employee is eligible to take Family Medical Leave. For example, the ADA states that conditions that are episodic or in remission are considered disabilities if the condition would substantially limit a major life activity (normal cell growth is considered a major life activity). Employers also need to be aware of what constitutes discrimination according to the ADA and prevent such issues from occurring. For women diagnosed with breast cancer, employers should provide information on the Women's Health & Cancer Rights Act, which provides protections to patients who choose to have breast reconstruction in connection with a mastectomy. However, employers and human resources professionals must go beyond the legislation and be aware of the support employees need when faced with such a stressful situation.

IMPACT OF CANCER ON EMPLOYEES

It is important to note that cancer does not discriminate—the impact of cancer on the diagnosed and those around them is similar in the United States, Canada, and Europe. Studies conducted in Great Britain, Belgium, and Canada have also found an increase in working-age cancer patients and survivors (Griffiths, 2011; Nowrousi, Lightfoot, Cote, & Watson, 2009; Tiedtke et al., 2012). Nowrousi et al. (2009) found that 62–84 percent of cancer survivors return to work after treatment. Working has been shown to be an important part of an individual's identity—work provides a distraction from the disease and allows the patient to return to some semblance of normalcy. However, there is a plethora of challenges that cancer patients and survivors face. Nowrousi et al. (2009) found in a review of the literature that issues such as job loss, problems with coworkers, and diminished work capacity materialize. Fesko (2001) cites a range of social problems, ranging from rejection to "smothering" by coworkers.

A cancer diagnosis undoubtedly produces feelings of fear, anxiety, and uncertainty. Tiedtke et al. (2012) found that Flemish women diagnosed with breast cancer had intense fears of dying, experienced extremely negative thoughts, and experienced a "disruption" period of loss and despair. Although research has shown that employment can play a significant role in maintaining one's self-esteem following a cancer diagnosis, one of the most difficult decisions an employee faces is if or when to disclose his or her condition. Fesko (2001) found that some cancer patients felt relief upon disclosing their condition and embraced the opportunity to educate coworkers about the importance of self-exams. Others found that upon disclosing their condition, they had to spend time dispelling myths and mitigating the fears of those they told.

Serious illnesses such as cancer will have a direct impact on an employee's work life. A diagnosis may impact people's choice of career, the way in which they view both their work and their employer, and in some cases, the scope of work they're able to perform. Griffiths (2011) found that initial reactions of employers are critical because many individuals afflicted by cancer harbor feelings of inadequacy and fear of discrimination, especially women afflicted with breast cancer. Concerns about one's appearance are also prevalent. These apprehensions are coupled with side effects such as fatigue, nausea, and mood swings that can affect their ability to work (Fesko, 2001). Employees who are experiencing such issues may doubt how accepting their employer and coworkers are (or will be). During a cancer experience, employees have overarching feelings of vulnerability. Munir and colleagues (2013) have suggested that employees with cancer utilize a "self-led intervention tool" that can assist them in taking control of their work lives and help in making informed decisions in regard to their treatment, employment, and support services. Some of the questions employees might consider asking include:

Questions for Physicians:

How much time will I need to take off for treatments?
Which treatment side effects are most likely to interfere with my work?
What support services are available to me?

Questions for Employer:

Where can I find company policies on disability and FMLA?
What support services are available to me?
What benefits do I have if I am unable to work?
What insurance/payment protections are available to me?
Is my job secure? (Munir et al., 2013, p. 9)

During treatment, employees may be forced by their condition to take time away from their employer through state disability or Family Medical Leave. While on leave, many employees experience fears of recurrence and are faced with the financial instability of being out of work (Tiedtke, et al., 2012). Concerns such as these compound the stress and anxiety that patients already are experiencing.

The decision to return to work is one that weighs heavily on those afflicted with cancer. After being away from the workplace, employees go through stages of change, including contemplation (beginning to consider returning to work) and preparation (making concrete plans to return) (Prochaska et al. [1992] as cited in Tiedtke et al., 2012). In studying breast cancer survivors, results indicated that women afflicted with breast cancer very carefully consider how to transition from "being ill" to "returning to work" (Tiedtke et al., 2012). As previously mentioned, returning to work is an important measure of health improvement and provides control over a situation that predominantly is left to medicine and chance. In a qualitative study of 22 women who had undergone breast cancer surgery, Tiedtke et al. (2012) found that a majority of women wanted to leave the "sick role." Returning to work after cancer is an opportunity to leave illness behind and return to a normal life. These women faced a multitude of unanswered questions, including if they were ready to return to work, if they were capable or going back to their old jobs, or if they should consider new positions. They also questioned whether it was worth the effort to return to work. As part of the women's considerations in returning to work, they not only thought about the medical aspects of their condition but also considered their social environment. Fear of recurrence was always on the women's minds, and each individual looked to various sources for cues on what action to take (e.g., family/friends, physicians, employers). Women described the conflicting messages received from employers (whether they would be accepted back into the workplace), doctors (advising against returning to work), insurance personnel (obligation to return to work sooner than ready), and spouses/partners. These uncertainties provide the perfect platform for employers and human resources professionals to be a source of support and act as a "beacon of stability" during such an upsetting time in an employee's life (Nowrousi et al., 2009).

STRATEGIES FOR EMPLOYERS

Cancer is a costly disease, both in actual dollars and from the emotional toll it takes on those affected. According to the National Institute of Health, the estimated annual costs of cancer in 2008 were $201.5 billion. Additionally, cancer was ranked as the leading cause of long-term disability for the ninth consecutive year—accounting for 11.8 percent of all claims (Nowrousi et al., 2009). This is an enormous amount of money—one that must be considered by employers and benefits administrators. One of the best ways to manage cancer and its subsequent costs is prevention and early detection. The National Business Group on Health in conjunction with the National Comprehensive Cancer Network have created a tool for employers, *An Employer's Guide to Cancer Treatment & Prevention*, intended to be a "plug and play" resource to help strategically reduce the costs associated with cancer claims in addition to increasing support for those diagnosed. One preventive suggestion is for employers to provide rewards for employees and dependents who adopt and maintain healthy habits, such as participating in routine cancer screenings. Promoting healthy behaviors, such as providing healthy food options in company break rooms, offering tobacco cessation programs, and combating issues such as obesity and alcohol misuse can go a long way in moderating future claims. The *Guide* also suggests a periodic review of a company's medical insurance and claims data, short-term and long-term disability plans, and employee assistance programs. If a company has a high incidence rate of cancer, it is recommended that an employer consider benefit plans that provide transplant services, lodging and travel assistance, and approval for participation in clinical studies. It also recommended that employers have specific policies on critical illness, setting out resources and support that are available. This will also ensure that employees are managed and treated in a consistent manner.

Griffiths (2011) found that women affected by cancer said the initial reactions of their employer were critical. Many women found a "culture of ignorance" in regard to their abilities and needs; they experienced great fear in disclosing their illness because they were afraid it would affect their career development. However, some felt they would not be able to hide the information indefinitely because of the need for time off for appointments (Griffiths, 2011). Employees that are diagnosed or are undergoing treatment for cancer must be treated with respect and sent a strong message that their employers care for and support them. *An Employer's Guide to Cancer Treatment & Prevention* suggests that for anyone applying for Family Medical Leave (for one's own serious diagnosis or that of a family member), information be given on employee assistance and work/life programs. It is also suggested that caregivers receive information on caregiver stress and support resources. Employers must also not forget managers and staff affected by the illness; resources should be provided to assist in coping with their coworkers' cancer.

Once an employer learns of a cancer diagnosis from an employee, he or she must keep any medical information confidential as well as provide reasonable accommodation for limitations caused by cancer, the side effects of medication or treatment, or both. The Job Accommodation Network suggests employers consider the following questions upon learning of a diagnosis:

What limitations is the employee with cancer experiencing?
How do these limitations affect the employee and his/her job performance?

What job tasks are problematic?

What accommodations are available to reduce/eliminate these problems?

Has the employee with cancer been consulted regarding possible accommodations?

Once accommodations are in place, would it be useful to meet with the employee to evaluate the effectiveness of the accommodations and to determine whether additional accommodations are needed?

Do supervisory employees and staff need training regarding cancer?

Reasonable accommodations are not only required by the Americans with Disabilities Act but also are measures that can assist employees in continuing to be productive, contributing members of the company. It should also be noted that employers have a responsibility to ensure that disabled persons do not face discrimination in the workplace. Below is a list of common accommodations that are generally easy to integrate:

Flexible scheduling—allowing patients to leave for doctors' appointments and/or recuperate from treatment

Permission to work from home/adjustments to the work schedule

Modification of office temperature

Placement of workstation near office equipment and supplies

Permission to use work phone to call doctors

Reallocation of marginal tasks to other employees

Reassignment to another job (If transferred, then the new position must be equivalent, or as close as possible, in terms of pay and status.)

Sensitivity training to coworkers (www.eeoc.gov)

It is important that employers and employees have open and clear lines of communication before, during, and after cancer treatment. Human resources professionals may want to consider offering periodic meetings to check in with employees and discuss any concerns they may have.

Employees diagnosed with (and recovering from) cancer need empowerment—it is clear that vulnerability is at an all-time high, and rebuilding a healthy lifestyle includes regaining confidence. Employees who are able to continue working during or after cancer treatment will feel accepted and supported. Simultaneously, employers will continue having productive and loyal employees at their firm.

REFERENCES

Family and Medical Leave (FMLA) of 1993. (2013). *SHRM Online-Society for Human Resources Management.* Retrieved from http://www.shrm.org/legalissues/federalresources/federalstatutesregulationsandguidanc/pages/familyandmedicalleaveactof1993.aspx.

Fesko, S. (2001). Workplace experiences of individuals who are HIV+ and individuals with cancer. *RCB, 45*, 2–11.

Finch, R., Kendall, D., Shebel, B., Danielson, E., & Goldsmith, P. (2012). *An employer's guide to cancer treatment & prevention*. Retrieved from https://www.businessgrouphealth.org/pub/f3128cb8-2354-d714-51c2-ae9436acf26a.

Griffiths, E. (2011). Focus on breast cancer and the workplace. *Occupational Health, 63*, 18–19.

Loy, B. (2013). Accommodation and compliance series: Employees with cancer. JAN-Job Accommodation Network. Retrieved from http://askjan.org/media/cancer.html.

Munir, F., Kalawsky, K., Wallis, D., & Donaldson-Feilder, E. (2013). Using intervention mapping to develop a work-related guidance tool for those affected by cancer. *BMC Public Health, 13*, 1–14.

Nowrousi, B., Lightfoot, N., Cote, K., & Watson, R. (2009). Workplace support for employees with cancer. *Current Oncology, 16*. Retrieved from http://www.current-oncology.com/index.php/oncology/article/view/381.

Tiedtke, C., de Rijk, A., Donceel, P., Christiaens, M., & Dierckx de Casterle, B. (2012). Survived but feeling vulnerable and insecure: A qualitative study of the mental preparation for RTW after breast cancer treatment. *BMC Public Health, 12*, 1–14.

U.S. Equal Employment Opportunity Commission. (2011). Questions and answers about cancer in the workplace and the Americans with Disabilities Act (ADA). Retrieved from http://www.eeoc.gov/facts/cancer.html.

Women's Health & Cancer Rights Act of 1998. (2007). *SHRM Online-Society for Human Resources Management*. Retrieved from http://www.shrm.org/legalissues/federalresources/federalstatutesregulationsandguidanc/pages/women's healthcancerrightsactof1998.aspx.

Appendix A: Organizations Concerned with Women's Cancers

Susan Strauss and Michele A. Paludi

Abramson Cancer Center
www.penncancer.org

Adjuvant! Online
www.adjuvantonline.com/index
.jsp

African Women's Cancer Awareness Association
www.awcaa.org

AlphaCancer Information Resource Center
www.alphacancer.com

American Cancer Society
www.cancer.org

American Pain Foundation
www.painfoundation.org

American Society of Clinical Oncology
www.asco.org

Association of Cancer Online Resources
www.acor.org

Athena Partners Cancer Resources
www.athenapartners.org

Avon Breast Cancer Awareness Crusade
www.avoncrusade.com

BC Cancer Agency
www.bccancer.bc.ca

Black Women's Health Imperative
www.blackwomenshealth.com

Breast Cancer Information Core National Human Genome Research Institute
http://research.nhgri.nih.gov/bic/
resources.shtml

Breast Cancer Net
www.breastcancer.net

Breast Cancer Online
www.bco.org

Breast Cancer Resource Center
www.healingwell.com/
breastcancer/

Breast Clinic
www.thebreastclinic.com

Bright Pink
www.bebrightpink.org

Canadian Breast Cancer
Network
www.cbcn.ca

Cancer and Careers
www.cancerandcareers.org

Cancer Care Inc.
www.cancercare.org

Cancer Genetics
www.cancergenetics.org

CancerGuide
www.cancerguide.org

Cancer Hope Network
www.cancerhopenetwork.org

Cancer Legal Resource Center
www.disabilityrightslegalcenter
.org

Cancer Links
www.cancerlinks.org

CancerQuest
www.cancerquest.org

The Cancer Support Community
www.cancersupportcommunity
.org

Cancer Wellness Center
www.cancerwellness.org

Centers for Disease Control and
Prevention
www.cdc.gov/cancer/knowledge/

Conversations: The
International Newsletter for
Those Fighting Ovarian Cancer
www.ovarian-news.org

Corporate Angel Network
www.corpangelnetwork.org

Family Caregiver Alliance
www.caregiver.org

Feminist Majority Foundation
www.feminist.org

Fertile Hope
www.fertilehope.org

Fighting Chance
www.fightingchance.org

FORCE: Facing Our Risk of
Cancer Empowered
www.facingourrisk.org

Foundation for Women's Cancer
www.foundationforwomen's
cancer.org

Friends of Cancer Research
www.focr.org

Gilda Radner Familial Ovarian
Cancer Registry
http://ovariancancer.com/app/
index/php

Guide to Internet Resources for
Cancer
www.ncl.ac.uk

Gynaecological Cancer Support
www.gynaecancersupport
.org.au

Health Finder
www.healthfinder.gov

Appendix A 417

Hystersisters
www.hystersisters.com

I'm Too Young for This! Cancer Foundation
www.i2y.com

Inflammatory Breast Cancer Information
www.infobreastcancer.cyberus.ca

Intercultural Cancer Council
www.iccnetwork.org

International Cancer Alliance
www.icare.org

International Union Against Cancer
www.uicc.org

Johns Hopkins Pathology's Ovarian Cancer Web
http://ovariancancer.jhml.edu

Kapi'olani Breast Center
www.kapiolaniwoman.org

Kapi'olani Women's Cancer Center
www.kapiolaniwoman.org

Kids Konnected: Special Support for Kids
www.kidskonnected.org

Know Cancer
www.knowcancer.com

Mautner Project
www.mautnerproject.org

M. D. Anderson Cancer Center
www.mdanderson.org/diseases/ovariancancer/

Minnesota Ovarian Cancer Alliance
www.mnovarian.org

National Action Plan on Breast Cancer
www.napbc.org

National Alliance of Breast Cancer
www.nationalbreastcancer.org

National Alliance of Breast Cancer Organizations
www.nabco.org

National Asian Women's Health Organization
www.nawho.org

National Breast Cancer Coalition
http://www.breastcancerdeadline2020.org/brest-cancer-information/

National Cancer Institute
www.cancer.gov

National Coalition for Cancer Survivorship
www.canceradvocacy.org

National Family Caregivers Association
www.nfcacares.org

National Institutes of Health
www.nih.gov

National Ovarian Cancer Coalition
www.ovarian.org

Native American Cancer Research
www.natamcancer.org

Native People's Circle of Hope
www.nativepeoplecoh.org

NCI, Genetics of Breast and Ovarian Cancer
http:/www.cancer.gov/cancertopics/pdq/genetics/

breast-and-ovarian/
healthprofessional/page1

NCI, Ovarian Cancer
http://www.cancer.gov/
cancertopics/types/ovarian

Oncolink
www.oncolink.com

**Online Management of Breast
Diseases**
www.breastdiseases.com

**Ovarian Cancer Alliance of
Florida**
www.ocaf.org

**Ovarian Cancer Alliance of
Nevada**
www.ocan.org

Ovarian Cancer Forum
www.medhelp.org

**Ovarian Cancer National
Alliance**
www.ovariancancer.org

Patient Advocate Foundation
www.patientadvocate.org

Peter MacCallum Cancer Center
www.petermac.org

Prevent Cancer Foundation
www.preventcancer.org

Research Advocacy Network
www.researchadvocacy.org

**SHARE: Self Help for Women
with Breast or Ovarian Cancer**
www.sharecancersupport.org

Sisters Network Inc.
www.sistersnetworkinginc.org

**Society for Women's Health
Research**
www.womenshealthresearch.org

**Society of Gynecologic
Oncologists**
www.sgo.org

South Carolina Cancer Alliance
www.sccanceralliance.org

Strength for Caring
www.strengthforcaring.com

**Susan G. Komen Breast Cancer
Foundation**
www.komen.org

Teens Living with Cancer
www.teenslivingwithcancer.org

**Ulman Cancer Fund for Young
Adults**
www.ulmanfund.org

Wellness Community
www.thewellnesscommunity.org

Well Spouse Association
www.wellspouse.org

Women's Cancer Network
www.wcn.org

Young Adult Cancer Canada
www.younadultcancer.ca

Young Adult Cancer Survivors
www.yacsdc.org

Young Cancer Spouses
www.youngcancerspouses.com

Young Empowered Survivors
www.youngempowered.org

Appendix B: Cancer Centers and Clinical Trials

Michele A. Paludi

CENTERS

Abramson Cancer Center
Philadelphia, PA
215-662-3929

M. D. Anderson Cancer Center
Houston, TX
713-792-2121

Arizona Cancer Center
Tucson, AZ
520-626-7685

The Cancer Institute of New Jersey
New Brunswick, NJ
732-235-8064

Cancer Therapy and Research Center
San Antonio, TX
210-450-1000

Case Comprehensive Cancer Center
Cleveland, OH
216-844-8562

Chao Family Comprehensive Cancer Center
Orange, CA
714-456-6310

City of Hope Comprehensive Cancer Center
Duarte, CA
626-301-8460

Cold Spring Harbor Laboratory Cancer Center
Cold Spring Harbor, NY
516-367-8383

Comprehensive Cancer Center—
James Cancer Hospital and
Solove Research Institute
Columbus, OH
614-293-7521

Dana-Farber/Harvard Cancer
Center
Boston, MA
617-632-2100

Duke Cancer Institute
Durham, NC
919-684-3052

Dan L. Duncan Cancer Center
Houston, TX
713-798-1354

Albert Einstein Cancer Center
Bronx, NY
718-430-2302

Eppley Cancer Center
Omaha, NE
402-559-4238

Fox Chase Cancer Center
Philadelphia, PA
215-728-3636

Fred Hutchinson/University of
Washington Cancer Consortium
Seattle, WA
206-667-4305

Georgetown Lombardi
Comprehensive Cancer Center
Washington, DC
202-687-2110

Greenebaum Cancer Center
Baltimore, MD
1-800-888-8823

Holden Comprehensive Cancer
Center
Iowa City, IA
319-353-8620

Hollings Cancer Center
Charleston, SC
843-792-8284

Huntsman Cancer
Institute
Salt Lake City, UT
801-585-0303

Indiana University Melvin
and Bren Simon Cancer Center
Indianapolis, IN
317-278-0070

Herbert Irving Comprehensive
Cancer Center
New York, NY
212-851-4680

The Jackson Laboratory Cancer
Center
Bar Harbor, ME
207-288-6841

Jonsson Comprehensive Cancer
Center
Los Angeles, CA
310-825-5268

The Barbara Ann Karmanos
Cancer Institute
Detroit, MI
313-576-8670

Kimmel Cancer Center
Philadelphia, PA
215-503-5692

Sidney Kimmel Comprehensive
Cancer Center
Baltimore, MD
410-955-8822

David H. Koch Institute for
Integrative Cancer Research at
MIT
Cambridge, MA
617-324-3533

Robert H. Lurie Comprehensive
Cancer Center
Chicago, IL
312-908-5250

Masonic Cancer Center
Minneapolis, MN
612-624-8484

Massey Cancer Center
Richmond, VA
804-828-0450

Mayo Clinic Cancer Center
Rochester, MN
507-266-4997

Memorial Sloan-Kettering
Cancer Center
New York, NY
212-639-2000

H. Lee Moffit Cancer Center and
Research Institute
Tampa, FL
813-745-1315

Moores Comprehensive Cancer
Center
La Jolla, CA
858-522-1222

New York University Cancer
Institute
New York, NY
212-263-3276

Norris Cotton Cancer Center
Lebanon, NH
603-653-9000

OHSU Knight Cancer Institute
Portland, OR
503-494-1617

Purdue University Center for
Cancer Research
West Lafayette, IN
765-494-9129

Roswell Park Cancer
Institute
Buffalo, NY
716-845-5772

St. Jude Children's Research
Hospital
Memphis, TN
901-595-3982

Salk Institute Cancer
Center
La Jolla, CA
858-453-4100

Sanford-Burnham Medical
Research Institute
La Jolla, CA
658-646-3100

Harold C. Simmons Cancer
Center
Dallas, TX
214-645-4673

Alvin J. Siteman Cancer Center
St. Louis, MO
314-362-8020

Stanford Cancer Institute
Stanford, CA
650-736-7716

University of Alabama
Comprehensive Cancer Center
Birmingham, AL
205-934-5077

University of California, Davis,
Comprehensive Cancer Center
Sacramento, CA
916-734-5800

University of California, San
Francisco, Helen Diller Family
Comprehensive Cancer Center
San Francisco, CA
415-502-1710

University of Chicago
Comprehensive Cancer Center
Chicago, IL
773-702-6180

University of Colorado Cancer
Center
Aurora, CO
303-724-7135

University of Hawaii Cancer
Center
Honolulu, HI
808-586-3010

University of Kansas Cancer
Center
Kansas City, KS
913-588-2568

University of Michigan
Ann Arbor, MI
734-936-1831

University of New Mexico
Cancer Research and Treatment
Center
Albuquerque, NM
505-272-5622

University of North Carolina
Lineberger Comprehensive
Cancer Center
Chapel Hill, NC
919-966-3036

University of Pittsburgh Cancer
Institute
Pittsburgh, PA
412-623-3205

University of Southern
California Norris
Comprehensive Cancer
Center
Los Angeles, CA
323-865-0816

University of Virginia
Cancer Center
Charlottesville, VA
434-924-5022

University of Wisconsin Paul P.
Carbone Cancer Center
Madison, WI
608-263-8610

Vanderbilt-Ingram Cancer
Center
Nashville, TN
615-936-1782

Wake Forest Comprehensive
Cancer Center
Winston-Salem, NC
336-716-7971

Winship Cancer Institute
Atlanta, GA
404-778-5669

The Wistar Institute
Philadelphia, PA
215-898-3926

Yale Cancer Center
New Haven, CT
203-785-4371

SAMPLE CLINICAL TRIALS

CancerCare
http://www.cancercare.org/
publications/146-clinical_
trials_for_women_with_
ovarian_cancer

Cedars-Sinai
http://www.cedars-sinai.edu/
Patients/Programs-and-Services/
Womens-Cancer-Program/
Research-and-Clinical-Trials/

Clinical Trials, National Institutes of Health
http://clinicaltrials.gov/show/
NCT01237067

Dana Farber/Brigham Women's Cancer Center
http://www.dfbwcc.org/clinical
-trials.html

Foundation for Women's Cancer
http://www.
foundationforwomenscancer.org/
breast-cancer/clinical-trials/

Hope Women's Cancer Centers
http://www.hopewcc.com/
research/

Magee Womens Hospital of UPMC
http://www.upmc.com/locations/
hospitals/Magee/womens-cancer/
breast-cancer/Pages/research.aspx

Medical College of Wisconsin
http://obgyn.mcw.edu/services/
gynecologic-oncology/
clinical-trials-for-womens-
cancers/

Memorial Sloan-Kettering Cancer Center
http://www.mskcc.org/cancer
-care/clinical-trials

National Breast Cancer Foundation Inc.
http://www.nationalbreastcancer.
org/breast-cancer-clinical-trials

National Cancer Institute at the National Institutes of Health
http://www.cancer.gov/
clinicaltrials/results/type/breast

Ovarian Cancer National Alliance
http://www.ovariancancer.org/
clinical-trials/

Appendix C: Legislation Regarding Women's Cancers

Michele A. Paludi

WOMEN'S HEALTH AND CANCER RIGHTS ACT OF 1998

Signed into law on October 21, 1998.

The U.S. Department of Labor and the U.S. Department of Health and Human Services oversee this federal legislation.

Requires group insurance plans, insurance companies, and health maintenance organizations (HMOs) (starting on or after October 21, 1998) that cover mastectomies to also cover services (e.g., reconstruction surgery, prostheses) and treatment of complications resulting from the mastectomy.

This legislation also applies to individual policies.

This legislation does not apply to Medicaid or to Medicare. However, Medicare does cover breast reconstruction following a mastectomy. Coverage varies by state.

Additional Information

Cancer Legal Resource Center
  www.disabilityrightslegalcenter.org
National Association of Insurance Commissioners
  www.naic.org/state_web_map.htm
United States Department of Labor
  dol/gov/ebsa/Publications/whcra.html

AMERICANS WITH DISABILITIES ACT

The Americans with Disabilities Act (ADA) was signed into law on July 26, 1990. The ADA was implemented on July 26, 1992.

Title I of the ADA prohibits discrimination in all employment practices, including recruitment and selection, training and development, compensation, layoff, fringe benefits, leave and other terms, and conditions and privileges of employment.

The ADA does not state that because individuals have physical or mental disabilities that they automatically qualify for a job. Rather, the act prohibits discrimination against "qualified individuals," individuals who, with or without a reasonable accommodation, can perform "essential functions" of the job.

Functions are essential when they are the reason the job exists or because the function is so highly specialized that the individual hired for the job is hired for his/her expertise in performing the specialized functions.

A modification or adjustment is "reasonable" by law if it "seems reasonable on its face, i.e., ordinarily or in the run of cases." Thus, the request is reasonable if it appears to be plausible or feasible. A reasonable accommodation enables an applicant/employee with a disability to have an equal opportunity to participate in the application process and to be considered for hire in an organization. In addition, a reasonable accommodation permits an employee with a disability the equal opportunity to enjoy the benefits and privileges of employment that employees enjoy.

Additional Information

Equal Employment Opportunity Commission
www.eeoc.gov

FAMILY AND MEDICAL LEAVE ACT

Passed into law in 1993.

Employers must provide up to 12 weeks of unpaid, job-protected leave to eligible employees for certain family and medical reasons. This legislation applies to employers with 50 or more employees. Employees must have worked at least 1,250 hours during the year prior to taking the leave.

BREAST AND CERVICAL CANCER PREVENTION AND TREATMENT ACT OF 2000

Signed into law on October 24, 2000.

Act gives states the option to provide Medicaid medical assistance to women who were screened through the Centers for Disease Control and

Prevention's Breast and Cervical Cancer Early Detection Program (NBC-CEDP) and have breast or cervical cancer.

Since 2007 NBCCEDP provides women with low-cost screening for breast and cervical cancer.

Appendix D: Sample of Popular Books on Women's Cancers

Michele A. Paludi

FOR CHILDREN, ADOLESCENTS, AND YOUNG ADULTS

Our Mom Has Cancer, by Abigail and Adrienne Ackermann. American Cancer Society (2000).

Staring Down the Dragon, by Dorothea N. Buckingham. Sydney Press (2007).

It's Not about You: A Mother and Daughter's Journey, by Cindy Daniel. Batelier Publishing (2007).

The Bald-Headed Princess: Cancer, Chemo, and Courage, by Maribeth R. Ditmars. Magination (2010).

Nana, What's Cancer? by Beverlye Hyman Fead and Tessa Mae Hamermesh. American Cancer Society (2009).

My One Night Stand with Cancer: A Memoir, by Tania Katan. Alyson Books (2005).

Grace: A Child's Intimate Journal through Cancer and Recovery, by Melinda Marchiano. Happy Quail Publishing (2010).

The Last Beach Bungalow, by Jennie Nash. Berkley Trade (2008).

Love in Bloom, by Sheila Roberts. St. Martin's Griffin (2009).

And Still They Bloom, by Amy Rovere. American Cancer Society (2012).

Faith, Hope, and Healing: Inspiring Lessons Learned from People Living with Cancer, by Bernie S. Siegel. Wiley (2009).

Teens with Cancer, by Gail B. Stewarat. Lucent (2001).

FOR ADULTS

Breast Cancer Clear and Simple. American Cancer Society (2007).

A Healing Journey: Writing Together through Breast Cancer, by Sharon Bray. Amherst Writers and Artists Press (2004).

Ovarian Cancer, by Kristine Conner and Lauren Langford. O'Reilly (2003).

Coping with Chemotherapy and Radiation Therapy, by Daniel Cukier. McGraw-Hill (2004).

Breast Cancer . . . You're Kidding . . . Right? by Catherine Doughty. Cancer Cat (2011).

Celebrating Life: African American Women Speak Out about Breast Cancer, by Sylvia Dunnavant and Nancy Wilson. USFI (1995).

Beyond Breast Cancer: Our Stories of Hope and Courage, by Alda Ellis. Harvest House Publishers (2002).

Reclaiming Our Lives after Breast and Gynecologic Cancer, by Kristine Falco. Jason Aronson (1998).

Couples Confront Cancer, by Joy L. Fincannon and Katherine V. Bruss. American Cancer Society (2002).

American Cancer Society Complete Guide to Nutrition for Cancer Survivors, by Barbara L. Grant, Abby S. Bloch, Kathyn Hamilton, and Cynthia Thomson. American Cancer Society (2010).

What to Say When You Don't Know What to Say, by Nancy Guilmartin. Jossey Bass (2002).

Mayo Clinic's Guide to Women's Cancers, by Lynn Hartmann and Charles L. Loprinzi. Mayo Clinic (2005).

No More Bad Hair Days: A Woman's Journey through Cancer, Chemotherapy, and Coping, by Susan Sturges Hyde. Taylor Trade Publishing (2001).

Woman Cancer Sex, by Anne Katz. Hygeia Media (2009).

Let Me Get This off My Chest: A Breast Cancer Survivor Overshares, by Margaret Lesh. StoryRhyme.com Publishing (2013).

The Cancer Journals, by Audre Lorde. Aunt Lute Books (2006).

Breast Cancer: Daughters Tell Their Stories, by Julianne S. Oktay. Haworth Press (2005).

I Am Not My Breast Cancer, by Ruth Peltason. William Morrow (2008).

Breast Cancer: Answers at Your Fingertips, by Emma Pennery, Val Speechley, and Maxine Rosenfield. Class Publishing (2008).

Before I Say Goodbye: Recollections and Observations from One Woman's Final Year, by Ruth Picardie. Henry Holt and Company (2000).

Abnormal Pap Smears: What Every Woman Needs to Know, by Lynda Rusing and Nancy Joste. Prometheus Books (2001).

A Caregiver's Challenge: Living, Loving, Letting Go, by Maryann Schacht. Feterson Press (2005).

What Helped Me Get Through: Cancer Survivors Share Wisdom and Hope, by
Julie K. Silver. American Cancer Society (2008).
Preventing Cervical Cancer: What Every Woman Should Know, by Anne Sza-
rewski. Altman Publishing (2007).
The Complete Cancer Survival Guide, by Peter Teeley and Philip Bashe. Dou-
bleday (2000).

Appendix E: Guidelines for Early Detection of Cancer Identified by the American Cancer Society

Summarized by Michele A. Paludi

BREAST CANCER

Annual mammograms recommended beginning at age 40.

Clinical breast exam every three years for women from age 20 to 39 and annually for women 40 and older.

Breast self-exam beginning for women at age 20.

Women with family history of breast cancer should be screened with an MRI as well as a mammogram.

CERVICAL CANCER

Cervical cancer screening beginning at age 21.

Screening every three years for women between 21 and 29.

Pap test and HPV test every five years, and Pap test alone every three years for women between 30 and 65.

Women 65 and older with normal screening results do not have to be tested.

Women 65 and older with a history of cervical precancer should be tested for 20 years after the diagnosis.

UTERINE CANCER

Endometrial biopsy annually for women, depending on history.
Additional information may be obtained from:

http://www.cancer.org/healthy/findcancerearly/cancerscreening
guidelines/american-cancer-society-guidelines-for-the-early-detection
-of-cancer

Appendix F: Legal and Financial Information for Cancer Patients

Michele A. Paludi

Bridge of Blessings
www.bridgeofblessings.org/index.html

Cancer Care
www.cancercare.org

Clinical Trials and Insurance Coverage: A Resource Guide
www.cancer.gov/clinicaltrials/learning/insurance-coverage

Corporate Angel Network
www.corpangelnetwork.org

Family and Medical Leave Act Advisor
www.dol.gov/compliance/laws/comp-fmla.htm

Look Good . . . Feel Better
www.lookgoodfeelbetter.org

Medicaid
www.cms.hhs.gov/home/medicaid.asp

Medicare
www.medicare.gov

National Collegiate Cancer Foundation
www.collegiatecancer.org

Patient Advocate Foundation
www.patientadvocate.org

Index

About the Editor and Contributors

EDITOR

MICHELE A. PALUDI, PhD, is the series editor for Women's Psychology and for Women and Careers in Management for Praeger. She is the author/editor of 50 college textbooks and more than 200 scholarly articles and conference presentations on sexual harassment, campus violence, psychology of women, gender, and discrimination. Her book *Ivory Power: Sexual Harassment on Campus* (1990, SUNY Press) received the 1992 Myers Center Award for Outstanding Book on Human Rights in the United States. Paludi served as chair of the U.S. Department of Education's Subpanel on the Prevention of Violence, Sexual Harassment, and Alcohol and Other Drug Problems in Higher Education. She was one of six scholars in the United States to be selected for this subpanel. She also was a consultant to and a member of former New York State governor Mario Cuomo's Task Force on Sexual Harassment. Paludi serves as an expert witness for court proceedings and administrative hearings on sexual harassment. She has had extensive experience in conducting training programs and investigations of sexual harassment and other Equal Employment Opportunity (EEO) issues for businesses and educational institutions. In addition, Paludi has held faculty positions at Franklin & Marshall College, Kent State University, Hunter College, Union College, Hamilton College, and Union Graduate College, where she directs the human resource management certificate program and is on the faculty in the School of Management. Paludi is also the Employee Relations Specialist/Title IX Coordinator/ADA/Section 504 Coordinator at Siena College.

CONTRIBUTORS

LAURIE A. BURKE is a clinical psychology intern at the Memphis Veterans Affairs Medical Center, Memphis, Tennessee, and a clinical psychology PhD candidate at the University of Memphis, where she is a bereavement researcher studying death, dying, loss, and grief. Her recent publications stem from her study of correlates of complicated grief, including negative social interactions, meaning making, risk factors of complicated bereavement, and complicated spiritual grief—a spiritual crisis following loss. Her recent projects include an ongoing examination of the African American grief experience; violent death bereavement; an extensive, empirical review of complicated grief in both civilian and military samples; developing and testing an intervention for complicated spiritual grief; and development and validation of the *Inventory of Complicated Spiritual Grief* (ICSG).

PHYLLIS BUTOW, BA (Hons) Dip Ed, MPH, M Clin Psych, PhD, has worked for more than 20 years in the area of psycho-oncology and has developed an international reputation in this and the area of health communication. She is currently Professor and NHMRC Senior Principal Research Fellow at the School of Psychology, University of Sydney. She directs the Centre for Medical Psychology and Evidence-based Decision-making (CeMPED), and chairs the Australian Psycho-Oncology Cooperative Research Group. She chairs the Communication Skills Advisory Group of the National Breast and Ovarian Cancer Centre and has taken a leading role in Australia in promoting and facilitating communication skills training for oncology health professionals. Much of her research concerns the impact of communication strategies on doctor and patient outcomes, and this has been translated into a number of communication skills modules for cancer health professions. Butow has more than 300 publications in peer-reviewed journals, most of which relate to psychological issues in cancer.

JOAN C. CHRISLER, PhD, is the Class of 1943 Professor of Psychology at Connecticut College, where she teaches courses on the psychology of women and health psychology. She has published extensively on the psychology of women and gender, and is especially known for her work on women's reproductive health and body image. Her most recent books are *Reproductive Justice: A Global Concern* (2012, Praeger), *Handbook of Gender Research in Psychology* (2010, Springer), and *Women over 50: Psychological Perspectives* (2007, Springer). She is the editor of *Women's Reproductive Health!*, an interdisciplinary, feminist journal, and she is currently working on a book about women's embodiment.

G. MICHELLE COLLINS-SIBLEY, PhD, joined the faculty at the University of Mount Union in 1994; professor of English, she directs the university's Integrative Core (general education curriculum) and chairs the newly implemented Department of Interdisciplinary and Liberal Studies. For nearly a decade she served as one of the lead faculty of the annual NEH Summer Seminar, ROOTS: African Dimensions of the History and Culture of the Americas through the Atlantic Slave Trade at the Virginia Foundation for the Humanities in Charlottesville, Virginia. Her teaching and research interests focus on Africana literatures, specifically women writers of the African diaspora, literary theory—womanist/feminist, postcolonial—contemplative and peace pedagogies, and comparative literature.

SAM M. DORROS received her MA and PhD from the Department of Communication at the University of Arizona. Her areas of research include interpersonal and health communication, cancer communication, and relational well-being. She is currently an assistant professor at Chapman University.

TINA C. ELACQUA has 20 years of teaching and research experience in the field of higher education, including the roles of research scientist, professor, consultant, and author. Elacqua teaches graduate-level business courses and undergraduate business and psychology courses for LeTourneau University. She enjoys teaching, writing, and publishing. Her scholarly productivity includes publications in journal articles, books, conference papers and presentations, technical reports, and technical presentations. Her research interests and publications are in the areas of management/leadership, career development, and faith-based bereavement post-violent death. Her most recent projects led to a book entitled *Hope Beyond Loss* and an intervention for counseling the bereaved through a biblical worldview.

JEANINE M. GALUSHA is a student in the PhD program at the University of Texas Southwestern. She is a 2010 graduate of the University of Texas at Tyler, where she earned a BS in psychology, and a 2013 graduate of the University of Texas at Tyler, where she earned an MS in clinical psychology. Her academic and research goals include completing her doctorate and continuing research in the field of neuropsychology. She is also an alumni member of the Honor Society of Phi Kappa Phi and Alpha Chi National Honor Society.

EMILEE GILBERT is a lecturer in the School of Social Sciences and Psychology, and a member of the Centre for Health Research at the University of Western Sydney. Her research focuses on gendered health behaviors and the application of poststructural theory to the analysis of issues surrounding gender, health, and sexuality. Gilbert's most recent projects have examined sexuality and intimacy post-cancer, the needs and concerns of cancer carers, and young women's construction and experience of cigarette smoking.

STEPHANIE M. KARWAN has had a long career in business and information technology, beginning in family businesses and segueing into private employment and eventually into the public sector, while pursuing studies in technology and management. Karwan is currently with the New York State Thruway Authority. Since joining the Thruway Authority in 1996, she has served in several capacities within the Department of Information Technology and is currently the senior project manager. She was the manager of technology administration for more than 13 years and also served as the manager of transportation systems. As senior project manager, Karwan is responsible for managing technology, administrative, and managerial projects. As the manager of technology administration, Karwan was responsible for managing IT administrative staff and technology business activities. Prior to joining the Thruway Authority, Karwan was an account manager with the former Keane Inc. and GE Consulting Services, as well as a software engineer for Keane, GE Consulting, and Mechanical Technology Incorporated. Karwan earned an associate's degree in applied science from Hudson Valley Community College in Troy, NY; a bachelor's degree in computer science from Union College; and an MBA from Union Graduate College's School of Management in Schenectady, NY.

BRIDGET R. KENNEDY earned her master of arts in counseling psychology from the University of Texas at Tyler in 2012. As a graduate student she conducted and assisted with research at the Clinical Psychophysiology Research (CPR) Laboratory. She earned her bachelor of arts in psychology from Humboldt State University. Her professional goals include earning a doctorate in counseling psychology, continuing psychological research, and counseling underserved populations.

ALICIA KRIKORIAN, Psychologist, MHSc (psycho-oncology), and PhD in health psychology. Krikorian works with the Pain and Palliative Care Group at the School of Health Sciences of the Universidad Pontificia Bolivariana (Medellín, Colombia). In addition, Krikorian is also part of the directive commission of the Latin American Association of Palliative Care. She actively works for the development of palliative care in the region.

ANNA-LENA LOPEZ, BPsych (Hons), has had more than eight years of research experience in the field of psycho-oncology. She is a psychologist and is currently a candidate for the doctor of clinical psychology and doctor of philosophy degrees at the University of Sydney, Australia. Her doctoral research is investigating the supportive care needs of women with gynecological cancer.

CECILY A. LUFT is a graduate student working on an MS in clinical neuropsychology at the University of Texas, Tyler. She has a BS in psychology from Texas A&M University, Commerce, and completed two years of graduate work in human development at Cornell University. She also spent a year as a Rotary Ambassadorial Scholar to Canterbury, England. Luft has worked directly with children and their families through Early Childhood Intervention in Tyler, TX, for the last seven years. Upon completing her master's degree, Luft plans to work as a counselor for children and adolescents in either public or private practice.

PAULA K. LUNDBERG-LOVE is a professor of psychology at the University of Texas at Tyler (UTT) and the Ben R. Fisch Endowed Professor in Humanitarian Affairs for 2001–2004. Her undergraduate degree was in chemistry, and she worked as a chemist at a pharmaceutical company for five years prior to earning her doctorate in physiological psychology with an emphasis in psychopharmacology. After a three-year postdoctoral fellowship in nutrition and behavior in the Department of Preventive Medicine at Washington University School of Medicine in St. Louis, she assumed her academic position at UTT, where she teaches classes in psychopharmacology, behavioral neuroscience, physiological psychology, sexual victimization, and family violence. Subsequent to her academic appointment, Lundberg-Love pursued postgraduate training and is a licensed professional counselor in Texas. She is a member of Tyler Counseling and Assessment Center, where she provides therapeutic services for victims of sexual assault, child sexual abuse, and domestic violence. She has conducted a long-term research study on women who were victims of childhood incestuous abuse, constructed a therapeutic program for their recovery, and documented its effectiveness upon their recovery. She is the author of nearly 100 publications and presentations and is coeditor of *Violence and Sexual Abuse at Home: Current Issues in Spousal Battering and Child Maltreatment, Intimate Violence against Women: When Spouses, Partners, or Lovers Attack,* and *Women and Mental Disorders.* As a result of her training in psychopharmacology and child maltreatment, her expertise has been sought as a consultant on various death penalty appellate cases in the state of Texas.

JENNIFER L. MARTIN, PhD, is an assistant professor of education at the University of Mount Union. Prior to working in higher education, Martin worked in public education for 17 years, 15 of those as the department head of English at an alternative high school for students labeled at-risk. Martin is the editor of the two-volume series *Women as Leaders in*

Education: Succeeding Despite Inequity, Discrimination, and Other Challenges (2011, Praeger), which examines the intersections of class, race, gender, and sexuality for current and aspiring leaders from a variety of perspectives. She has conducted research and published numerous peer-reviewed articles and book chapters on bullying and harassment, peer sexual harassment, gender equity, mentoring, issues of social justice, service-learning, and teaching at-risk students. Her other current research interests include culturally responsive pedagogy, school reform for social justice, and women and leadership.

ALLISON MARZILIANO, MA, is a doctoral student in the area of social and health psychology in the Department of Psychology at Stony Brook University. She is interested in the psychosocial issues surrounding cancer and cancer treatment.

SILVIA L. MAZZULA, PhD, NCC, LPC, is an assistant professor at John Jay College of Criminal Justice in the Department of Psychology. She received her PhD in counseling psychology from Columbia University (BS and MA, The College of New Jersey; MPhil, Columbia University) and completed her formal clinical training at the University of Medicine and Dentistry of New Jersey-UBHC Newark Campus. Her research interests focus primarily on multicultural issues in psychology, including multicultural competencies in research and practice, immigrant issues, and mental health/health disparities, particularly among Latino(a) Americans. She is a member of the American Psychological Association, the National Latino Psychological Association, and the Latino Psychological Association of New Jersey.

MEAGAN A. MEDINA is a graduate student in the MS clinical neuropsychology program at the University of Texas at Tyler. She is a 2009 graduate of the University of Texas at Tyler, where she earned a BBA in management and graduated summa cum laude. She spent 2011 in Lima, Peru, serving as a Rotary Ambassadorial Scholar. Her academic and professional goals include earning a doctorate in clinical psychology, working in private practice, and yearly joining psychological missions that serve people in areas without access to mental health care.

ANDREA L. MELTZER is on the faculty at Southern Methodist University. Her research examines how intimate relationships affect individual health and how individual health affects intimate relationships. Because the prevalence of overweight and obese individuals is growing at an alarming rate, and because body weight is a significant predictor of a variety of health outcomes, one line of her research focuses on the role of intimate relationships in shaping body weight and vice versa. Through the use of large longitudinal studies of newlyweds, Meltzer works to understand the dyadic effects of numerous relationship factors (e.g., satisfaction, support) on physical health. A second line of her research examines the way health and markers of health, such as weight, sex, and physical appearance, affect intimate relationship functioning. Together, these lines of research can inform interventions aimed at maintaining physical health in the context of intimate relationships.

ANNE MOYER, PhD, is an associate professor of social and health psychology in the Department of Psychology at Stony Brook University. She studies psychosocial issues surrounding cancer and cancer risk. She is also interested in research methodology and methods of synthesizing research.

ROBERT A. NEIMEYER, PhD, is a professor in the Department of Psychology at the University of Memphis and is the editor of the international journal *Death Studies*. Neimeyer has published 27 books, including *Techniques of Grief Therapy: Creative Practices for Counseling the Bereaved* and *Grief and the Expressive Arts: Practices for Creating Meaning*, as well as more than 400 articles and chapters, many of which explore grieving as a process of reconstruction of a world of meaning that has been challenged by loss. He has served as past president of the Association for Death Education and Counseling, which has presented him with both its Research Recognition and Clinical Practice Awards, as well as served as chair of the International Work Group on Death, Dying, and Bereavement. Most recently, he has been made an honored associate of the Viktor Frankl Association, in recognition of his career contributions to the study of human meaning.

JESSICA R. NEWTON is an MA candidate in psychology at Connecticut College, where she is focusing on social psychology and the psychology of gender. Topics of particular interest to her are body image, stereotype threat, and applications of psychology to social issues.

ALEXANDRA M. NOBEL earned her MA in psychology at Connecticut College, where she focused on clinical health psychology and the psychology of gender. Her master's thesis was on oncologists' and oncology nurses' attitudes toward fertility preservation for adolescent cancer patients. She is now a doctoral student in clinical psychology at the University of Rhode Island.

MARIA DA GRACA PEREIRA is an associate professor in the School of Psychology at University of Minho, in Portugal. She graduated from the University of Oporto in psychology (FPCE), did her master's degree in the field of marital and family therapy at Montana State University (MSU), and completed her doctoral dissertation in family systems medicine and the practice of medical family therapy at Florida State University (FSU). She is a certified psychotraumatologist by the Traumatology Institute and a fellow of the Family Institute at FSU. Her area of expertise is centered on family, health, and illness in terms of the psychosocial impact of chronic illness on patients and caregivers/family members; the physical and clinical impact of traumatic stress on patients/at-risk populations and their families; and individual/family health promotion, particularly the promotion of healthier lifestyles in vulnerable groups as well as in chronic patients. She has several books and papers, published nationally and internationally, on these topics.

JANETTE PERZ is an associate professor in the Centre for Health Research at the University of Western Sydney. She researches in the field of reproductive and sexual health with a particular focus on gendered experiences, subjectivity, and identity. She has undertaken a significant research program in psycho-oncology, including the evaluation of gendered experiences and interventions for cancer carers; research on sexual experiences and interventions for people facing cancer; and an examination of changes to fertility across a range of cancer types.

KATIE L. PUSTOLKA, PHR, is the human resources generalist at Ballston Spa National Bank, a community bank located in Saratoga County, NY. She is primarily responsible for the overall staffing and recruitment initiatives for the bank, benefits administration, and employee health and wellness initiatives. Pustolka is a certified professional in human resources and holds a bachelor of science degree in psychology with a minor in classics from Union College, as well as a certificate in human resources management from Union Graduate College. She is a member of the Society of Human Resource Management's national and local chapter. Pustolka has published several chapters and writing pieces and recently acted as a panel moderator on a human resources roundtable discussion for the 2013 conference of the International Coalition Against Sexual Harassment.

REBECCA RANGEL, MA, ATR-BC, earned her master's degree in expressive therapy with a specialization in art therapy and mental health counseling from Lesley University and is currently a PhD candidate at Teachers College, Columbia University. Rebecca has worked with children, adolescents, and families in school-based and outpatient settings. She currently treats monolingual Spanish-speaking and English-speaking patients with severe mental illness in the outpatient Rafael Tavares clinic and women's program at Columbia Presbyterian Medical Center. Her research interests include internalized oppression and discrimination, psychopathology in women of color, mind-body connections, creative arts therapy, loss/grief, stress, and trauma.

LORENE PALUDI RICHARDSON began her career at the New York State Department of Law steno pool in Albany, NY, and left as secretary to the assistant attorney general. Recruited by IBM in 1966, she held several positions in her 30 years there, retiring as senior administrative analyst. She also taught several secretarial, personnel, and benefits classes at IBM's headquarters in White Plains and the IBM regional offices in New York City and Boston. She was the winner of several prestigious awards throughout her IBM career. She joined the Golub Corporation in Schenectady, where she took part in several telethons for M.D.A. and St. Jude's Children's Research Hospital, retiring in 2008. She is an avid worker for the FESTA Finance Committee for her parish each year, as well as eucharistic minister, secretary of the parish "seniors" group, and past president of the Parish Council. She is also a member of the Rotterdam Seniors Association and Sergeant at Arms for the Abruzzese Women's Auxiliary (part of the Abruzzese Men's Society), an organization promoting Italian heritage, which her grandfather helped found.

She is from Schenectady, NY, the granddaughter of Italian immigrants whose family learned very early in life about determination and hope. She's written several poems for family and friends. Her Mother's Day tribute was published in the *Schenectady Gazette* in 2013.

ELISBETH SANTORE earned her master's in social work with a focus on health and mental health from Rutgers University in 2011. She is a residence hall director at Stony Brook University. Her interests include college students who are affected by cancer. She has experience with counseling people affected by cancer and has been an advocate for the Leukemia Lymphoma Society.

MEG STEITZ has been the executive director of HERA Women's Cancer Foundation since 2010. She was formerly the director of the Humanities Institute at the University of Denver.

SUSAN STRAUSS has worked as a registered nurse (RN) in the operating room, pediatrics, medical-surgical, psychiatry, and public health. She is a seasoned health educator working with a variety of community, education, and professional groups. She has also been the director of health care quality improvement and director of education and development, and has held other health care leadership roles. She researched physician abuse to RNs in the operating room to determine if the abuse varied based on the gender of the nurse. Strauss has authored more than

30 books, book chapters, and articles, as well as written curriculum and training manuals. She has been featured on *20/20*, *CBS Evening News*, and other television and radio programs, and has been interviewed for newspaper and journal articles in such publications as the *Times of London*, *Lawyers Weekly*, and *Harvard Education Newsletter*. Strauss has presented at international conferences in Botswana, Egypt, Thailand, Israel, and the United States, and conducted sex discrimination research in Poland. She has consulted with professionals from other countries, such as Israel, England, Australia, Canada, and St. Maarten. In addition to her RN, Susan has a master's degree in community health science and holds a doctorate in organizational leadership.

KATHERINE SWAINSTON is a senior lecturer in psychology based at Teesside University. She is a chartered psychologist on the register of the British Psychological Society (BPS), a health psychologist (Health Professions Council Registered), and an associate fellow of the British Psychological Society. She is a researcher within the Social Futures Institute at Teesside University, is a full member of the British Psychological Society Division of Health Psychology, and is a founding member of the Qualitative Methods in Psychology Section. Swainston is a registered applied psychology supervisor (BPS) and has been teaching undergraduate and postgraduate psychology since 2005. She has been researching women's longitudinal experiences of breast cancer since 2004 and has led service evaluations within the UK National Health Service in the areas of cardiothoracics and chronic pain management. Past projects include a series of systematic rapid reviews evaluating the effectiveness of community engagement methods/approaches in primary health promotion.

RICARDO JOAO TEXEIRA graduated in psychology with a prespecialization in clinical and health psychology. He received his PhD in health psychology from the University of Minho, in Portugal. For his dissertation in psycho-oncology, he was granted a scholarship by the Portuguese Foundation for Science and Technology. He completed postgraduate studies in health psychology, cognitive-behavior therapies, and palliative care. Since 2010 he has been a board member of the Portuguese Society for Studies in Psycho-Oncology. He has received several national and international scientific awards in the field of psycho-oncology, is an award-winning member of the Stress Oncology, and has been collaborating with various institutions of higher education. He currently works as an invited assistant lecturer at the Department of Human and Social Sciences, School of Allied Health Sciences—Polytechnic Institute of Porto, and in a support center for patients with breast cancer (MamaHelp). His special research interests are caregiving in oncology, distress-screening programs for cancer patients, acceptance-focused therapies, and mindfulness, as well as emotional regulation toward health promotion. He has published several scientific articles and book chapters on these topics.

CHERYL BROWN TRAVIS is a professor in the Department of Psychology at the University of Tennessee, Knoxville, and chair of the women's studies program. Her work on women and health care issues has focused on gender and race disparities in the treatment of heart disease. Her latest books include an edited volume on evolution, gender, and rape and a coedited volume on sexuality, society, and feminism.

JANE M. USSHER is professor of women's health psychology, at the University of Western Sydney, Australia. She has published widely on the construction and lived experience of health, in particular women's mental health, the reproductive body, and sexuality. She is editor of Routledge's Women and Psychology book series and is author of a number of books, including *The Psychology of the Female Body* (Routledge), *Women's Madness: Misogyny or Mental Illness?* (Harvester Wheatsheaf), *Fantasies of Femininity: Reframing the Boundaries of Sex* (Penguin), *Managing the Monstrous Feminine: Regulating the Reproductive Body* (Routledge), and *The Madness of Women: Myth and Experience* (Routledge). Her current research is on sexuality and fertility in the context of cancer, and women's premenstrual experiences.

ANNA VAN WERSCH is professor of psychology, a chartered psychologist on the register of the British Psychological Society (BPS), and a health psychologist on the register of the Health Professions Council (HPC). Since 1998 she has served as the program director of the accredited master's program in health psychology at Teesside University and is a qualified supervisor for the second stage BPS Health Psychology Award. Since 1997 she has been teaching undergraduate and postgraduate modules, and has supervised 9 clinical doctorate theses, and more than 130 undergraduate and 110 postgraduate dissertations. She has been external examiner for 8 PhDs and acts currently as external examiner for the doctorate health psychology qualification at the University of Surrey and Staffordshire University, and the master's program in health psychology at Sheffield Hallam University. In March 2012 van Wersch received the prestigious title of Fellow of the British Psychological Society (BPS) to distinguish her as an internationally respected expert in health and in sports and exercise psychology.